SPRINGHOUSE NOTES

Medical- Surgical Nursing

Third Edition

Mildred Wernet Boyd, RN, MSN, MSA

Associate Professor of Nursing
Essex Community College
Baltimore

Barbara L. Tower, RN, MSN, MA, CCRN

Professor of Nursing
Essex Community College
Baltimore

Springhouse Corporation
Springhouse, Pennsylvania

Staff

Executive Director
Matthew Cahill

Editorial Director
June Norris

Art Director
John Hubbard

Managing Editor
David Moreau

Acquisitions Editors
Patricia Kardish Fischer, RN, BSN;
Louise Quinn

Clinical Consultant
Maryann Foley, RN, BSN

Editor
Karyn C. Newell

Copy Editors
Cynthia C. Breuninger (manager),
Christine Cunniffe, Brenna Mayer,
Patrice E. Polgar

Designers
Arlene Putterman (associate art
director), Lesley Weissman-Cook
(book designer), Diane Armento-
Feliz, Joseph Clark, Jacalyn
Facciolo, Linda Franklin, Donald
G. Knauss, Kaaren Mitchel, Mary
Stangl

Typographers
Diane Paluba (manager), Joyce Rossi
Biletz, Phyllis Marron, Valerie
Rosenberger

Production Coordinator
Margaret Rastiello

Editorial Assistants
Beverly Lane, Mary Madden, Jeanne
Napier

Manufacturing
Debbie Meiris (director), Pat Dor-
shaw (manager), Anna Brindisi, T.A.
Landis

Printed in the United States of America.
SNMS3- D
02 01 00 99   10 9 8 7 6 5 4 3 2
Ⓡ A member of the Reed Elsevier plc group

Library of Congress Cataloging-in-Publication Data
Boyd, Mildred W.
    Medical surgical nursing / Mildred Warnet Boyd,
    Barbara L. Tower–3rd ed.
        p. cm.–(Springhouse Notes)
    Includes bibliographical references and index.
    1. Nursing–Outlines, syllabi, etc. 2. Surgical nursing–
    outlines, syllabi, etc. I. Tower, Barbara L. II. Title
    III. Series
    [DNLM: 1. Nursing Care–Outlines. 2. Perioperative
    Nursing–outlines. WY 18.2 B789m 1997]
RT52.B64 1997
610.73'02–dc20
DNLM/DLC   96-29017
ISBN 0-87434-861-7 (alk.paper)   CIP

Contents

Advisory Board and Reviewers

How to Use
Springhouse Notes

Springhouse Notes is a multivolume study guide series developed especially for nursing students. Each volume provides essential course material in an outline format, enabling the student to review information efficiently.

Special features appear in every chapter to make information accessible and easy to remember. **Learning objectives** encourage the student to evaluate knowledge before and after study. **Chapter overview** highlights the chapter's major concepts. Within the outlined text, key points are highlighted in shaded blocks to facilitate a quick review of critical information. Key points may include cardinal signs and symptoms, current theories, important steps in a nursing procedure, critical assessment findings, crucial nursing interventions, or successful therapies and treatments. **Points to remember** summarize each chapter's major themes. **Study questions** then offer another opportunity to review material and assess knowledge gained before moving on to new information. **Critical thinking and application exercises** conclude each chapter, challenging students to expand on knowledge gained.

Other features appear throughout the book to facilitate learning: **Teaching tips** highlight key areas to address with patient teaching. **Clinical alerts** point out essential information on how to provide safe, effective care. **Decision trees** promote critical thinking. Difficult, frequently used, or sometimes misunderstood terms are indicated by SMALL CAPITAL LETTERS in the outline and defined in the glossary, Appendix A; answers to the study questions appear in Appendix B. Finally, a brand-new Windows-based software program (see diskette on inside back cover) poses 100 multiple-choice questions in random or sequential order to assess your knowledge.

The Springhouse Notes volumes are designed as learning tools, not as primary information sources. When read conscientiously as a supplement to class attendance and textbook reading, Springhouse Notes can enhance understanding and help improve test scores and final grades.

CHAPTER

1

Cardiovascular System

Learning objectives

After studying this chapter, you should be able to:

♦ Describe the psychosocial impact of cardiovascular disorders.

♦ Differentiate between modifiable and nonmodifiable risk factors in the development of a cardiovascular disorder.

♦ List three probable and three possible nursing diagnoses for a patient with any cardiovascular disorder.

♦ Identify nursing interventions for a patient with a cardiovascular disorder.

♦ Write three teaching goals for a patient with a cardiovascular disorder.

Chapter overview

Caring for the patient with a cardiovascular disorder requires a sound understanding of cardiovascular anatomy and physiology and hemodynamic function. A thorough assessment is essential to planning and implementing appropriate patient care. The assessment includes a complete history, physical examination, diagnostic testing, identification of modifiable and nonmodifiable risk factors, and information related to the psychosocial impact of the disorder on the patient. Nursing diagnoses focus primarily on altered tissue perfusion and decreased cardiac output. Nursing interventions are designed to decrease the cardiac workload and increase blood supply, thereby improving tissue perfusion. Patient teaching, a crucial nursing activity, involves information about medical follow-up, medication regimens, signs and symptoms of possible complications, and reduction of modifiable risk factors through weight control, activity and diet restrictions, stress management, and smoking cessation.

◆ I. Anatomy and physiology review

    A. Cardiac structures

        1. The heart is a muscular organ composed of two atria and two ventricles

        2. It is surrounded by a pericardial sac that consists of two layers

            a. Visceral (inner) layer

            b. Parietal (outer) layer

        3. The heart wall has three layers

            a. Epicardium (visceral pericardium)

            b. Myocardium

            c. Endocardium

        4. The heart has four valves

            a. Tricuspid (atrioventricular valve)

            b. Mitral (atrioventricular valve)

            c. Pulmonary (semilunar valve)

            d. Aortic (semilunar valve)

    B. Myocardial blood supply

        1. The left coronary artery branches into the left anterior descending artery (LAD) and the circumflex artery

            a. The LAD artery supplies blood to the anterior wall of the left ventricle, the anterior ventricular septum, and the bundle branches

            b. The circumflex artery provides blood to the lateral and posterior portions of the left ventricle

        2. The right coronary artery (RCA) fills the groove between the atria and ventricles and gives rise to the acute marginal artery, ending as the posterior descending artery

            a. The RCA sends blood to the sinus and atrioventricular nodes and to the right atrium

            b. The posterior descending artery supplies the posterior and inferior wall of the left ventricle and the posterior portion of the right ventricle

        3. Coronary arteries receive blood primarily during ventricular relaxation (diastole)

        4. Blood is pumped out to the systemic circulation during contraction of the ventricles (systole)

C. Circulation
1. From the inferior and superior venae cavae to the right atrium
2. Through the tricuspid valve to the right ventricle
3. Through the pulmonic valve to the pulmonary artery, to the lungs where blood is oxygenated, through the pulmonary veins to the left atrium
4. Through the mitral valve to the left ventricle
5. Through the aortic valve to the aorta and the systemic circulation
6. The goal of nursing management in cardiovascular disorders is to reduce oxygen demand and increase blood supply; thus increasing oxygenation to the tissues

D. Electrical conduction
1. The heart contains specialized muscle fibers that spontaneously generate and conduct their own electrical impulses
2. The sinoatrial (SA) node, internodal tracts, atrioventricular (AV) node, bundle of His, right and left bundle branches, and Purkinje fibers make up the system that conducts electrical impulses and coordinates chamber contraction
3. Impulses follow a right-to-left, top-to-bottom path
4. A normal electrical impulse is initiated at the SA node, the heart's intrinsic pacemaker
5. Once generated, the normal impulse must move forward through the conduction system to the ventricles
6. Numerous events occur almost simultaneously in the following order after initiation of the impulse at the SA node
   a. Atrial depolarization
   b. Atrial contraction
   c. Impulse transmission to the AV node
   d. Impulse transmission to the Bundle of His, bundle branches, and Purkinje fibers
   e. Ventricular depolarization
   f. Ventricular contraction
   g. Ventricular repolarization

E. Cardiac function
1. Cardiac output (CO) is the total amount of blood ejected per minute
2. Stroke volume (SV) is the amount of blood ejected with each beat
3. Cardiac output equals stroke volume times heart rate (CO = SV × HR)
4. Alterations in CO affect every body system
5. Ejection fraction is the percent of left ventricular end-diastolic volume ejected during systole (60% to 70% normal)

F. Blood vessels
1. Arteries are three-layered vessels (intima, media, adventitia) that carry oxygenated blood from the heart to the tissues
2. Arterioles are small-resistance vessels that feed into capillaries
3. Capillaries join arterioles to venules (larger, lower-pressured vessels than arterioles), where nutrients and wastes are exchanged
4. Venules join capillaries to veins
5. Veins are large-capacity, low-pressure vessels that return unoxygenated blood to the heart

◆ **II. Physical assessment findings**

A. History
1. Dyspnea
2. PAROXYSMAL NOCTURNAL DYSPNEA (PND)
3. ORTHOPNEA
4. Chest pain
5. Fatigue and weakness
6. Cough
7. Syncope
8. Palpitations
9. Leg pain

B. Physical examination
1. Blood pressure changes
2. Pulse changes including rate, rhythm, and quality
3. Skin color and temperature
4. Abnormal heart sounds
5. Edema
6. Arrhythmias
7. JUGULAR VENOUS DISTENTION (JVD)
8. Respiratory distress
9. Vascular BRUITS
10. POINT OF MAXIMAL IMPULSE alterations
11. Pruritus

◆ **III. Diagnostic tests and procedures**

A. Electrocardiography (ECG)
1. Definition and purpose
   a. Noninvasive test of the heart
   b. Graphical representation of the heart's electrical activity
2. Nursing interventions
   a. Determine the patient's ability to lie still
   b. Reassure the patient that electrical shock will not occur
   c. Interpret ECG for changes, such as life-threatening arrhythmias

B. Ambulatory electrocardiography (Holter monitoring)
   1. Definition and purpose
      a. Noninvasive test of the heart
      b. Recording of the heart's electrical activity and cardiac events for 24 hours
   2. Nursing interventions
      a. Instruct the patient to keep an activity diary
      b. Advise the patient not to bathe or shower, operate machinery, or use a microwave oven or an electric shaver while wearing the monitor

C. Cardiac catheterization
   1. Definition and purpose
      a. Fluoroscopic procedure using a radiopaque dye
      b. Examination of the intracardiac structures, pressures, oxygenation, and cardiac output after the dye is injected
   2. Nursing interventions before the procedure
      a. Withhold the patient's food and fluids after midnight
      b. Take baseline vital signs (VS) and peripheral pulses
      c. Obtain written, informed consent
      d. Inform the patient about possible nausea, chest pain, flushing of the face, or throat irritation from the injection of radiopaque dye

CLINICAL ALERT

      e. Note the patient's allergies to seafood, iodine, or radiopaque dyes
   3. Nursing interventions after the procedure
      a. Monitor VS, peripheral pulses, and the injection site for bleeding
      b. Maintain a pressure dressing and bed rest
      c. Force fluids unless contraindicated

CLINICAL ALERT

      d. Allay the patient's anxiety
      e. Monitor for complaints of chest pain and report immediately; possible sign of myocardial infarction (MI), a serious complication of cardiac catheterization

D. Echocardiography
   1. Definition and purpose
      a. Noninvasive examination of the heart
      b. Test that uses echoes from sound waves to visualize intracardiac structures and direction of blood flow
   2. Nursing interventions
      a. Determine the patient's ability to lie still
      b. Explain the procedure

E. Exercise testing (stress)
   1. Definition and purpose
      a. Noninvasive test of the heart
      b. Study of the heart's electrical activity and ischemic events during prescribed levels of exercise

    2. Nursing interventions
      a. Withhold food and fluids for 1 hour before the test
      b. Instruct the patient to wear loose-fitting clothing and supportive shoes
      c. Explain the procedure

F. Nuclear cardiology
    1. Definition and purpose
      a. Visual examination of the heart using radioisotopes
      b. Imaging of myocardial perfusion and contractility after I.V. injection of isotopes
    2. Nursing interventions
      a. Explain the procedure
      b. Allay the patient's anxiety
      c. Determine the patient's ability to lie still during the procedure

G. Coronary arteriography
    1. Definition and purpose
      a. Fluoroscopic procedure using a radiopaque dye
      b. Examination of the coronary arteries

CLINICAL ALERT

    2. Nursing interventions before the procedure
      a. Note the patient's allergies to iodine, seafood, or radiopaque dyes
      b. Monitor the patient's VS
      c. Allay the patient's anxiety
      d. Inform the patient about possible flushing of the face or throat irritation from the injection
    3. Nursing interventions after the procedure
      a. Check the insertion site for bleeding
      b. Assess peripheral pulses
      c. Maintain a pressure dressing and bed rest

H. Digital subtraction angiography
    1. Definition and purpose
      a. Invasive procedure using a computer system and fluoroscopy with an image intensifier
      b. Complete visualization of the arterial blood supply to a specific area
    2. Nursing interventions before the procedure
      a. Obtain written, informed consent
      b. Monitor the patient's VS
    3. Nursing interventions after the procedure
      a. Check the insertion site for bleeding
      b. Instruct the patient to drink at least 1 liter of fluid

I. Hemodynamic monitoring (single procedure or continuous monitoring)
   1. Definition and purpose
      a. Procedure using a balloon-tipped, flow-directed catheter (Swan-Ganz)
      b. Examination of intracardiac pressures and cardiac output
   2. Nursing interventions before the procedure
      a. Obtain written, informed consent
      b. Explain the procedure and its purpose to the patient
   3. Nursing interventions after the procedure
      a. Check the insertion site for signs of infection
      b. Monitor the pressure tracings and record readings

J. Chest X-ray
   1. Definition and purpose
      a. Noninvasive examination of the heart and lungs
      b. Radiographic picture of the heart and lungs
   2. Nursing interventions
      a. Determine the patient's ability to hold the breath
      b. Ensure that the patient removes jewelry

K. Blood chemistries
   1. Definition and purpose
      a. Laboratory test of a blood sample
      b. Analysis for sodium, potassium, magnesium, calcium, glucose, phosphorus, cholesterol, triglycerides, uric acid, bicarbonate, creatinine, blood urea nitrogen (BUN), bilirubin, creatinine kinase (CK), CK isoenzymes, lactic dehydrogenase (LDH), LDH isoenzymes, aspartate aminotransferase (AST), and alanine aminotransferase
   2. Nursing interventions
      a. Note any drugs that may alter test results
      b. Restrict the patient's exercise before the blood sample is drawn
      c. Withhold intramuscular injections or note the time of the injection on the laboratory slip (alter CK levels)
      d. Withhold food and fluids, as ordered
      e. Assess the venipuncture site for bleeding

L. Hematologic studies
   1. Definition and purpose
      a. Laboratory test of a blood sample
      b. Analysis for red blood cells, white blood cells (WBCs), erythrocyte sedimentation rate (ESR), prothrombin time (PT), partial thromboplastin time (PTT), platelets, hemoglobin, and hematocrit (HCT)

      2. Nursing interventions
         a. Note any drugs that might alter test results before the procedure
         b. Assess the venipuncture site for bleeding after the procedure

M. Arterial blood gas (ABG) analysis
      1. Definition and purpose
         a. Test of arterial blood
         b. Assessment of tissue oxygenation, ventilation, and acid-base status
      2. Nursing interventions before the procedure
         a. Document the patient's temperature
         b. Note whether the patient needs supplemental oxygen or mechanical ventilation
      3. Nursing interventions after the procedure
         a. Check the site for bleeding
         b. Maintain a pressure dressing

N. Doppler ultrasound
      1. Definition and purpose
         a. Noninvasive procedure that transforms echoes from sound waves into audible sounds
         b. Examination of blood flow in peripheral circulation
      2. Nursing interventions
         a. Determine the patient's ability to lie still
         b. Explain the procedure

O. Venogram
      1. Definition and purpose
         a. Visualization of the veins after I.V. injection of a dye
         b. Diagnosis of deep vein thrombosis or incompetent valves
      2. Nursing interventions before the procedure
         a. Withhold food and fluids after midnight
         b. Record the patient's baseline VS and peripheral pulses

CLINICAL ALERT

         c. Obtain written, informed consent
         d. Note the patient's allergies to seafood, iodine, or radiopaque dyes
         e. Inform the patient about possible flushing of the face or throat irritation from the injection
      3. Nursing interventions after the procedure
         a. Check the injection site for bleeding and hematoma
         b. Force fluids unless contraindicated

P. Pulse oximetry
      1. Definition and purpose
         a. Noninvasive procedure using infrared light to measure arterial oxygen saturation (SaO_2) in the blood
         b. Continuous measurement of SaO_2 assists in pulmonary assessment of patient and weaning patient from a ventilator

2. Nursing interventions
   a. Do not place the sensor on an extremity that has impeded blood flow
   b. Protect the sensor from bright light

   c. Attach the monitoring sensor to a fingertip, ear lobe, or toe.
   d. Remove artificial nails or nail tips; may interfere with light transmission (some sensors can accurately read through these as long as polish is removed, but this is not recommended)

◆ IV. Psychosocial impact of cardiovascular disorders

A. Developmental impact
  1. Fear of rejection
  2. Lowered self-esteem
  3. Fear of dying
  4. Role conflict

B. Economic impact
  1. Disruption or loss of employment
  2. Cost of hospitalization, medications, and special diets

C. Occupational and recreational impact
  1. Restrictions in work activity
  2. Changes in leisure activity
  3. Restrictions in physical activity (walking, climbing stairs)
  4. Restrictions in activity related to environmental temperature; for example, hot or cold weather may interfere with the patient's ability to take walks or go outside

D. Social impact
  1. Changes in dietary habits, such as dining out
  2. Changes in sexual function
  3. Changes in role performance, including work and family roles
  4. Social isolation

◆ V. Risk factors for developing cardiovascular disorders

A. Modifiable risk factors (impact of cardiovascular disorders can be reduced by altering these)
  1. Smoking
  2. Hypertension
  3. Hypercholesterolemia
  4. Obesity
  5. Physical inactivity
  6. Emotional stress

B. Nonmodifiable risk factors
  1. Gender
  2. Family history of cardiovascular illness

3. Childhood history of cardiovascular illness
4. Ethnicity
5. Race
6. Aging

♦ VI. Nursing diagnostic categories for a patient with a cardiovascular disorder

A. Probable nursing diagnostic categories
   1. Decreased cardiac output
   2. Pain, chronic pain
   3. Altered cardiopulmonary tissue perfusion
   4. Altered peripheral tissue perfusion
   5. Altered cerebral tissue perfusion
   6. Risk for peripheral neurovascular dysfunction

B. Possible nursing diagnostic categories
   1. Fluid volume excess
   2. Activity intolerance
   3. Fear
   4. Anxiety
   5. Ineffective individual coping
   6. Ineffective family coping: compromised
   7. Self-esteem disturbance
   8. Altered role performance
   9. Body image disturbance
   10. Sexual dysfunction
   11. Noncompliance
   12. Chronic low self-esteem
   13. Situational low self-esteem
   14. Fatigue

♦ VII. Cardiac surgery

A. Description
   1. Coronary artery bypass graft (CABG)—surgical revascularization of the coronary arteries using the saphenous veins or the internal mammary artery to bypass an obstruction caused by atherosclerosis
   2. Valve replacement—surgical replacement of stenotic or incompetent valves with a mechanical or bioprosthetic valve, such as Starr-Edwards "ball-in-cage" valves, porcine valves, or Bjork-Shiley "tilting disk" valves
   3. Valvular annuloplasty—surgical repair or reconstruction of the leaflets and annulus of the valve
   4. Mitral valve commissurotomy—surgical opening of the fused portion of the mitral valve leaflets, using a dilator

5. Valvuloplasty—surgical repair or reconstruction of the valve
6. Percutaneous transluminal valvuloplasty—dilation of calcified and stenotic valvular leaflets, using a balloon catheter
7. Percutaneous transluminal coronary angioplasty (PTCA)—dilation of a coronary artery using a balloon-tipped catheter to compress plaque against the vessel wall

B. Preoperative nursing interventions
1. Complete patient and family preoperative teaching
   a. Determine the patient's understanding of the procedure
   b. Describe the operating room (OR), postanesthesia care unit (PACU), and preoperative and postoperative routines
   c. Demonstrate postoperative turning, coughing, and deep-breathing (TCDB), splinting, leg exercises, and range-of-motion (ROM) exercises
   d. Explain the postoperative need for drainage tubes, surgical dressings, oxygen therapy, I.V. therapy, and pain control
2. Allay the patient's and family's anxiety about surgery
3. Document the patient's history and physical assessment data base
4. Obtain baseline hemodynamic variables, ECG readings, and ABG studies
5. Complete a preoperative checklist
6. Administer preoperative medications

C. Postoperative nursing interventions
1. Assess cardiac, respiratory, and neurologic status
2. Assess fluid balance
3. Assess pain and administer analgesics, as prescribed
4. Administer oxygen and maintain an endotracheal tube to the ventilator
5. Monitor VS, urine output (UO), intake/output (I/O), laboratory studies, ECG, hemodynamic variables, daily weight, and pulse oximetry
6. Monitor and maintain the water-seal chest drainage system for mediastinal and pleural chest tubes
7. Monitor and maintain the position and patency of drainage tubes and catheters, such as a nasogastric (NG) tube, indwelling urinary catheter, and wound drainage and chest tubes
8. Administer I.V. fluids and transfusion therapy, as prescribed
9. Inspect and change the surgical dressing, as directed
10. Keep the patient in semi-Fowler's position
11. Provide incentive spirometry after extubation or endotracheal suction
12. Reinforce TCDB and splinting of the incision

13. Administer antiarrhythmics, anticoagulants, vasopressors, beta adrenergics, diuretics, or cardiac glycosides, as prescribed
14. Monitor the patient for arrhythmias
15. Check peripheral circulation: color, temperature, pulses, and complaints of abnormal sensations, such as numbness or tingling
16. Insulate epicardial pacing wires; have temporary pacemaker available
17. Administer antibiotics, as prescribed
18. Assess for return of peristalsis
19. Provide the prescribed diet, as tolerated
20. Assist the patient with active and passive ROM and isometric exercises, as tolerated
21. Allay the patient's anxiety
22. Encourage the patient to express feelings about changes in body image or a fear of dying
23. Provide information about support groups, such as Mended Hearts
24. Individualize home care instructions
    a. Avoid driving and heavy lifting for 6 weeks
    b. Complete incision care daily
    c. Elevate the leg with the saphenous graft when seated
    d. Wear antiembolism stockings
    e. Follow a low-sodium diet

D. Possible surgical complications
   1. Bleeding from the mediastinal tube
   2. MI
   3. Decreased cardiac output
   4. Arrhythmias
   5. Cardiac tamponade
   6. Heart block
   7. Embolism
   8. Valve malfunction

♦ VIII. Pacemaker therapy

A. Description—electronic device which stimulates the heart to contract when the intrinsic pacemaker or conduction system fails

B. Types of pacemakers
   1. Demand (Synchronous, non-competitive)—pacemaker fires when inherent heart rate falls below predetermined set rate
   2. Fixed rate (Asynchronous, competitive)—pacemaker fires at a constant, preset rate

Pacemaker codes

CHAMBER PACED	CHAMBER SENSED	RESPONSE TO SENSING	PROGRAMMABLE FUNCTIONS AND RATE MODULATION	ANTITACHY-ARRHYTHMIA FUNCTIONS
V (ventricle)	V (ventricle)	T (triggers pacing)	P (programmable rate, output, or both)	P (pacing)
A (atrium)	A (atrium)	I (inhibits pacing)	M (multiprogrammable rate, output, sensitivity)	S (shock)
D (dual, A + V)	D (dual, A + V)	D (dual, T + I)	C (communicating functions, such as telemetry)	D (dual, P + S)
O (none)	O (none)	O (none)	R (rate modulation) O (none)	O (none)

3. Temporary—pulse generator is attached to pacemaker wires which are inserted temporarily
   a. Transvenous
   b. Epicardial
   c. Transcutaneous
4. Permanent—pulse generator implanted in subcutaneous tissue in right or left pectoral area

C. Pacemaker components
   1. Pulse generator—power source of pacemaker which is electronically controlled
      a. Plutonium—lasts 20+ years
      b. Lithium—lasts 10 years
      c. Mercury-zinc—lasts 3 to 4 years
   2. Lead—insulated wire implanted in the heart and connected to pulse generator to transmit electrical impulses from the pulse generator to the heart
   3. Controls
      a. Sensitivity
      b. Rate
      c. Output

D. Classification system — International Pacemaker Code
   (See *Pacemaker codes*)

E. Preoperative nursing interventions
   1. Complete patient and family preoperative teaching
      a. Determine the patient's understanding of the procedure
      b. Describe the OR, PACU, and preoperative and postoperative routines
      c. Demonstrate postoperative TCDB, splinting, and leg and ROM exercises
      d. Explain the postoperative need for surgical dressings, oxygen therapy, I.V. therapy, and pain control
   2. Complete a preoperative checklist
   3. Administer preoperative medications, as prescribed
   4. Allay the patient's and family's anxiety about surgery
   5. Document the patient's history and physical assessment data base
   6. Obtain a baseline assessment of heart rhythm and rate, peripheral circulation
   7. Administer antibiotics, as prescribed

F. Postoperative nursing interventions
   1. Assess cardiac status: heart sounds, rhythm
   2. Assess pain and administer analgesics as prescribed
   3. Monitor VS, UO, I/O, neurovascular checks, pulse oximetry
   4. Obtain a 12-lead ECG as ordered
   5. Protect control settings if temporary pacer
   6. Change dressing as ordered
   7. Monitor insertion site for signs of infection
   8. Immobilize upper extremity if used for insertion of temporary pacer
   9. Individualize home care instructions

CLINICAL ALERT

      a. Recognize signs of pacemaker malfunction
      b. Carry pacemaker ID card at all times
      c. Perform active ROM to upper extremity on side of insertion
      d. Check pulse daily
      e. Avoid physical contact sports
      f. Recognize signs of electrical interference
      g. Know the rate and battery life of pacemaker

G. Possible surgical complications
   1. Pneumothorax
   2. Perforation of heart
   3. Infection
   4. Breakage of a lead
   5. Migration of a lead

♦ IX. Abdominal aneurysm resection

A. Description—surgical removal of a portion of weakened arterial wall with an end-to-end anastomosis to a prosthetic graft

B. Preoperative nursing interventions
1. Complete patient and family preoperative teaching
   a. Determine the patient's understanding of the procedure
   b. Describe the OR, PACU, and preoperative and postoperative routines
   c. Demonstrate postoperative TCDB, splinting, and leg and ROM exercises
   d. Explain the postoperative need for drainage tubes, surgical dressings, oxygen therapy, I.V. therapy, and pain control
2. Complete a preoperative checklist
3. Administer preoperative medications, as prescribed
4. Allay the patient's and family's anxiety about surgery
5. Document the patient's history and physical assessment data base
6. Assess renal status and urine output

C. Postoperative nursing interventions
1. Assess cardiac, respiratory, and neurologic status
2. Assess fluid balance
3. Assess pain and administer analgesics, as prescribed
4. Administer I.V. fluids and transfusion therapy, as prescribed
5. Administer oxygen and maintain an endotracheal tube to the ventilator
6. Provide incentive spirometry after extubation or endotracheal suction
7. Reinforce TCDB and splinting of the incision
8. Monitor VS, UO, I/O, central venous pressure (CVP), laboratory studies, ECG, hemodynamic variables, and pulse oximetry
9. Monitor and maintain the position and patency of NG tubes and indwelling urinary catheters
10. Administer antibiotics, as prescribed
11. Assess for scrotal and retroperitoneal bleeding
12. Check peripheral circulation: color, temperature, complaints of abnormal sensation, and pulses in extremities
13. Inspect and change the surgical dressing, as directed
14. Keep the patient flat; set up a turning schedule, turning from side to side regularly
15. Assist the patient with active and passive ROM and isometric exercises, as tolerated
16. Assess for return of peristalsis
17. Provide the prescribed diet, as tolerated
18. Measure and record the patient's abdominal girth

CLINICAL ALERT

19. Allay the patient's anxiety
20. Individualize home care instructions
    a. Avoid lifting, bending, and driving for 6 weeks or as allowed by the doctor
    b. Monitor blood pressure daily
    c. Identify ways to reduce stress
    d. Complete incision care daily

D. Possible surgical complications
   1. Renal failure
   2. Atelectasis
   3. Graft hemorrhage

♦ X. Vascular grafting

A. Description-surgical revascularization of an artery
   1. Uses a synthetic or autogenous graft
   2. Bypasses or resects the diseased segment

B. Types of revascularization
   1. Femoropopliteal
   2. Aortofemoral
   3. Aortoiliac
   4. Femorofemoral
   5. Axillofemoral

C. Preoperative nursing interventions
   1. Complete patient and family preoperative teaching
      a. Determine the patient's understanding of the procedure
      b. Describe the OR, PACU, and preoperative and postoperative routines
      c. Demonstrate postoperative TCDB, splinting, and leg and ROM exercises
      d. Explain the postoperative need for drainage tubes, surgical dressings, oxygen therapy, I.V. therapy, and pain control
   2. Complete a preoperative checklist
   3. Administer preoperative medications, as prescribed
   4. Allay the patient's and family's anxiety about surgery
   5. Document the patient's history and physical assessment data base
   6. Obtain a baseline assessment of peripheral circulation
   7. Administer antibiotics, as prescribed

D. Postoperative nursing interventions
   1. Assess cardiac and neurovascular status
   2. Assess pain and administer analgesics, as prescribed
   3. Administer I.V. fluids and transfusion therapy, as prescribed

4. Monitor VS, UO, I/O, laboratory studies, neurovascular checks, and pulse oximetry
5. Monitor and maintain the position and patency of NG tubes and indwelling urinary catheters
6. Administer anticoagulants, as prescribed

7. Inspect and change the surgical dressing, as directed
8. Keep the patient in semi-Fowler's position; avoid positioning on or flexion at the graft site
9. Provide a bed cradle
10. Check peripheral circulation: temperature, color, pulses, and complaints of abnormal sensations in extremities distal to the graft site
11. Measure and record the patient's ankle, calf, and thigh circumferences
12. Provide incentive spirometry
13. Reinforce TCDB and splinting of the incision
14. Assess for return of peristalsis
15. Provide the prescribed diet, as tolerated
16. Measure and record the patient's abdominal girth
17. Assist the patient with active and passive ROM and isometric exercises, as tolerated
18. Allay the patient's anxiety
19. Encourage the patient to express feelings about changes in body image
20. Increase ambulation, as tolerated
21. Individualize home care instructions
    a. Avoid pressure or flexion at the graft site
    b. Avoid wearing constrictive clothing
    c. Complete incision care daily
    d. Check pulses distal to the graft site daily
    e. Adhere to long-term anticoagulant therapy
    f. Provide proper foot care daily

E. Possible surgical complications
   1. Thrombosis
   2. Embolism
   3. Graft rejection
   4. Hemorrhage

♦ XI. Hypertension

A. Definition—constant elevation of systolic or diastolic blood pressure (greater than 140/90 mm Hg)
   1. Stage 1 (mild) — 140-159/90-99 mm Hg
   2. Stage 2 (moderate) — 160-179/100-109 mm Hg

     3. Stage 3 (severe) — 180-209/110-119 mm Hg

     4. Stage 4 (very severe) — 210/120 mm Hg

B. Possible etiology

     1. Primary hypertension - unknown etiology

     2. Secondary hypertension

       a. Renal disease

       b. Pheochromocytoma

       c. Cushing's disease

C. Pathophysiology

     1. Blood pressure = Cardiac output × peripheral resistance

     2. Narrowing of the arterioles, which increases peripheral resistance

     3. Increased force needed to circulate blood, which elevates blood pressure

D. Possible assessment findings

     1. Asymptomatic

     2. Elevated blood pressure

     3. Headache

     4. Visual disturbances

     5. Left ventricular hypertrophy

     6. Renal failure

     7. Dizziness

     8. Papilledema

     9. Congestive heart failure (CHF)

    10. Cerebral ischemia

E. Possible diagnostic test findings

     1. Blood pressure: sustained readings greater than 140/90 mm Hg

     2. ECG: left ventricular hypertrophy

     3. Chest X-ray: cardiomegaly

     4. Ophthalmoscopic examination: retinal changes, such as severe vasoconstriction, papilledema, and retinopathy

     5. Blood chemistry: elevated sodium, BUN, creatinine, and cholesterol levels

F. Medical management

     1. Diet: low-sodium, low-calorie, low-cholesterol, and low-fat; restrict alcohol and caffeine

     2. I.V. therapy: heparin lock

     3. Activity: as tolerated

     4. Monitoring: VS, ECG, UO, and I/O

     5. Laboratory studies: sodium, potassium, and cholesterol

     6. Diuretics: furosemide (Lasix), spironolactone (Aldactone), hydrochlorothiazide (HydroDIURIL), bumetanide (Bumex)

TEACHING TIPS
Patients with cardiovascular disorders

Be sure to include the following topics when teaching patients with cardiovascular disorders.
- Smoking cessation
- Regular exercise
- Optimal weight maintenance
- Medication therapy, including the action, adverse effects, and scheduling
- Dietary recommendations and restrictions
- Stress reduction
- Rest and activity patterns
- Frequent blood pressure monitoring
- Risk factor modification

 7. Antihypertensives: methyldopa (Aldomet), hydralazine (Apresoline), prazosin (Minipress), doxazosin mesylate (Cardura)

 8. Vasodilators: sodium nitroprusside (Nipride)

 9. Calcium blockers: nifedipine (Procardia), verapamil (Calan), diltiazem (Cardizem), nicardipine (Cardene)

 10. Beta-adrenergic blockers: propranolol (Inderal), metoprolol (Lopressor), carteolol hydrochloride (Cartrol), penbutolol sulfate (Levatol)

 11. ACE inhibitors: captopril (Capoten), enalapril (Vasotec), lisinopril (Prinivil)

G. Nursing interventions

 1. Maintain the patient's prescribed diet

 2. Assess cardiovascular status

 3. Monitor and record VS, UO, I/O, laboratory studies, and daily weight

 4. Administer medications, as prescribed

 5. Encourage the patient to express feelings about daily stress

 6. Maintain a quiet environment

 7. Provide information about the American Heart Association

CLINICAL ALERT

 8. Take an average of two or more blood pressure readings rather than relying on one single abnormal reading

 9. Individualize home care instructions (For more information about teaching, see *Patients with cardiovascular disorders*)

  a. Take blood pressure daily

  b. Start an exercise program

H. Possible complications

 1. Cerebrovascular accident (CVA)

 2. Visual changes

3. Renal failure
4. CHF
5. Hypertensive crisis

I. Possible surgical interventions: none

◆ **XII. Coronary artery disease (CAD): Arteriosclerosis and atherosclerosis**

A. Definitions
   1. Arteriosclerosis—loss of elasticity of the arteries' intimal layer (sometimes called hardening of the arteries)
   2. Atherosclerosis—accumulation in the arteries of fatty plaque made of lipids

B. Possible etiology
   1. Aging
   2. Stress
   3. Genetics
   4. Depletion of estrogen post-menopause
   5. High-fat, high-cholesterol diet

C. Pathophysiology
   1. Narrowing or obstruction of the coronary arteries by an embolus, vasospasm, or accumulated plaque
   2. Decreased perfusion and inadequate myocardial oxygen supply

D. Possible assessment findings
   1. Hypertension
   2. Angina
   3. MI
   4. CHF

E. Possible diagnostic test findings
   1. ECG or Holter monitoring: ST depression, T wave inversion
   2. Stress test: elevated ST segment, multiple premature ventricular contractions (PVCs) on ECG, chest pain
   3. Coronary arteriography: plaque formation
   4. Blood chemistry: increased cholesterol (decreased high-density lipoproteins, increased low-density lipoproteins)

F. Medical management
   1. Diet: low-calorie, low-sodium, low-cholesterol, and low-fat; increased dietary fiber
   2. I.V. therapy: heparin lock
   3. Oxygen therapy
   4. Monitoring: VS, UO, CVP, ECG, hemodynamic variables, I/O, and neurovascular checks

    5. Laboratory studies: sodium, potassium, cholesterol, CK, LDH, AST, CK isoenzymes, LDH isoenzymes, and ABGs

    6. Weight reduction

    7. Arterial line for blood pressure monitoring

    8. Intraaortic balloon pump (IABP)

    9. Thrombolytic therapy: streptokinase (Streptase)

    10. PTCA

    11. Indwelling urinary catheter

    12. Antihyperlipidemic agents: cholestyramine (Questran), lovastatin (Mevacor), nicotinic acid (Niacin), gemifibrozil (Lopid), colestipol hydrochloride (Colestid)

    13. Nitrates: nitroglycerin (Nitro-Bid), isosorbide dinitrate (Isordil)

    14. Beta-adrenergic blockers: propranolol (Inderal), nadolol (Corgard)

    15. Calcium blockers: nifedipine (Procardia), verapamil (Calan), diltiazem (Cardizem)

    16. Analgesic: morphine sulfate (I.V.)

    17. Antianxiety agent: diazepam (Valium)

    18. Laser angioplasty

    19. Atherectomy

G. Nursing interventions

    1. Maintain the patient's prescribed diet

    2. Administer oxygen and medications, as prescribed

    3. Assess cardiovascular status

    4. Monitor and record VS, UO, hemodynamic variables, I/O, ECG, and laboratory studies

    5. Encourage the patient to express anxiety, fears, or concerns

    6. Provide information about the American Heart Association

    7. Individualize home care instructions

        a. Adhere to activity limitations

        b. Limit daily alcohol intake to 2 ounces

        c. Limit dietary fat intake

H. Possible complications

    1. Angina

    2. MI

    3. CHF

    4. Arrhythmias

I. Possible surgical interventions: CABG (see page 10)

◆ XIII. Angina

A. Definition

    1. Angina is chest pain caused by inadequate myocardial oxygen supply

        a. Stable angina — consistent symptoms with pain relieved by rest

      b. Unstable angina — increase in severity, duration, and frequency of pain which is eventually relieved by nitroglycerin

      c. Prinzmetal angina — pain which occurs at rest

    2. Complaints of chest pain have increased significance in a patient with a peripheral vascular problem

B. Possible etiology

    1. Atherosclerosis

    2. Vasospasm

    3. Aortic stenosis

    4. Activity or disease that increases metabolic demands

C. Pathophysiology

    1. Narrowing of the coronary arteries, which results from plaque accumulation in the intimal lining

    2. Obstruction of blood flow, which diminishes myocardial oxygen supply

D. Possible manifestations

    1. Substernal, crushing, compressing pain

      a. May radiate to the arms

      b. Usually lasts 3 to 5 minutes

      c. Usually occurs after exertion, emotional excitement, or exposure to cold but also can develop when the patient is at rest

    2. Dyspnea

    3. Palpitations

    4. Epigastric distress

    5. Tachycardia

    6. Diaphoresis

    7. Anxiety

CLINICAL ALERT

E. Possible diagnostic test findings

    1. ECG: ST depression, T wave inversion during acute pain

    2. Stress test: abnormal ECG, chest pain

    3. Coronary arteriography: plaque accumulation

    4. Blood chemistry: increased cholesterol

    5. Cardiac enzymes: within normal limits

    6. Holter monitoring: ST depression, T wave inversion

F. Medical management

    1. Diet: low-calorie, low-sodium, and low-cholesterol

    2. I.V. therapy: heparin lock

    3. Oxygen therapy

    4. Position: semi-Fowler's

    5. Monitoring: VS, UO, ECG, hemodynamic variables, I/O, and neurovascular checks

   6. Laboratory studies: ABGs, sodium, potassium, CK with isoenzymes, LDH with isoenzymes, and AST
   7. PTCA
   8. Arterial line for blood pressure monitoring
   9. Nitrates: nitroglycerin (Nitrostat), isosorbide dinitrate (Isordil)
   10. Beta-adrenergic blockers: propranolol (Inderal), nadolol (Corgard), atenolol (Tenormin), metoprolol (Lopressor)
   11. Calcium channel blockers: verapamil (Calan), diltiazem (Cardizem), nifedipine (Procardia), nicardipine (Cardene)

G. Nursing interventions
   1. Maintain the patient's prescribed diet (low-fat, low-sodium, and low-cholesterol)
   2. Administer oxygen and medications, as prescribed
   3. Assess cardiovascular status
   4. Monitor and record VS, UO, hemodynamic variables, I/O, and laboratory studies
   5. Assess for chest pain
   6. Encourage the patient to express anxiety, fears, or concerns
   7. Advise the patient to rest if pain begins
   8. Obtain an ECG reading during an acute attack
   9. Keep the patient in semi-Fowler's position
   10. Provide information about the American Heart Association
   11. Individualize home care instructions
       a. Discard nitroglycerin tablets after 6 months
       b. Know the difference between angina and MI
       c. Avoid activities or situations that cause angina, such as exertion, heavy meals, emotional upsets, and exposure to cold
       d. Seek medical attention if pain lasts more than 20 minutes

H. Possible complications
   1. Arrhythmias
   2. CHF
   3. MI

I. Possible surgical interventions: CABG (see page 10)

♦ XIV. Myocardial infarction

A. Definition—death of a portion of the myocardial muscle cells caused by a lack of oxygen from inadequate perfusion

B. Possible etiology
   1. Atherosclerosis
   2. Inadequate perfusion to meet metabolic demands
   3. Embolism or thrombus
   4. Coronary artery spasm

C. Pathophysiology
   1. Narrowing and eventual obstruction of the coronary arteries from plaque accumulation
   2. Death of the myocardial cells from inadequate perfusion and oxygenation

D. Possible assessment findings
   1. Crushing substernal pain
      a. May radiate to the jaw, back, and arms
      b. Lasts longer than anginal pain
      c. Is unrelieved by rest or nitroglycerin
      d. May not be present (asymptomatic, or "silent," MI)
   2. Dyspnea
   3. Nausea and vomiting
   4. Anxiety
   5. Diaphoresis
   6. Pallor
   7. Arrhythmias
   8. Elevated temperature

E. Possible diagnostic test findings
   1. ECG: enlarged Q wave, elevated ST segment, T wave inversion
   2. Blood chemistry: increased CK, LDH, AST, lipids; positive CK-MB fraction; flipped LDH-1 (LDH-1 levels exceed LDH-2 levels, the reversal of their normal patterns)
   3. Hematology: increased WBC count

F. Medical management
   1. Diet: low-calorie, low-cholesterol, low-fat
   2. Antiarrhythmics: quinidine gluconate (Quinaglute), lidocaine (Xylocaine), procainamide (Pronestyl)
   3. Anticoagulant: aspirin
   4. Antihypertensives: hydralazine (Apresoline), methyldopa (Aldomet)
   5. Angiotensin-converting enzyme (ACE) inhibitors: captopril (Capoten), enalaprilat (Vasotec)

   6. Nitrates: nitroglycerin (I.V.)
   7. Beta-adrenergic blockers: propranolol (Inderal), nadolol (Corgard), metoprolol tartrate (Lopressor); beta blockers contraindicated if patient also has CHF, hypotension, or bronchospasm
   8. Calcium channel blockers: verapamil (Calan), diltiazem (Cardizem), nifedipine (Procardia), nicardipine (Cardene)
   9. IABP
   10. Left ventricular assist device (LVAD)
   11. Thrombolytic therapy: anistreplase (Eminase), anisoylated plasminogen-streptokinase activator complex, streptokinase (Streptase)
   12. Monitoring: VS, UO, ECG, and hemodynamic variables

13. Oxygen therapy
14. Laboratory studies: ABGs, CK, CK isoenzymes, LDH, LDH isoenzymes, AST, WBC, sodium, potassium, and glucose
15. Position: semi-Fowler's
16. I.V. therapy: heparin lock
17. PTCA
18. Arterial line for blood pressure monitoring
19. Laser angioplasty
20. Vascular stents
21. Atherectomy

G. Nursing interventions
   1. Maintain the patient's prescribed diet
   2. Assess cardiovascular and respiratory status
   3. Monitor and record VS, UO, I/O, hemodynamic variables, laboratory studies, and ECG results
   4. Maintain bed rest

CLINICAL
ALERT

   5. Administer oxygen and medications, as prescribed
   6. Obtain an ECG reading during acute pain
   7. Allay the patient's anxiety
   8. Keep the patient in semi-Fowler's position
   9. Provide information about the American Heart Association
   10. Individualize home care instructions
      a. Participate in a cardiac rehabilitation program
      b. Maintain a low-cholesterol, low-fat, low-sodium diet
      c. Know the difference between the pain of angina and MI
      d. Alternate rest periods with activity

H. Possible complications
   1. Arrhythmias
   2. Cardiogenic shock
   3. CHF
   4. Papillary muscle rupture
   5. Pericarditis
   6. Thromboembolism

I. Possible surgical interventions: CABG (see page 10)

◆ **XV. Congestive heart failure: Left-sided**

A. Definition—failure of the left side of the heart to pump enough blood to meet metabolic demands

B. Possible etiology
   1. Atherosclerosis
   2. Fluid overload
   3. MI

      4. Valvular stenosis

      5. Valvular insufficiency

      6. Hypertension

      7. Cardiac conduction defects

C. Pathophysiology

      1. Decreased myocardial contractility or increased myocardial work-load, either of which increases left ventricular pressure and left atrial pressure and reduces cardiac output

      2. Impaired oxygenation and respiratory manifestations of fluid over-load

D. Possible assessment findings

      1. Dyspnea

      2. PND

      3. Crackles

      4. Cough

      5. Gallop rhythm: S_3, S_4

      6. Arrhythmias

      7. Fatigue

      8. Anxiety

      9. Orthopnea

    10. Tachycardia

    11. Tachypnea

E. Possible diagnostic test findings

      1. Chest X-ray: increased pulmonary congestion, left ventricular hypertrophy

      2. Echocardiography: increased size of cardiac chambers and decreased wall motion

      3. Hemodynamic monitoring: increased pulmonary capillary wedge pressure (PCWP), CVP, and pulmonary artery pressure (PAP); decreased cardiac output

      4. ABGs: hypoxemia, hypercapnia

      5. ECG: left ventricular hypertrophy

      6. Blood chemistry: decreased potassium, sodium; increased BUN, creatinine

F. Medical management

      1. Diet: low-sodium; limit fluids

      2. I.V. therapy: electrolyte replacement, heparin lock

      3. Oxygen therapy

      4. Position: semi-Fowler's

      5. Activity: bed rest; active ROM and isometric exercises

      6. Monitoring: VS, UO, I/O, ECG, and hemodynamic variables

      7. Laboratory studies: ABGs, sodium, potassium, BUN, and creatinine

      8. Indwelling urinary catheter

9. IABP
10. LVAD
11. Analgesic: morphine sulfate (I.V.)
12. Diuretics: furosemide (Lasix), bumetanide (Bumex), metolazone (Zaroxolyn)
13. Vasodilator: sodium nitroprusside (Nipride)
14. Cardiac inotropes: dopamine hydrochloride (Intropin), dobutamine (Dobutrex)
15. Cardiac glycoside: digoxin (Lanoxin)
16. Nitrates: isosorbide dinitrate (Isordil), nitroglycerin (Nitro-Bid)
17. ACE inhibitors: captopril (Capoten), enalapril (Vasotec), lisinopril (Prinivil)
18. Phosphodiesterase inhibitor: amrinone lactate (Inocor)
19. Specialized bed: active or static, low air loss (Kin Air, Flexicair)

G. Nursing interventions
1. Maintain the patient's prescribed diet
2. Restrict oral fluids
3. Administer I.V. fluids, oxygen, and medications, as prescribed
4. Provide suctioning and TCDB
5. Assess cardiovascular and respiratory status
6. Weigh the patient daily
7. Keep the patient in semi-Fowler's position
8. Monitor and record VS, UO, CVP, hemodynamic variables, I/O, and laboratory studies
9. Assess peripheral edema
10. Encourage the patient to express feelings, such as a fear of dying
11. Provide information about the American Heart Association
12. Individualize home care instructions
   a. Limit sodium intake
   b. Supplement the diet with foods high in potassium
   c. Recognize the signs and symptoms of fluid overload

H. Possible complications
1. Digoxin toxicity
2. Fluid overload
3. Cardiogenic shock
4. Pulmonary edema
5. Hypokalemia

I. Possible surgical interventions: none

♦ **XVI. Congestive heart failure: Right-sided**

A. Definition—failure of the right side of the heart to pump enough blood to meet metabolic demands

B. Possible etiology

    1 Atherosclerosis

    2. Left-sided CHF

    3. Chronic obstructive pulmonary disease

    4. Valvular stenosis

    5. Valvular insufficiency

    6. Pulmonary hypertension

C. Pathophysiology

    1. Increased pressure from left-sided CHF

    2. Increased venous congestion in the systemic circulation with fluid overload

    3. Increased resistance in lungs

D. Possible assessment findings

    1. JVD

    2. Anorexia

    3. Nausea

    4. Ascites

    5. Hepatomegaly

    6. Dependent edema

    7. Weight gain

    8. Signs of left-sided CHF

    9. Gallop rhythm: S_3, S_4

    10. Tachycardia

    11. Fatigue

E. Possible diagnostic test findings

    1. Chest X-ray: pulmonary congestion, cardiomegaly, pleural effusions

    2. Echocardiogram: increased size of chambers, decrease in wall motion

    3. Hemodynamic monitoring: increased PCWP, PAP, CVP; decreased cardiac output

    4. ABGs: hypoxemia

    5. ECG: left and right ventricular hypertrophy

    6. Blood chemistry: decreased sodium, potassium; increased BUN, creatinine

F. Medical management

    1. Diet: low-sodium; limit fluids

    2. I.V. therapy: electrolyte replacement, heparin lock

    3. Oxygen therapy

    4. Position: semi-Fowler's

    5. Activity: bed rest, active ROM and isometric exercises

    6. Monitoring: VS, UO, I/O, ECG, and hemodynamic variables

    7. Laboratory studies: ABGs, sodium, potassium, BUN, and creatinine

    8. Indwelling urinary catheter

     9. IABP

   10. Thoracentesis

   11. Paracentesis

   12. Analgesic: morphine sulfate (I.V.)

   13. Diuretics: furosemide (Lasix), bumetanide (Bumex), metolazone (Zaroxolyn)

   14. Vasodilator: sodium nitroprusside (Nipride)

   15. Cardiac inotropes: dopamine hydrochloride (Intropin), dobutamine (Dobutrex)

   16. Cardiac glycoside: digoxin (Lanoxin)

   17. Nitrates: isosorbide dinitrate (Isordil), nitroglycerin (Nitro-Bid)

G. Nursing interventions

    1. Maintain the patient's prescribed diet (low-sodium, low-cholesterol, no caffeine)

    2. Restrict oral fluids

    3. Administer I.V. fluids, oxygen, and medications, as prescribed

    4. Provide suctioning and TCDB

    5. Assess cardiovascular and respiratory status

    6. Assess peripheral edema

    7. Keep the patient in semi-Fowler's position

    8. Monitor and record VS, UO, I/O, hemodynamic variables, and laboratory studies

    9. Weigh the patient daily

   10. Encourage the patient to express feelings, such as a fear of dying

   11. Measure and record the patient's abdominal girth

   12. Individualize home care instructions

      a. Elevate legs when seated

      b. Limit sodium intake

      c. Supplement the diet with foods high in potassium

      d. Recognize the signs and symptoms of fluid overload

H. Possible complications

    1. Digoxin toxicity

    2. Fluid overload

    3. Cardiogenic shock

    4. Pulmonary edema

    5. Hypokalemia

    6. Hypernatremia

I. Possible surgical interventions: none

◆ XVII. Acute pulmonary edema

A. Definition—complication of left-sided heart failure; results in increased pressure in the capillaries of the lungs and acute transudation of fluid

B. Possible etiology
   1. Atherosclerosis
   2. MI
   3. Myocarditis
   4. Valvular disease
   5. Smoke inhalation
   6. Drug overdose: heroin, barbiturates, morphine sulfate
   7. Overload of I.V. fluids
   8. CHF
   9. Adult respiratory distress syndrome

C. Pathophysiology
   1. Pulmonary capillary pressure exceeds intravascular osmotic pressure
   2. Alveolar and interstitial edema result from the heart's failure to pump adequately
   3. Impaired oxygenation and hypoxia result

D. Possible assessment findings
   1. Dyspnea
   2. Paroxysmal cough
   3. Blood-tinged, frothy sputum
   4. Orthopnea
   5. Tachypnea
   6. Agitation
   7. Restlessness
   8. Intense fear
   9. Chest pain
   10. Syncope
   11. Tachycardia
   12. Cold, clammy skin
   13. Gallop rhythm: S_3, S_4
   14. JVD

E. Possible diagnostic test findings
   1. Chest X-ray: interstitial edema
   2. ABGs: respiratory alkalosis or acidosis
   3. ECG: tachycardia, ventricular enlargement
   4. Hemodynamic monitoring: increased PCWP, CVP, PAP; decreased cardiac output

F. Medical management
   1. Diet: low-sodium; limit fluids
   2. I.V. therapy: electrolyte replacement, heparin lock
   3. Oxygen therapy
   4. Intubation and mechanical ventilation
   5. Tourniquets: rotating
   6. Position: high-Fowler's

7. Activity: bed rest; active ROM and isometric exercises

8. Monitoring: VS, UO, I/O, ECG, and hemodynamic variables

9. Laboratory studies: sodium, potassium, ABGs, BUN, and creatinine

10. Indwelling urinary catheter, endotracheal tube suctioning

11. Analgesic: morphine sulfate (I.V.)

12. Diuretics: furosemide (Lasix), bumetanide (Bumex), metolazone (Zaroxolyn)

13. Vasodilator: sodium nitroprusside (Nipride)

14. Cardiac inotropes: dopamine hydrochloride (Intropin), dobu- tamine (Dobutrex)

15. Cardiac glycoside: digoxin (Lanoxin)

16. Nitrates: isosorbide dinitrate (Isordil), nitroglycerin (Nitro-Bid)

17. Bronchodilators: aminophylline (Somophyllin)

18. Pulse oximetry

G. Nursing interventions

1. Withhold food and fluids, as directed

2. Administer I.V. fluids, oxygen, and medications, as prescribed

3. Provide suctioning and TCDB

4. Assess cardiovascular and respiratory status

5. Keep the patient in high-Fowler's position

6. Monitor and record VS, UO, I/O, hemodynamic variables, labora- tory studies, and daily weight

7. Allay the patient's anxiety

8. Encourage the patient to express feelings, such as a fear of suffoca- tion

9. Note the color, amount, and consistency of sputum

10. Apply rotating tourniquets

11. Individualize home care instructions

   a. Weigh daily

   b. Recognize the signs of fluid overload

   c. Sleep with the head of the bed elevated

   d. Recognize the signs and symptoms of respiratory distress

   e. Supplement the diet with foods high in potassium

H. Possible complications

1. Digoxin toxicity

2. Fluid overload

3. Pulmonary embolism

4. Hypokalemia

5. Hypernatremia

I. Possible surgical interventions: none

♦ **XVIII. Cardiogenic shock**

    A. Definition—failure of the heart to pump adequately, thereby reducing cardiac output and compromising tissue perfusion

    B. Possible etiology

       1. MI

       2. Myocarditis

       3. Advanced heart block

       4. CHF

    C. Pathophysiology

       1. Decreased stroke volume and cardiac output; increased left ventricular volume, increased peripheral resistance due to increased sympathetic nervous system activity

       2. Compensatory increases in heart rate and contractility, which raise the demand for myocardial oxygen

       3. Imbalance between oxygen supply and demand, which increases myocardial ischemia and further compromises the heart's pumping action

    D. Possible assessment findings

       1. Hypotension (systolic pressure of less than 90 mm Hg)

       2. Oliguria (urine output of less than 30 ml/hour)

       3. Cold, clammy skin

       4. Tachycardia

       5. Restlessness

       6. Hypoxia

       7. Tachypnea

       8. Anxiety

       9. Arrhythmias

     10. Disorientation and confusion

    E. Possible diagnostic test findings

       1. ABGs: metabolic acidosis, hypoxemia

       2. ECG: MI (enlarged Q wave, ST elevation)

       3. Blood chemistry: increased BUN, creatinine

       4. Hemodynamic monitoring: decreased stroke volume and cardiac output; increased PCWP, CVP, PAP

    F. Medical management

       1. Diet: withhold food and fluids

       2. I.V. therapy: electrolyte replacement, heparin lock

       3. Oxygen therapy

       4. Intubation and mechanical ventilation

       5. Position: semi-Fowler's

       6. Activity: bed rest; passive ROM and isometric exercises

    7. Monitoring: VS, UO, I/O, ECG, hemodynamic variables, and level of consciousness

    8. Laboratory studies: potassium, sodium, BUN, creatinine, and ABGs

    9. Indwelling urinary catheter, endotracheal tube suction

  10. IABP

  11. Diuretics: furosemide (Lasix), bumetanide (Bumex), metolazone (Zaroxolyn)

  12. Vasodilator: sodium nitroprusside (Nipride)

  13. Cardiac inotropes: dopamine hydrochloride (Intropin), dobutamine (Dobutrex), amrinone lactate (Inocor)

  14. Cardiac glycoside: digoxin (Lanoxin)

  15. Vasopressor: norepinephrine (Levophed)

  16. Adrenergic agent: epinephrine hydrochloride (Adrenalin)

  17. Hemopump

  18. Pulse oximetry

G. Nursing interventions

    1. Withhold food and fluids, as directed

    2. Administer I.V. fluids, oxygen, and medications, as prescribed

    3. Provide suctioning and TCDB

    4. Assess cardiovascular and respiratory status and fluid balance

    5. Keep the patient in semi-Fowler's position

    6. Monitor and record VS, UO, I/O, hemodynamic variables, level of consciousness, and laboratory studies

    7. Encourage the patient to express feelings, such as a fear of dying

    8. Allay the patient's anxiety

    9. Individualize home care instructions

      a. Recognize the signs and symptoms of fluid overload

      b. Adhere to activity limitations

      c. Alternate rest periods with activity

      d. Maintain low-fat, low-sodium diet

H. Possible complications

    1. Arrhythmias

    2. Cardiac arrest

    3. Infection

I. Possible surgical interventions: CABG (see page 10)

◆ XIX. Mitral stenosis

A. Definition—narrowing of the mitral valve opening

B. Possible etiology: rheumatic endocarditis, congenital

C. Pathophysiology
  1. Thickening and calcification of valvular tissue, thereby narrowing the mitral valve opening and limiting blood flow from the left atrium to the left ventricle
  2. Increased pressure in the left atrium, leading to pulmonary hypertension and left atrial hypertrophy
  3. Right ventricular failure, producing pulmonary congestion

D. Possible assessment findings
  1. Fatigue
  2. Low cardiac output
  3. Dyspnea on exertion
  4. Right-sided heart failure
  5. Cough
  6. Peripheral edema
  7. Atrial fibrillation
  8. Orthopnea
  9. JVD
  10. Tachycardia
  11. PND
  12. Hemoptysis
  13. Murmurs, clicks

E. Possible diagnostic test findings
  1. Chest X-ray: enlargement of the left atrium and right ventricle; pulmonary congestion
  2. Echocardiogram: thickening of the mitral valve and left atrial enlargement
  3. Cardiac catheterization: increased left atrial pressure, PCWP; decreased cardiac output
  4. Angiography: mitral stenosis

F. Medical management
  1. Diet: low-sodium; limit fluids
  2. I.V. therapy: heparin lock
  3. Oxygen therapy
  4. Position: semi-Fowler's
  5. Activity: bed rest; active ROM and isometric exercises
  6. Monitoring: VS, UO, I/O, ECG, and hemodynamic variables
  7. Laboratory studies: sodium, potassium, PT, PTT, and ABGs
  8. Indwelling urinary catheter
  9. Cardiac glycoside: digoxin (Lanoxin)
  10. Nitrates: isosorbide dinitrate (Isordil), nitroglycerin (Nitro-Bid)
  11. Diuretics: furosemide (Lasix), bumetanide (Bumex)
  12. Antiarrhythmics: quinidine (Cardioquin), procainamide (Pronestyl)
  13. Anticoagulants: warfarin sodium (Coumadin)

14. Antibiotics: penicillin G potassium (Pentids)
15. Percutaneous transluminal valvuloplasty

G. Nursing interventions
1. Maintain the patient's prescribed diet; restrict oral fluids
2. Administer I.V. fluids, oxygen, and medications, as prescribed
3. Assess cardiovascular and respiratory status
4. Keep the patient in semi-Fowler's position
5. Monitor and record VS, UO, I/O, hemodynamic variables, laboratory studies, and ECG readings
6. Encourage the patient to express feelings, such as a fear of dying
7. Assess pain
8. Allay the patient's anxiety
9. Assess peripheral edema
10. Individualize home care instructions
    a. Recognize the signs and symptoms of CHF
    b. Adhere to activity limitations; alternate rest periods with activity
    c. Monitor for infection, avoid exposure to people with infections, and seek treatment if infection develops
    d. Test stools for occult blood

H. Possible complications
1. Thrombosis
2. Embolism
3. CHF
4. Atrial fibrillation

I. Possible surgical interventions
1. Valve replacement (see page 10)
2. Open mitral commissurotomy (see page 10)

◆ XX. Mitral regurgitation (mitral insufficiency)

A. Definition—incomplete closure of the mitral valve

B. Possible etiology
1. Congenital defect
2. Rheumatic fever
3. Trauma
4. Papillary muscle dysfunction
5. Bacterial endocarditis

C. Pathophysiology
1. Valvular incompetence
2. Backflow of blood to the left atrium
3. Increased left atrial pressure, pulmonary hypertension, and left atrial hypertrophy

D. Possible assessment findings
1. Shortness of breath
2. Cough
3. Fatigue
4. Dyspnea on exertion
5. Peripheral edema
6. Atrial fibrillation
7. Angina pectoris
8. Orthopnea
9. Hemoptysis
10. Murmurs and clicks

E. Possible diagnostic test findings
1. Chest X-ray: enlargement of the left atrium and the left ventricle
2. ECG: atrial fibrillation, left atrial hypertension, and left ventricular hypertrophy
3. Echocardiogram: enlargement of the left atrium, abnormal movement of the mitral valve
4. Cardiac catheterization: increased left atrial and left ventricular pressure
5. Angiography: regurgitation

F. Medical management
1. Diet: low-sodium; limit fluids
2. I.V. therapy: heparin lock
3. Oxygen therapy
4. Position: semi-Fowler's
5. Monitoring: VS, UO, I/O, ECG, and hemodynamic variables
6. Laboratory studies: sodium, potassium, BUN, creatinine, and ABGs
7. Indwelling urinary catheter
8. Cardiac glycoside: digoxin (Lanoxin)
9. Nitrates: isosorbide dinitrate (Isordil), nitroglycerin (Nitro-Bid)
10. Diuretics: furosemide (Lasix), bumetanide (Bumex)
11. Antiarrhythmics: quinidine (Cardioquin), procainamide (Pronestyl)
12. Anticoagulants: warfarin sodium (Coumadin)

G. Nursing interventions
1. Maintain the patient's prescribed diet; limit oral fluids
2. Administer I.V. fluids, oxygen, and medications, as prescribed
3. Assess cardiovascular and respiratory status
4. Keep the patient in semi-Fowler's position
5. Monitor and record VS, UO, I/O, hemodynamic variables, laboratory studies, and ECG readings
6. Encourage the patient to express feelings, such as a fear of dying
7. Assess pain
8. Assess peripheral edema
9. Allay the patient's anxiety

10. Provide information about the American Heart Association
11. Individualize home care instructions
    a. Test stools for occult blood
    b. Adhere to activity limitations; alternate rest periods with activity
    c. Monitor for infection, avoid exposure to people with infections, and seek treatment if infection develops

H. Possible complications
   1. Embolism
   2. Thrombosis
   3. CHF
   4. Ruptured papillary muscle

I. Possible surgical interventions
   1. Mitral valve replacement (see page 10)
   2. Valvuloplasty (see page 11)

◆ XXI. Aortic stenosis

A. Definition—narrowing of the aortic valve

B. Possible etiology
   1. Syphilis
   2. Rheumatic fever
   3. Atherosclerosis
   4. Congenital malformations

C. Pathophysiology
   1. Fibrosis and calcification of valvular tissue, which narrows the valve opening and limits blood flow
   2. Increased left ventricular pressure, which causes hypertrophy of the left ventricle and lowers cardiac output
   3. Increased congestion in the lungs, resulting in right ventricular failure

D. Possible assessment findings
   1. Angina pectoris
   2. Syncope
   3. Pulmonary hypertension
   4. Left-sided heart failure
   5. Fatigue
   6. Orthopnea
   7. PND
   8. Murmurs and clicks

E. Possible diagnostic test findings
   1. Chest X-ray: aortic valve calcification, left ventricular enlargement
   2. ECG: left bundle branch block, first-degree heart block, left ventricular hypertrophy

     3. Echocardiogram: thickened left ventricular wall, thickened aortic valve that moves abnormally

     4. Cardiac catheterization: increased left ventricular pressure

F. Medical management

     1. Diet: low-sodium; limit fluids

     2. I.V. therapy: heparin lock

     3. Monitoring: VS, UO, I/O, ECG, and hemodynamic variables

     4. Laboratory studies: sodium, potassium, BUN, creatinine, and ABGs

     5. Cardiac glycoside: digoxin (Lanoxin)

     6. Nitrates: isosorbide dinitrate (Isordil), nitroglycerin (Nitro-Bid)

     7. Diuretics: furosemide (Lasix), bumetanide (Bumex)

     8. Percutaneous transluminal valvuloplasty

G. Nursing interventions

     1. Maintain the patient's prescribed diet; limit fluids

     2. Assess cardiovascular and respiratory status

     3. Monitor and record VS, UO, I/O, hemodynamic variables, laboratory studies, and ECG readings

     4. Administer I.V. therapy and medications, as prescribed

     5. Encourage the patient to express feelings, such as a fear of dying

     6. Assess pain

     7. Allay the patient's anxiety

     8. Provide information about the American Heart Association

     9. Individualize home care instructions

       a. Recognize the signs and symptoms of CHF

       b. Adhere to activity limitations; alternate rest periods with activity

       c. Follow dietary restrictions and recommendations

H. Possible complications

     1. CHF

     2. Pulmonary edema

I. Possible surgical interventions

     1. Aortic valve replacement (see page 10)

     2. Commissurotomy (see page 10)

♦ XXII. Aortic regurgitation (aortic insufficiency)

A. Definition—incomplete closure of the aortic valve

B. Possible etiology

     1. Rheumatic fever

     2. Infective endocarditis

     3. Syphilis

     4. Atherosclerosis

     5. Congenital defect

C. Pathophysiology
  1. Retrograde flow of blood from the aorta to the left ventricle
  2. Left ventricular hypertrophy

D. Possible assessment findings
  1. Signs of left-sided heart failure
  2. Dyspnea on exertion
  3. Dizziness
  4. Neck pain
  5. Orthopnea
  6. Angina pectoris
  7. Tachycardia
  8. PND
  9. Murmurs and clicks

E. Possible diagnostic test findings
  1. Chest X-ray: enlarged left ventricle, aortic valve calcification
  2. ECG: left ventricular hypertrophy, sinus tachycardia
  3. Echocardiogram: left ventricular enlargement, abnormal valve movement
  4. Cardiac catheterization: increased left atrial and left ventricular pressures
  5. Cardiac angiography: regurgitation

F. Medical management
  1. Diet: low-sodium; limit fluids
  2. I.V. therapy: heparin lock
  3. Monitoring: VS, UO, I/O, ECG, and hemodynamic variables
  4. Laboratory studies: ABGs, sodium, potassium, BUN, and creatinine
  5. Indwelling urinary catheter
  6. Antibiotic: penicillin G potassium (Pentids)
  7. Cardiac glycoside: digoxin (Lanoxin)
  8. Nitrates: isosorbide dinitrate (Isordil), nitroglycerin (Nitro-Bid)
  9. Diuretics: furosemide (Lasix), bumetanide (Bumex)
  10. Vasodilators: hydralazine (Apresoline), nifedipine (Procardia)
  11. ACE inhibitors: captopril (Capoten), enalapril (Vasotec), lisinopril (Prinivil)

G. Nursing interventions
  1. Maintain the patient's prescribed diet; restrict oral fluids
  2. Administer I.V. fluids and medications, as prescribed
  3. Assess cardiovascular and respiratory status
  4. Monitor and record VS, UO, I/O, hemodynamic variables, and laboratory studies
  5. Assess pain
  6. Encourage the patient to express feelings, such as a fear of dying
  7. Allay the patient's anxiety

8. Provide information about the American Heart Association
9. Individualize home care instructions
    a. Recognize the signs and symptoms of CHF
    b. Adhere to activity limitations; alternate rest periods with activity
    c. Monitor for infection

H. Possible complications
    1. CHF
    2. Thrombosis
    3. Embolism
    4. Infection

I. Possible surgical interventions
    1. Valvuloplasty (see page 11)
    2. Valve replacement (see page 10)

♦ XXIII. Peripheral vascular disease (PVD)

A. Definition—chronic inadequate blood flow in the lower extremities

B. Types
    1. Arteriosclerosis obliterans—sclerosis of arterioles resulting in thickening of the walls and occlusion
    2. Raynaud's phenomenon—intermittent vasoconstriction and ischemia of fingers and toes accompanied by pallor and cyanosis
    3. Buerger's disease (Thromboangiitis obliterans)—inflammation of blood vessels resulting in occlusion of the vessel

C. Possible etiology
    1. Atherosclerosis
    2. Vasospasm
    3. Inflammation

D. Pathophysiology
    1. Arterial thickening and loss of elasticity, narrowing the diameter of the artery
    2. Decreased perfusion and blood clot formation, causing arterial blockage and ischemia (common sites are the femoral, popliteal, and iliac arteries and the aorta)

CLINICAL ALERT

E. Possible assessment findings
    1. INTERMITTENT CLAUDICATION
    2. Pain in extremities at rest
    3. Trophic changes: thickened nails; absence of hair; taut, shiny skin
    4. Diminished or absent pulses in extremities (a unilateral finding has greater significance than bilateral findings) (See *Managing diminished or absent pulse,* pages 42 to 43)
    5. Temperature changes in extremities
    6. Color changes in extremities: rubor, cyanosis, pallor

    7. Ulcerations in extremities

F. Possible diagnostic test findings

    1. Arteriography: location of obstructing plaque

    2. Doppler studies: decreased blood flow and arterial pressure

    3. Blood chemistry: increased lipids

G. Medical management

    1. Diet: low-fat, low-calorie

    2. Activity: active ROM and isometric exercises, as tolerated

    3. Monitoring: VS, I/O, and neurovascular checks

    4. Laboratory studies: serum lipids, PTT, and PT

    5. Bed cradle

    6. Antiplatelet: aspirin

    7. Vasodilators: pentoxifylline (Trental)

    8. Anticoagulants: warfarin sodium (Coumadin)

    9. Lipid reducers: cholestyramine (Questran), lovastatin (Mevacor)

    10. Percutaneous transluminal angioplasty

    11. Laser angioplasty

    12. Vascular stents

    13. Thrombolytic therapy: streptokinase (Streptase)

H. Nursing interventions

    1. Maintain the patient's prescribed diet

    2. Assess cardiovascular status

    3. Monitor and record VS, UO, I/O, and laboratory studies

    4. Administer medications, as prescribed

    5. Encourage the patient to express feelings about changes in body image

    6. Check peripheral circulation: pulses, color, temperature, and complaints of abnormal sensations, such as numbness or tingling

    7. Encourage walking and other leg exercises

    8. Provide daily foot care

    9. Individualize home care instructions

        a. Recognize the symptoms of decreased peripheral circulation

        b. Monitor for skin breakdown

CLINICAL ALERT

        c. Care for the feet daily

        d. Avoid activities or situations that will exacerbate the condition, such as temperature extremes, prolonged standing, constrictive clothing, or crossing the legs at the knee when seated

I. Possible complications

    1. Gangrene

    2. Septicemia

    3. Pressure sores

    4. Acute vascular occlusion

Text continues on page 44.

DECISION TREE

Managing diminished or absent pulse

A diminished or absent pulse can result from several life-threatening disorders. Your assessment and interventions will vary depending on whether the diminished or absent pulse is localized to one extremity or generalized. They will also depend on associated signs and symptoms. Use the decision tree below to help you establish priorities for managing this problem.

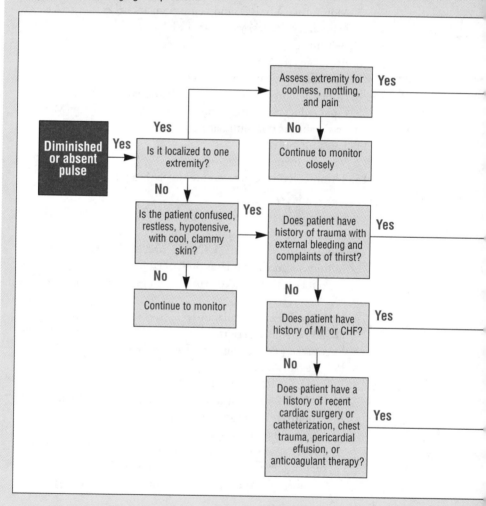

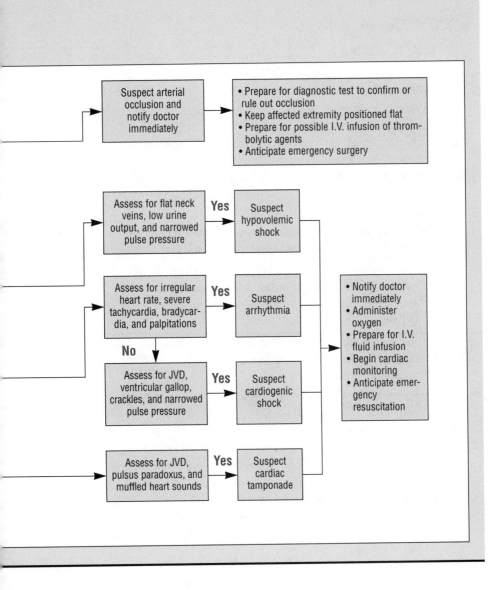

J. Possible surgical interventions
  1. Bypass grafting (see page 16)
  2. Endarterectomy (see page 96)
  3. SYMPATHECTOMY
  4. Amputation (see page 289)
  5. Embolectomy (see page 64)

♦ **XXIV. Thrombophlebitis**

A. Definition—inflammation of the venous wall, resulting in clot formation

B. Possible etiology
  1. Venous stasis (from varicose veins, pregnancy, CHF, prolonged bed rest)
  2. Hypercoagulability (from cancer, blood dyscrasias, oral contraceptives)
  3. Injury to the venous wall (from I.V. injections, fractures, antibiotics)

C. Pathophysiology
  1. Massing of red blood cells in a fibrin network
  2. Obstruction by enlarged thrombus, leading to venous insufficiency (common sites are deep veins and superficial veins)

D. Possible assessment findings
  1. Superficial veins: red, warm skin that is tender to touch
  2. Deep veins: edema, positive Homans' sign, tender to touch, cramping pain

E. Possible diagnostic test findings
  1. Venography: venous-filling defects
  2. Ultrasound: decreased blood flow
  3. Phlebography: venous-filling defects
  4. Hematology: increased WBC count

F. Medical management
  1. Position: elevation of the affected extremity
  2. Activity: bed rest; active and passive ROM and isometric exercises
  3. Monitoring: VS and neurovascular checks
  4. Laboratory studies: WBC, PT, and PTT
  5. Antiembolism stockings; warm, moist compresses
  6. Anticoagulants: warfarin sodium (Coumadin), heparin sodium (Lipo-Hepin)
  7. Fibrinolytic agents: streptokinase (Streptase)
  8. Anti-inflammatory agent: aspirin

G. Nursing interventions
  1. Assess cardiovascular status
  2. Keep the patient in bed, and elevate the affected extremity

3. Monitor and record VS, neurovascular checks, and laboratory studies
4. Administer medications, as prescribed
5. Assess for Homans' sign
6. Assess for bleeding

CLINICAL
ALERT

7. Apply warm, moist compresses
8. Measure and record the circumference of thighs and calves
9. Individualize home care instructions
   a. Recognize the signs and symptoms of bleeding
   b. Avoid prolonged sitting or standing, constrictive clothing, or crossing the legs when seated
   c. Do not take oral contraceptives

H. Possible complications
   1. Pulmonary embolism
   2. CVA

I. Possible surgical interventions
   1. Vena cava filter (plication of inferior vena cava; see page 65)
   2. Vein ligation and stripping
   3. Thrombectomy

♦ XXV. Bacterial endocarditis

A. Definition—inflammation and infection of the endocardial lining

B. Possible etiology
   1. Bacterial infection: Beta-hemolytic streptococcus, *Staphylococcus aureus*
   2. Rheumatic heart disease
   3. Dental extractions
   4. Invasive monitoring
   5. I.V. drug abuse

C. Pathophysiology
   1. Formation of bacterial colonies on the endocardial lining, destroying heart valve leaflets
   2. Disrupted blood flow, resulting in murmurs
   3. Vegetations that seed the bloodstream with bacteria

D. Possible assessment findings
   1. Elevated temperature
   2. Heart murmur
   3. Diaphoresis
   4. Malaise
   5. Dyspnea
   6. Tachycardia
   7. Clubbing of fingers and toes
   8. Petechiae

9. Night sweats
10. Splinter hemorrhages in nail beds

E. Possible diagnostic test findings
 1. Blood cultures: positive for specific organism
 2. Hematology: increased WBCs, ESR; decreased HCT
 3. Echocardiography: valvular damage, vegetations

F. Medical management
 1. I.V. therapy: hydration, heparin lock
 2. Oxygen therapy
 3. Activity: bed rest
 4. Monitoring: VS, UO, I/O, and neurovascular checks
 5. Laboratory studies: blood cultures, WBC, and HCT
 6. Antibiotics: penicillin G potassium (Pentids), vancomycin hydro-chloride (Vancocin), cefazolin sodium (Ancef)
 7. Positive inotropic agents: digoxin (Lanoxin), dobutamine hydro-chloride (Dobutrex)
 8. Fluids: increased intake
 9. Antipyretic: aspirin
10. Anticoagulant: warfarin sodium (Coumadin)

G. Nursing interventions
 1. Force fluids
 2. Administer I.V. fluids, oxygen, and medications, as prescribed
 3. Assess cardiovascular status
 4. Monitor and record VS, UO, I/O, and laboratory studies
 5. Encourage the patient to express feelings, such as a fear of dying
 6. Allay the patient's anxiety
 7. Individualize home care instructions
  a. Recognize the signs and symptoms of endocarditis
  b. Follow activity limitations; alternate rest periods with activity, and adhere to the prescribed exercise regimen
  c. Avoid exposure to people with infections; monitor self for infection, particularly after a dental or gynecologic exam, and seek treatment if infection develops
  d. Wear a medical identification bracelet

H. Possible complications
 1. Embolism
 2. CHF
 3. Mycotic aneurysm

I. Possible surgical intervention: valve replacement (see page 10)

♦ XXVI. Abdominal aortic aneurysm

A. Definition—dilation of or localized weakness in the medial layer of an abdominal artery

B. Possible etiology
1. Atherosclerosis
2. Congenital defect
3. Trauma
4. Syphilis
5. Hypertension
6. Infection
7. Marfan's syndrome

C. Pathophysiology
1. Degenerative changes from atherosclerosis, weakening the medial layer
2. Continued weakening from the force of blood flow, resulting in outpouching of the artery
3. Four types: saccular, fusiform, dissecting, false

D. Possible assessment findings
1. Asymptomatic
2. Lower abdominal pain, low back pain
3. Abdominal mass to the left of the midline
4. Abdominal pulsations
5. Bruits
6. Diminished femoral pulses
7. Systolic blood pressure in the legs lower than that in the arms

E. Possible diagnostic test findings
1. Chest X-ray: aneurysm
2. ECG: differentiation of aneurysm from MI
3. Abdominal ultrasound: aneurysm
4. Aortography: aneurysm

F. Medical management
1. Activity: bed rest
2. Monitoring: VS, UO, I/O, and neurovascular checks
3. Analgesic: oxycodone (Tylox)
4. Beta-adrenergic blocker: propranolol (Inderal)
5. Antihypertensives: methyldopa (Aldomet), hydralazine (Apresoline), prazosin (Minipress)

G. Nursing interventions
1. Assess cardiovascular status
2. Monitor and record VS, UO, I/O, neurovascular checks, and laboratory studies

      3. Administer medications, as prescribed

      4. Encourage the patient to express feelings, such as a fear of dying

      5. Assess pain

      6. Check peripheral circulation: pulses, temperature, color, and complaints of abnormal sensations

      7. Allay the patient's anxiety

      8. Observe the patient for signs of shock, such as anxiety; restlessness; decreased pulse pressure; increased thready pulse; and pale, cool, moist, clammy skin

      9. Palpate the abdomen for distention

    10. Individualize home care instructions

        a. Recognize the signs and symptoms of decreased peripheral circulation, such as change in skin color or temperature, complaints of numbness or tingling, and absent pulses

        b. Adhere to activity limitations; alternate rest periods with activity, and adhere to prescribed exercise regimen

        c. Maintain a quiet environment

H. Possible complication: rupture of aneurysm

I. Possible surgical intervention: resection of aneurysm (see page 15)

◆ XXVII. Cardiomyopathy

A. Definition

    1. Disease of the muscle of the heart impacting the structure and function of the ventricle

    2. Types

      a. Congestive (dilated)

      b. Hypertrophic (obstructive)

      c. Restrictive (obliterative)

B. Etiology

    1. Infection

    2. Metabolic and immunologic disorders

    3. Pregnancy and postpartum disorders

    4. Congenital

    5. Chronic alcoholism (congestive)

    6. Idiopathic hypertrophic subaortic stenosis (hypertrophic)

    7. Amyloidosis (restrictive)

    8. Cancer and other infiltrative diseases (restrictive)

C. Pathophysiology

    1. Cardiac function is altered, resulting in decreased cardiac output

    2. Increased heart rate and increased muscle mass compensate in early stages

3. Heart failure develops in later stages
4. Myocardium becomes flabby

D. Possible assessment findings
1. Signs and symptoms of heart failure
2. Dyspnea
3. PND
4. Cough
5. Fatigue
6. JVD
7. Dependent pitting edema
8. Enlarged liver
9. Murmur
10. Rales
11. S_3, S_4 heart sounds

E. Possible diagnostic test findings
1. ECG: left ventricular hypertrophy
2. Echocardiogram: decreased myocardial function
3. Cardiac catheterization: rule out CAD
4. Chest X-ray: cardiomegaly

F. Medical management
1. Diet: low-sodium, vitamin supplements
2. I.V. therapy
3. Oxygen therapy
4. Position: semi-Fowler's
5. Monitoring: VS, UO, ECG, hemodynamic variables, I/O
6. Laboratory studies: ABGs, sodium, potassium, CK and LDH with isoenzymes
7. Left ventricular assist device
8. Intraaortic balloon pump
9. Arterial line for blood pressure monitoring
10. Diuretics: furosemide (Lasix), bumetanide (Bumex), metolazone (Zaroxolyn)
11. Beta-adrenergic blockers: propranolol (Inderal), nadolol (Corgard), metoprolol (Lopressor)
12. Calcium channel blockers: verapamil (Calan), diltiazem (Cardizem), nifedipine (Procardia), nicardipine (Cardene)

G. Nursing interventions
1. Maintain the patient's prescribed diet
2. Assess cardiovascular and respiratory status

3. Monitor and record VS, UO, I/O, hemodynamic variables, laboratory studies, and ECG results
4. Maintain bed rest
5. Administer oxygen and medications, as prescribed
6. Allay the patient's anxiety
7. Keep the patient in semi-Fowler's position
8. Provide information about the American Heart Association
9. Individualize home care instructions
   a. Recognize signs and symptoms of CHF
   b. Avoid straining during bowel movements
   c. Monitor pulses and blood pressure
   d. Weigh daily and report increases over 3 pounds
   e. Demonstrate exercises to increase cardiac output (raising arms)
   f. Refrain from smoking and drinking alcohol

H. Possible complications
   1. Heart failure
   2. Arterial emboli

I. Possible surgical interventions
   1. Ventricular myomectomy
   2. Heart transplant

POINTS TO REMEMBER

♦ The focus of nursing management in cardiovascular disorders is to increase blood supply—and thus oxygenation—to tissues.

♦ Alterations in cardiac output affect every system in the body.

♦ The impact of cardiovascular disease can be reduced by altering modifiable risk factors.

♦ Complaints of chest pain have increased significance in a patient with peripheral vascular disorders.

♦ A unilateral finding in the assessment of peripheral circulation has greater significance than bilateral findings.

STUDY QUESTIONS

To evaluate your understanding of this chapter, answer the following questions in the space provided; then compare your responses with the correct answers in Appendix B, page 382.

1. What is the formula for calculating cardiac output? _____

_____

_____

2. Which nursing interventions are appropriate after cardiac catheterization?

_____

_____

3. Which risk factors for cardiovascular disorders can be modified? _____

_____

_____

4. What are key postoperative assessments of circulation for a patient who had vascular graft surgery? _____

_____

_____

5. What should the patient be taught about dietary modifications for hypertension? _____

_____

_____

6. How would a patient with angina describe the pain? _____

_____

_____

7. What are the assessment findings in the patient with acute pulmonary edema? _____

_____

_____

8. What are three possible assessment findings in the patient with PVD?

_____

_____

CRITICAL THINKING AND APPLICATION EXERCISES

1. Observe a cardiac catheterization. Prepare an oral presentation for your fellow students, describing the procedure and patient care before, during, and after the procedure.

2. Develop a chart comparing the major drug classes used for treating angina.

3. Draw a diagram showing the stepped care approach to antihypertensive treatment.

4. Obtain a 3-day food history from a fellow student. Evaluate the information for possible cardiovascular risk factors and identify ways to modify them.

5. Follow a patient with a cardiovascular disorder from admission through discharge. Develop a patient-specific plan of care, including any needs for follow-up and home care.

CHAPTER

2

Respiratory System

LEARNING OBJECTIVES

After studying this chapter, you should be able to:

♦ Describe the psychosocial impact of respiratory disorders.

♦ Differentiate between modifiable and nonmodifiable risk factors in the development of a respiratory disorder.

♦ List three probable and three possible nursing diagnoses for a patient with any respiratory disorder.

♦ Identify the nursing interventions for a patient with a respiratory disorder.

♦ Write three goals for teaching a patient with a respiratory disorder.

CHAPTER OVERVIEW

Caring for the patient with a respiratory disorder requires a sound understanding of respiratory anatomy and physiology and diffusion of oxygen. A thorough assessment is essential to planning and implementing appropriate patient care. The assessment includes a complete history, physical examination, diagnostic testing, identification of modifiable and nonmodifiable risk factors, and information related to the psychosocial impact of respiratory dysfunction on the patient. Nursing diagnoses focus primarily on ineffective breathing patterns and impaired gas exchange. Patient teaching, a crucial nursing activity, involves information about medical follow-up, medication regimens, signs and symptoms of possible complications, and reduction of modifiable risk factors through avoiding people with infections, activity and diet restrictions, stress management, and smoking cessation

♦ I. Anatomy and physiology review

A. Nares
   1. Filters out particles
   2. Humidifies inspired air
   3. Contains olfactory receptor sites

B. Paranasal sinuses
   1. Air-filled, cilia-lined cavities
   2. Function: to trap particles

C. Pharynx
   1. Serves as a passageway to digestive and respiratory tracts
   2. Maintains air pressure in the middle ear
   3. Contains mucosal lining that humidifies and warms inspired air and traps particles

D. Larynx
   1. Known as the "voice box"
   2. Connects the upper and lower airways
   3. Contains vocal cords that produce sounds and initiate the cough reflex

E. Trachea
   1. Consists of smooth muscle
   2. Contains C-shaped cartilaginous rings
   3. Connects the larynx to the bronchi

F. Bronchi and bronchioles
   1. Bronchi and bronchioles are formed by branching of the trachea
   2. Right main bronchus is slightly larger and more vertical than the left
   3. Bronchioles branch into terminal bronchioles, which end in alveoli

G. Alveoli
   1. Clustered microscopic sacs enveloped by capillaries
   2. Gases exchange in the alveoli
   3. Coating of surfactant reduces surface tension to keep alveoli from collapsing
   4. Diffusion of gases occurs across the alveolar-capillary membrane

H. Lungs
   1. Composed of three lobes on the right side and two lobes on the left side

       2. Covered by pleura

       3. Regulate air exchange by concentration gradient

  I. Pleura

       1. Visceral pleura covers the lungs

       2. Parietal pleura lines the thoracic cavity

       3. Pleural fluid lubricates the pleura to reduce friction during respiration

◆ II. Assessment findings

A. History

       1. Difficulty breathing, shortness of breath, DYSPNEA

       2. Chest pain

       3. Voice change

       4. Dysphagia

       5. Fatigue

       6. Weight change

       7. Cough

B. Physical examination

       1. Respiratory system changes

         a. Nasal flaring

         b. Decreased respiratory excursion

         c. Accessory muscle use

         d. Retractions

       2. Sputum characteristics

       3. Clubbing of fingers

       4. Adventitious sounds: CRACKLES, RHONCHI, wheezing, and pleural friction rub

       5. Fremitus

       6. Crepitus

       7. Pattern and character of respirations

       8. Shape of thoracic anatomy (for example, barrel chest)

       9. Change in mentation

     10. Skin color and temperature

◆ III. Diagnostic tests and procedures

A. Bronchoscopy

       1. Definition and purpose

         a. Procedure using a bronchoscope for direct visualization of the trachea and bronchial tree

         b. Biopsies may be taken and deep tracheal suctioning performed

       2. Nursing interventions before the procedure

         a. Withhold food and fluids

         b. Allay the patient's anxiety

3. Nursing interventions after the procedure
   a. Check cough and gag reflex; minimizes risk of aspiration
   b. Assess sputum
   c. Assess respiratory status
   d. Withhold food and fluids until gag reflex returns
   e. Check vasovagal response

B. Chest X-ray
   1. Definition and purpose
      a. Noninvasive examination
      b. Radiographic picture of lung tissue
   2. Nursing interventions
      a. Determine the patient's ability to inhale and hold breath
      b. Ensure that the patient removes jewelry

C. Pulmonary angiography
   1. Definition and purpose
      a. Procedure using an injection of a radiopaque dye through a catheter
      b. Radiographic examination of the pulmonary circulation

   2. Nursing interventions before the procedure
      a. Note the patient's allergies to iodine, seafood, and radiopaque dyes
      b. Instruct the patient about possible flushing of the face or burning in the throat after dye is injected
   3. Nursing interventions after the procedure
      a. Assess peripheral neurovascular status
      b. Check the insertion site for bleeding

D. Sputum studies
   1. Definition and purpose
      a. Laboratory test
      b. Microscopic evaluation of sputum that includes culture and sensitivity, Gram's stain, and acid-fast bacillus
   2. Nursing interventions: obtain early-morning sterile specimen from suctioning or expectoration

E. Thoracentesis
   1. Definition and purpose
      a. Procedure using needle aspiration of intrapleural fluid under local anesthesia
      b. Specimen examination or removal of pleural fluid
   2. Nursing interventions during the procedure
      a. Reassure the patient
      b. Place the patient in the proper position (either sitting on the edge of the bed or lying partially on the side, partially on the back)

3. Nursing interventions after the procedure
   a. Assess the patient's respiratory status
   b. Monitor vital signs frequently
   c. Position the patient on the affected side, as ordered, for at least 1 hour to seal the puncture site
   d. Check the puncture site for fluid leakage
   e. Auscultate lungs to assess for pneumothorax

F. Pulmonary function tests (PFTs)
   1. Definition and purpose
      a. Noninvasive test
      b. Measurement of lung volume, ventilation, and diffusing capacity
   2. Nursing interventions
      a. Document bronchodilators or narcotics used before testing
      b. Allay the patient's anxiety during testing

G. Arterial blood gases (ABGs)
   1. Definition and purpose
      a. Laboratory test
      b. Assessment of arterial blood for tissue oxygenation, ventilation, and acid-base status
   2. Nursing interventions before the procedure
      a. Note temperature
      b. Document oxygen and assisted mechanical ventilation used
   3. Nursing interventions after the procedure
      a. Apply pressure to the site for 5 minutes
      b. Apply a pressure dressing

H. Lung scan
   1. Definition and purpose
      a. Procedure using visual inhalation or I.V. injection of radioisotopes
      b. Imaging of distribution and blood flow in the lungs
   2. Nursing interventions
      a. Allay the patient's anxiety
      b. Determine the patient's ability to lie still during procedure
      c. Check the catheter insertion site for bleeding after the procedure

I. Mantoux intradermal skin test
   1. Definition and purpose
      a. Procedure involving the administration of tuberculin
      b. Detection of tuberculosis antibodies
   2. Nursing interventions
      a. Document current dermatitis or rashes
      b. Document history of positive results in past skin testing
      c. Circle and record test site
      d. Note date for follow-up reading (48 to 72 hours after injection)

J. Laryngoscopy
   1. Definition and purpose
      a. Procedure using a laryngoscope
      b. Direct visualization of the larynx
   2. Nursing interventions before the procedure
      a. Withhold food or fluids for 6 to 8 hours before the test
      b. Explain that the patient will receive a sedative to promote relaxation
      c. Make sure a consent form has been signed
   3. Nursing interventions after the procedure
      a. Assess respiratory status
      b. Allay the patient's anxiety
      c. Withhold food and fluids until gag reflex returns

CLINICAL ALERT

K. Lung biopsy
   1. Definition and purpose
      a. Procedure involving the percutaneous removal of a small amount of lung tissue
      b. Histologic evaluation
   2. Nursing interventions before the procedure
      a. Withhold food and fluids
      b. Obtain written, informed consent
   3. Nursing interventions after the procedure
      a. Observe the patient for signs of pneumothorax and air embolism
      b. Check the patient for HEMOPTYSIS and hemorrhage
      c. Monitor and record vital signs (VS)
      d. Check the insertion site for bleeding

L. Hematologic studies
   1. Definition and purpose
      a. Laboratory test of a blood sample
      b. Analysis for red blood cells (RBCs), white blood cells (WBCs), prothrombin time (PT), partial thromboplastin time (PTT), erythrocyte sedimentation rate (ESR), platelets, hemoglobin (Hgb), and hematocrit (HCT)
   2. Nursing interventions
      a. Note current drug therapy before the procedure
      b. Check the site for bleeding after the procedure

M. Blood chemistry
   1. Definition and purpose
      a. Laboratory test of a blood sample
      b. Analysis for potassium, sodium, calcium, phosphorus, glucose, bicarbonate, blood urea nitrogen, creatinine, protein, albumin, osmolality, and alpha$_1$-antitrypsin

2. Nursing interventions
  a. Withhold food and fluids before the procedure, as directed
  b. Check the site for bleeding after the procedure

◆ IV. Psychosocial impact of respiratory disorders

A. Developmental impact
  1. Decreased self-esteem
  2. Fear of dying

B. Economic impact
  1. Disruption or loss of employment
  2. Cost of hospitalizations and home health care

C. Occupational and recreational impact
  1. Restrictions in work activity
  2. Changes in leisure activities

D. Social impact
  1. Changes in sexual function
  2. Social isolation
  3. Changes in role performance

◆ V. Possible risk factors

A. Modifiable risk factors
  1. Crowded living conditions
  2. Inadequate knowledge of risk factors
  3. Exposure to chemical and environmental pollutants
  4. Cigarette or pipe smoking
  5. Use of chewing tobacco
  6. Alcohol abuse

B. Nonmodifiable risk factors
  1. Aging
  2. History of allergies
  3. Previous respiratory illness
  4. Family history of respiratory illness
  5. Family history of allergies

◆ VI. Nursing diagnostic categories for a patient with a respiratory disorder

A. Probable nursing diagnostic categories
  1. Impaired physical mobility
  2. Ineffective breathing patterns
  3. Impaired gas exchange
  4. Ineffective airway clearance

5. Sleep pattern disturbance
6. Activity intolerance

B. Possible nursing diagnostic categories
1. Inability to sustain spontaneous ventilation
2. Dysfunctional ventilatory weaning response
3. Anxiety
4. Fear
5. Altered nutrition: less than body requirements
6. Impaired verbal communication
7. Noncompliance
8. Risk for aspiration

♦ VII. Laryngectomy

A. Description
1. Partial laryngectomy: surgical excision of a lesion on one vocal cord
2. Total laryngectomy: surgical removal of the larynx, hyoid bone, and tracheal rings with closure of the pharynx and formation of a permanent tracheostomy

B. Preoperative nursing interventions
1. Complete patient and family preoperative teaching
   a. Determine the patient's understanding of the procedure
   b. Describe the operating room (OR), postanesthesia care unit (PACU), and preoperative and postoperative routines
   c. Demonstrate postoperative turning, coughing, and deep breathing (TCDB), splinting, leg exercises, and range-of-motion (ROM) exercises
   d. Explain the postoperative need for drainage tubes, surgical dressings, oxygen therapy, I.V. therapy, and pain control
2. Complete a preoperative checklist
3. Administer preoperative medications, as prescribed
4. Allay the patient's and family's anxiety about surgery

CLINICAL ALERT

5. Document the patient's history and physical assessment database
6. Establish methods of communication: writing, call bell, "magic slate," picture board
7. Encourage the patient to express feelings about changes in body image and loss of voice

C. Postoperative nursing interventions
1. Assess respiratory status
2. Assess pain and administer postoperative analgesics, as prescribed
3. Assess for return of peristalsis; provide solid foods and liquids, as tolerated
   a. Increase calories
   b. Increase protein

4. Administer I.V. fluids and nasogastric (NG) tube feedings
5. Allay the patient's anxiety
6. Inspect the surgical dressing and change, as directed
7. Reinforce TCDB
8. Keep the patient in semi-Fowler's position
9. Provide tracheal suction
10. Increase activity, as tolerated
11. Administer oxygen via high humidity tracheostomy mask
12. Monitor and record VS, urinary output (UO), intake and output (I/O), laboratory studies, and pulse oximetry
13. Monitor and maintain position and patency of drainage tubes: wound drainage
14. Assess the color, amount, and consistency of sputum
15. Encourage the patient to express feelings about changes in body image and loss of voice
16. Provide oral hygiene
17. Reinforce method of communication established preoperatively

18. Reinforce speech therapy
19. Assess gag and cough reflex and ability to swallow
20. Provide stoma and laryngectomy care
21. Reinforce increased intake of fluids
22. Observe for hemorrhage and edema in the neck
23. Arrange referrals to community agencies
24. Individualize home care instructions
    a. Communicate using esophageal speech or artificial larynx
    b. Avoid swimming, showering, and using aerosol sprays
    c. Complete stoma and laryngectomy care daily
    d. Suction laryngectomy using clean technique

    e. Protect the neck from injury
    f. Demonstrate ways to prevent debris from entering the stoma

D. Possible surgical complications
    1. Hemorrhage
    2. Atelectasis
    3. Pneumonia
    4. Aspiration

◆ VIII. Radical neck dissection

A. Description—surgical excision of the sternocleidomastoid and omohyoid muscles, muscles of the floor of the mouth, submaxillary gland, internal jugular vein, external carotid artery, and cervical chain of lymph nodes in addition to laryngectomy

B. Preoperative nursing interventions
   1. Complete patient and family preoperative teaching
      a. Determine the patient's understanding of the procedure
      b. Describe the OR, PACU, and preoperative and postoperative routines
      c. Demonstrate postoperative TCDB, splinting, and leg and ROM exercises
      d. Explain the postoperative need for drainage tubes, surgical dressings, oxygen therapy, I.V. therapy, and pain control
   2. Complete a preoperative checklist
   3. Administer preoperative medications, as prescribed
   4. Allay the patient's and family's anxiety about surgery
   5. Document the patient's history and physical assessment database
   6. Establish methods of communication: writing, call bell, "magic slate," picture board

C. Postoperative nursing interventions
   1. Assess cardiac, respiratory, and neurologic status
   2. Assess pain and administer postoperative analgesics, as prescribed
   3. Assess for the return of peristalsis; provide solid foods and liquids, as tolerated
   4. Administer I.V. fluids, NG tube feedings, and transfusion therapy, as prescribed
   5. Allay the patient's anxiety
   6. Inspect the surgical dressing and change, as directed
   7. Reinforce TCDB
   8. Keep the patient in high-Fowler's position
   9. Provide tracheal suction
   10. Maintain activity: active and passive ROM and isometric exercises, as tolerated
   11. Administer oxygen via high humidity tracheostomy mask
   12. Monitor and record VS, UO, I/O, laboratory studies, and pulse oximetry
   13. Monitor and maintain position and patency of drainage tubes: NG, indwelling urinary catheter, and wound drainage

CLINICAL ALERT

   14. Assess gag and cough reflex and ability to swallow
   15. Encourage the patient to express feelings about changes in body image and loss of voice
   16. Provide stoma and laryngectomy care; arrange for referrals to community agencies for follow-up care
   17. Reinforce increased intake of fluids
   18. Observe the patient for hemorrhage and edema in the neck
   19. Provide suture line care
   20. Reinforce method of communication established preoperatively
   21. Reinforce speech therapy

22. Individualize home care instructions
    a. Communicate using esophageal speech or artificial larynx
    b. Recognize the signs and symptoms of tracheostomy stenosis
    c. Avoid swimming, showers, and using aerosol sprays
    d. Protect the neck from injury
    e. Suction laryngectomy using clean technique
    f. Complete incision, stoma, and laryngectomy care daily
    g. Demonstrate ways to prevent debris from entering the stoma
    h. Complete ROM exercises for arms, shoulders, and neck daily

D. Possible surgical complications
    1. Tracheostomy stenosis
    2. Aspiration
    3. Pneumonia
    4. Hemorrhage

♦ IX. Pulmonary resections

A. Description
    1. Lobectomy: surgical removal of one lobe of the lung
    2. Wedge resection: surgical removal of a wedge-shaped section of a lobe
    3. Pneumonectomy: surgical removal of a lung

B. Preoperative nursing interventions
    1. Complete patient and family preoperative teaching
        a. Determine the patient's understanding of the procedure
        b. Describe the OR, PACU, and preoperative and postoperative routines
        c. Demonstrate postoperative TCDB, splinting, and leg and ROM exercises
        d. Explain the postoperative need for drainage tubes, chest tubes, surgical dressings, oxygen therapy, I.V. therapy, and pain control
    2. Complete a preoperative checklist
    3. Administer preoperative medications, as prescribed
    4. Allay the patient's and family's anxiety about surgery
    5. Document the patient's history and physical assessment database

C. Postoperative nursing interventions
    1. Assess cardiac and respiratory status
    2. Assess pain and administer postoperative analgesics, as prescribed
    3. Assess for return of peristalsis; provide solid foods and liquids, as tolerated
    4. Administer I.V. fluids
    5. Allay the patient's anxiety
    6. Inspect the surgical dressing and change, as directed

7. Reinforce TCDB and splinting of incision
8. Maintain the patient's position: for pneumonectomy patient, on the back or the side of the surgery; for lobectomy or wedge resection patient, on the back or the side opposite the surgery
9. Provide incentive spirometry, suction, chest physiotherapy (CPT), postural drainage
10. Maintain activity: active and passive ROM and isometric exercises, as tolerated
11. Administer oxygen and maintain endotracheal tube to ventilator
12. Monitor and record VS, UO, I/O, laboratory studies, electrocardiogram (ECG), hemodynamic variables, and pulse oximetry

13. Monitor and maintain position and patency of drainage tubes: NG, indwelling urinary, chest tube
14. Assess chest tube insertion site for subcutaneous air and drainage (except pneumonectomy)
15. Encourage the patient to express feelings about a fear of dying
16. Administer antibiotics, as prescribed
17. Individualize home care instructions
    a. Recognize the signs and symptoms of respiratory distress
    b. Complete incision care daily
    c. Maintain active ROM exercises to operative shoulder

D. Possible surgical complications
  1. Hemorrhage
  2. Pneumonia

♦ X. Embolectomy

A. Description—removal of an embolus from an artery using a balloon-tipped catheter

B. Preoperative nursing interventions
  1. Complete patient and family preoperative teaching
     a. Determine the patient's understanding of the procedure
     b. Describe the OR, PACU, and preoperative and postoperative routines
     c. Demonstrate postoperative TCDB, splinting, and leg and ROM exercises
     d. Explain the postoperative need for drainage tubes, surgical dressings, oxygen therapy, I.V. therapy, and pain control
  2. Complete a preoperative checklist
  3. Administer preoperative medications, as prescribed
  4. Allay the patient's and family's anxiety about surgery
  5. Document the patient's history and physical assessment database
  6. Obtain a baseline vascular assessment
  7. Administer anticoagulants, as prescribed

    8. Maintain extremity in slightly dependent position
    9. Administer thrombolytics, as prescribed
  10. Provide a bed cradle
  11. Avoid bumping the bed

C. Postoperative nursing interventions
    1. Assess cardiac, respiratory, and neurologic status
    2. Assess pain and administer postoperative analgesics, as prescribed
    3. Assess for return of peristalsis; provide solid foods and liquids, as tolerated
    4. Administer I.V. fluids
    5. Allay the patient's anxiety
    6. Inspect the surgical dressing and change, as directed
    7. Reinforce TCDB
    8. Keep the patient in semi-Fowler's position
    9. Provide incentive spirometry
  10. Maintain activity: active and passive ROM and isometric exercises, as tolerated
  11. Administer oxygen
  12. Monitor and record VS, UO, I/O, laboratory studies, neurovascular checks, and pulse oximetry
  13. Administer anticoagulants, as prescribed

  14. Provide bed cradle
  15. Check site for bleeding
  16. Maintain pressure dressing
  17. Individualize home care instructions

    a. Recognize the signs and symptoms of bleeding
    b. Avoid prolonged sitting
    c. State cautions of long-term anticoagulant therapy
    d. Complete incision care daily

D. Possible surgical complications
    1. Hemorrhage
    2. Embolism
    3. Thrombosis

◆ XI. Vena caval filter and plication of inferior vena cava

A. Description
    1. Vena caval filter (for example, Greenfield filter): surgical insertion of an intracaval filter (umbrella) to partially occlude the inferior vena cava and prevent pulmonary emboli
    2. Plication: surgical suturing and placement of Teflon clips to partially occlude the inferior vena cava and prevent pulmonary emboli

CLINICAL ALERT

CLINICAL ALERT

B. Preoperative nursing interventions
 1. Complete patient and family preoperative teaching
    a. Determine the patient's understanding of the procedure
    b. Describe the OR, PACU, and preoperative and postoperative routines
    c. Demonstrate postoperative TCDB, splinting, and leg and ROM exercises
    d. Explain the postoperative need for drainage tubes, surgical dressings, oxygen therapy, I.V. therapy, and pain control
 2. Complete a preoperative checklist
 3. Administer preoperative medications, as prescribed
 4. Allay the patient's and family's anxiety about surgery
 5. Document the patient's history and physical assessment database

C. Postoperative nursing interventions
 1. Assess cardiac and respiratory status
 2. Assess pain and administer postoperative analgesics, as prescribed
 3. Assess for return of peristalsis; provide solid foods and liquids, as tolerated
 4. Administer I.V. fluids
 5. Allay the patient's anxiety
 6. Inspect the surgical dressing and change, as directed
 7. Reinforce TCDB
 8. Keep the patient in semi-Fowler's position, with the foot of the bed elevated
 9. Provide incentive spirometry
 10. Maintain activity: active and passive ROM, and isometric exercises, as tolerated
 11. Administer oxygen
 12. Monitor and record VS, UO, I/O, laboratory studies, neurovascular checks, and pulse oximetry

CLINICAL ALERT

 13. Check the insertion site for bleeding and hematoma
 14. Assess peripheral edema
 15. Apply antiembolism stockings
 16. Avoid hip flexion
 17. Individualize home care instructions
    a. Recognize the signs and symptoms of infection and edema
    b. Avoid prolonged sitting or crossing legs when sitting
    c. Complete incision care daily
    d. Walk daily
    e. Elevate legs when sitting
    f. Wear antiembolism stockings
    g. Adhere to long-term anticoagulant therapy

D. Possible surgical complications
   1. Embolism
   2. Infection

◆ **XII. Pneumonia**

   A. Definition—bacterial, viral, parasitic, or fungal infection that causes inflammation of the alveolar spaces

   B. Possible etiology
      1. Organisms: *E. coli, H. influenzae, S. aureus, Pneumocystis carinii, Pneumococcal,* and *Pseudomonas*
      2. Aspiration of food
      3. Aspiration of fluid
      4. Chemical irritants

   C. Pathophysiology
      1. Microorganisms enter the alveolar spaces by droplet inhalation
      2. Inflammation occurs and alveolar fluid increases
      3. Ventilation decreases as secretions thicken

   D. Possible assessment findings
      1. Cough
      2. Malaise
      3. Chills
      4. Shortness of breath
      5. Dyspnea
      6. Elevated temperature
      7. Crackles
      8. Rhonchi
      9. Pleural friction rub
      10. Pleuritic pain
      11. Sputum production

CLINICAL ALERT

   -a. Rusty, green, or bloody (pneumococcal pneumonia)
   b. Yellow-green (bronchopneumonia)

   E. Possible diagnostic test findings
      1. Sputum studies: identification of organism
      2. Chest X-ray: pulmonary infiltrates
      3. Hematology: increased WBCs, ESR
      4. ABGs: hypoxemia, respiratory alkalosis

   F. Medical management
      1. Diet: high-calorie, high-protein
      2. Dietary recommendation: force fluids
      3. I.V. therapy: hydration, heparin lock
      4. Oxygen therapy
      5. Intubation and mechanical ventilation

6. Position: semi-Fowler's
7. Activity: bed rest, active and passive ROM and isometric exercises
8. Monitoring: VS, UO, and I/O
9. Laboratory studies: WBCs, sputum culture, blood culture, and throat culture
10. Nutritional support: total parental nutrition (TPN)
11. Treatments: indwelling urinary catheter, CPT, postural drainage, and incentive spirometry
12. Antibiotics: penicillin G potassium (Pentids), ampicillin (Omnipen), pentamidine isethionate (NebuPent)
13. Antipyretics: aspirin, acetaminophen (Tylenol)
14. Bronchodilators: metaproterenol sulfate (Alupent), isoetharine (Bronkosol), albuterol (Proventil)
15. Specialized bed: rotation (Rotorest)
16. Pulse oximetry

G. Nursing interventions
1. Maintain the patient's diet
2. Force fluids to 3 to 4 liters/day
3. Administer I.V. fluids
4. Administer oxygen
5. Provide suction, TCDB
6. Assess respiratory status
7. Keep the patient in semi-Fowler's position
8. Monitor and record VS, UO, I/O, laboratory studies, and pulse oximetry
9. Administer medications, as prescribed
10. Encourage the patient to express feelings about fear of suffocation
11. Monitor and record color, consistency, and amount of sputum
12. Allay the patient's anxiety
13. Prevent spread of infection
14. Provide oral hygiene
15. Provide information about the American Lung Association
16. Individualize home care instructions (For more information about teaching, see *Patients with respiratory disorders,* page 69)
   a. Recognize the signs and symptoms of respiratory infections
   b. Avoid exposure to people with infections
   c. Increase fluid intake to 3,000 ml/day

H. Possible complications
1. Congestive heart failure (CHF)
2. Pulmonary edema
3. Respiratory failure

I. Possible surgical interventions: none

TEACHING TIPS
Patients with respiratory disorders

Be sure to include the following topics in your teaching plan for the patient with a respiratory disorder.
- Follow-up appointments
- Smoking cessation; avoidance of irritants
- Self-monitoring for infection, including avoiding exposure to people with infections
- Signs of infection and respiratory distress
- Optimal weight maintenance
- Medication therapy including action, adverse effects, and scheduling of medications
- Dietary recommendations and restrictions
- Rest and activity patterns
- Community agencies and resources

◆ XIII. Chronic obstructive pulmonary disease (COPD)

A. Definition
 1. COPD is group of diseases that result in persistent obstruction of bronchial air flow
 2. Diseases include emphysema, asthma, bronchiectasis, and chronic bronchitis

CLINICAL ALERT

 3. In emphysema the stimulus to breathe is low P_{O_2} instead of increased P_{CO_2}

B. Possible etiology
 1. Congenital weakness
 2. Respiratory irritants: smoke, polluted air, chemical irritants
 3. Respiratory tract infections
 4. Genetic predisposition

C. Pathophysiology
 1. Bronchiectasis: infection destroys the bronchial mucosa, which is replaced by fibrous scar tissue; loss of resilience and dilation of airways causes pooling of secretions, obstruction of air flow, and decreased perfusion
 2. Asthma: irritants to bronchial tree cause bronchoconstriction, resulting in narrowed inflamed airways, dyspnea, and mucus production which is all reversible
 3. Bronchitis: excessive bronchial mucus production causes chronic or recurrent productive cough

4. Emphysema: destruction of elastin alters alveolar walls and narrows airways, resulting in enlargement of air spaces distal to terminal bronchioles, trapped air, and coalesced alveoli

D. Possible assessment findings
1. Cough
2. Dyspnea
3. Sputum production
4. Weight loss
5. Barrel chest (emphysema)
6. Hemoptysis
7. Exertional dyspnea
8. Clubbing of fingers
9. Malaise
10. Wheezes
11. Crackles
12. Anemia
13. Anxiety
14. Diaphoresis
15. Use of accessory muscles
16. Orthopnea

E. Possible diagnostic test findings
1. Chest X-ray: congestion, hyperinflation
2. ABGs: respiratory acidosis, hypoxemia
3. Sputum studies: positive identification of organism
4. PFTs: increased residual volume, increased functional residual capacity, decreased vital capacity

F. Medical management
1. Diet: high in protein, vitamin C, calories, and nitrogen
2. Dietary recommendation: force fluids to 3,000 ml/day as tolerated
3. I.V. therapy: heparin lock
4. Oxygen therapy: 2 to 3 liters/minute
5. Intubation and mechanical ventilation
6. Position: high-Fowler's
7. Activity: as tolerated
8. Monitoring: VS, UO, and I/O
9. Laboratory studies: ABGs, WBCs, and sputum studies
10. Treatments: CPT, postural drainage, intermittent positive pressure breathing (IPPB), and incentive spirometry
11. Antibiotics: ampicillin (Omnipen), tetracycline (Achromycin), cefixime (Suprax)
12. Antacid: aluminum hydroxide gel (AlternaGEL)
13. Bronchodilators: terbutaline (Brethine), aminophylline (Aminophyllin), isoproterenol (Isuprel), theophylline (Theo-Dur); via ne-

bulizer: albuterol (Proventil), Ipratropium bromide (Atrovent), metaproterenol sulfate (Alupent)

14. Steroids: hydrocortisone (Solu-Cortef), methylprednisolone sodium succinate (Solu-Medrol)
15. Expectorant: guaifenesin (Robitussin)
16. Beta-adrenergic drug: epinephrine hydrochloride (Adrenalin)
17. Respiratory inhalant: cromolyn sodium (Intal)

G. Nursing interventions
   1. Maintain the patient's diet
   2. Administer small, frequent feedings
   3. Force fluids
   4. Administer low-flow oxygen
   5. Provide CPT, IPPB, TCDB, postural drainage, incentive spirometry, and suction

   6. Assess respiratory status
   7. Reinforce pursed-lip breathing
   8. Keep the patient in high-Fowler's position
   9. Monitor and record VS, UO, I/O, and laboratory studies
   10. Administer medications, as prescribed
   11. Encourage the patient to express feelings about fear of suffocation
   12. Allow activity, as tolerated
   13. Monitor and record the color, amount, and consistency of sputum
   14. Allay the patient's anxiety
   15. Weigh the patient daily
   16. Provide information about the American Lung Association
   17. Individualize home care instructions
       a. Identify ways to reduce stress
       b. Recognize the signs and symptoms of respiratory infection and hypoxia
       c. Adhere to activity limitations
       d. Know proper use of home oxygen
       e. Demonstrate pursed-lip and diaphragmatic breathing
       f. Avoid exposure to chemical irritants and pollutants
       g. Demonstrate deep-breathing and coughing exercises
       h. Avoid eating gas-producing foods, spicy foods, and extremely hot or cold foods

H. Possible complications
   1. From emphysema
      a. Pulmonary hypertension
      b. Right-sided CHF
      c. Spontaneous pneumothorax
   2. Carbon dioxide narcosis
   3. Acute respiratory failure

4. Pneumonia

I. Possible surgical interventions: none

◆ XIV. Respiratory distress syndrome (ARDS, shock lung)

A. Definition—clinical syndrome of respiratory insufficiency

B. Possible etiology

1. Viral pneumonia
2. Fat emboli
3. Sepsis
4. Decreased surfactant production
5. Fluid overload
6. Shock
7. Trauma
8. Neurologic injuries
9. Oxygen toxicity

C. Pathophysiology

1. Damaged capillary membranes cause interstitial edema and intra-alveolar hemorrhage
2. Decreased gas exchange results
3. Cellular damage causes decreased surfactant production, resulting in hypoxemia

D. Possible assessment findings

1. Dyspnea
2. TACHYPNEA
3. Cyanosis
4. Cough
5. Crackles
6. RHONCHI
7. Anxiety
8. Restlessness
9. Decreased breath sounds

E. Possible diagnostic test findings

1. ABGs: respiratory acidosis, hypoxemia that does not respond to increased percentage of oxygen
2. Chest X-ray: interstitial edema
3. Sputum studies: organism
4. Blood cultures: organism

F. Medical management

1. Diet: restrict fluid intake
2. I.V. therapy: heparin lock

3. Oxygen therapy
4. Intubation and mechanical ventilation using positive end expiratory pressure
5. Position: high-Fowler's
6. Activity: bed rest; active ROM and isometric exercises
7. Monitoring: VS, UO, I/O, central venous pressure (CVP), ECG, and hemodynamic variables
8. Laboratory studies: ABGs, sputum studies, blood cultures, Hgb, and HCT
9. Nutritional support: TPN
10. Treatments: indwelling urinary catheter, CPT, postural drainage, and suction
11. Transfusion therapy: platelets, packed RBCs
12. Antibiotics: amoxicillin (Amoxil), ampicillin (Omnipen)
13. Analgesic: morphine sulfate
14. Diuretics: furosemide (Lasix), ethacrynic acid (Edecrin)
15. Anticoagulant: heparin (Lipo-Hepin)
16. Steroids: hydrocortisone (Solu-Cortef), methylprednisolone sodium succinate (Solu-Medrol)
17. Antacid: aluminum hydroxide gel (AlternaGEL)
18. Neuromuscular blocking agents: pancuronium bromide (Pavulon), vecuronium bromide (Norcuron)
19. Mucosal barrier fortifier: sucralfate (Carafate)
20. Pulse oximetry

G. Nursing interventions
1. Maintain fluid restrictions
2. Administer I.V. fluids
3. Monitor mechanical ventilation
4. Provide suction, TCDB, and postural drainage
5. Assess respiratory status
6. Keep the patient in high-Fowler's position
7. Monitor and record VS, UO, CVP, hemodynamic variables, I/O, specific gravity, laboratory studies, and pulse oximetry
8. Administer TPN
9. Administer medications, as prescribed
10. Encourage the patient to express feelings about fear of suffocation
11. Organize nursing care to allow rest periods
12. Weigh the patient daily
13. Allay the patient's anxiety
14. Maintain bed rest
15. Individualize home care instructions
    a. Recognize the signs and symptoms of respiratory distress
    b. Demonstrate deep breathing and coughing exercises
    c. Avoid exposure to chemical irritants and pollutants

H. Possible complications
   1. Pulmonary edema
   2. Atelectasis

I. Possible surgical interventions: none

♦ XV. Tuberculosis (TB), pulmonary

A. Definition—airborne, infectious, communicable disease that can occur acutely or chronically

B. Possible etiology: *Mycobacterium tuberculosis*

C. Pathophysiology
   1. Alveoli become the focus of infection from inhaled droplets containing bacteria
   2. Tubercle bacilli multiply, spread through the lymphatics, and drain into the systemic circulation
   3. In the lung tissue, macrophages surround the bacilli and form tubercles
   4. Tubercles go through the process of caseation, liquefaction, and cavitation

D. Possible assessment findings
   1. Fatigue
   2. Malaise
   3. Irritability
   4. Night sweats
   5. Tachycardia
   6. Weight loss
   7. Anorexia
   8. Cough
   9. Yellow and mucoid sputum
   10. Dyspnea
   11. Hemoptysis
   12. Crackles
   13. Elevated temperature

E. Possible diagnostic test findings
   1. Chest X-ray: active or calcified lesions
   2. Sputum cultures: positive acid-fast bacillus; positive *M. tuberculosis*
   3. Hematology: increased WBCs, ESR
   4. Mantoux skin test: positive

F. Medical management
   1. Diet: high-carbohydrate, high-protein, high-vitamin B6 and C, high-calorie
   2. I.V. therapy: heparin lock
   3. Activity: bed rest, active ROM and isometric exercises

   4. Monitoring: VS, UO, and I/O
   5. Laboratory studies: ABGs and sputum studies
   6. Treatments: CPT, postural drainage, and incentive spirometry
   7. Precautions: universal
   8. Antibiotic: streptomycin
   9. Antituberculosis: isoniazid, ethambutol (Myambutol), rifampin (Rifadin), pyrazinamide (pms-Pyrazinamide)

G. Nursing interventions
   1. Maintain the patient's diet
   2. Provide small frequent meals
   3. Provide suction, TCDB, CPT, and postural drainage
   4. Assess respiratory status
   5. Monitor and record VS, UO, I/O, and laboratory studies
   6. Administer medications, as prescribed
   7. Allay the patient's anxiety
   8. Maintain infection control precautions
   9. Force fluids
   10. Maintain bed rest
   11. Instruct the patient to cover nose and mouth when sneezing
   12. Provide frequent oral hygiene
   13. Provide ultraviolet light or well-ventilated room
   14. Provide information about the American Lung Association
   15. Individualize home care instructions
      a. Demonstrate methods to prevent spread of droplets of sputum
      b. Provide adequate air ventilation in rooms
      c. Reinforce need to finish entire course of medication (6 to 18 months)

CLINICAL ALERT

H. Possible complications
   1. Atelectasis
   2. Spontaneous pneumothorax

I. Possible surgical intervention: lobectomy (see page 63)

◆ XVI. Pneumothorax

A. Definition
   1. Loss of negative intrapleural pressure results in collapse of the lung
   2. Types include spontaneous, open, tension

B. Possible etiology
   1. Blunt chest trauma
   2. Rupture of a bleb
   3. CVP line insertion
   4. Thoracentesis

    5. Penetrating chest injuries

    6. Thoracic surgeries

C. Pathophysiology

    1. The loss of negative intrapleural pressure causes the collapse of the lung

    2. Surface area for gas exchange is reduced, resulting in hypoxia and hypercarbia

    3. Spontaneous pneumothorax occurs with the rupture of a bleb

    4. Open pneumothorax occurs when an opening through the chest wall allows the entrance of positive atmospheric pressure into the pleural space

    5. Tension pneumothorax occurs when there is a buildup of positive pressure in the pleural space

D. Possible assessment findings

    1. Sharp pain that increases with exertion

    2. Diminished or absent breath sounds unilaterally

    3. Dyspnea

    4. Tracheal shift

    5. Anxiety

    6. Diaphoresis

    7. Tachycardia

    8. Tachypnea

    9. Decreased chest expansion unilaterally

    10. Subcutaneous emphysema

    11. Pallor

    12. Cough

E. Possible diagnostic test findings

    1. Chest X-ray: pneumothorax

    2. ABGs: respiratory acidosis, hypoxemia

    3. Ventilation-perfusion scintigraphy: decreased

    4. Ventilation-perfusion (V/Q) defects: V/Q mismatches

F. Medical management

    1. Oxygen therapy

    2. Position: high-Fowler's

    3. Activity: out of bed to chair, active ROM exercises to affected arm

    4. Monitoring: VS and I/O

    5. Laboratory studies: ABGs

    6. Treatments: incentive spirometry

    7. Insertion: chest tube to water-seal drainage

    8. Thoracentesis

    9. Analgesic: oxycodone hydrochloride (Tylox)

G. Nursing interventions
 1. Administer oxygen
 2. Provide TCDB and incentive spirometry
 3. Assess respiratory status
 4. Maintain chest tube to water-seal drainage
 5. Keep the patient in high-Fowler's position
 6. Monitor and record VS, chest tube drainage, air leak or subcutaneous emphysema, and laboratory studies
 7. Administer medications, as prescribed
 8. Allay the patient's anxiety
 9. Assess the patient's pain
 10. Individualize home care instructions
   a. Recognize the signs and symptoms of pneumothorax and respiratory infection
   b. Avoid heavy lifting

H. Possible complications
 1. Mediastinal shift
 2. Respiratory insufficiency
 3. Infection

I. Possible surgical interventions: none

♦ XVII. Pulmonary embolism

A. Definition
 1. Undissolved substance in the pulmonary vasculature that obstructs blood flow
 2. Three types
   a. Fat
   b. Air
   c. Thrombus

B. Possible etiology
 1. Flat, long bone fractures
 2. Thrombophlebitis
 3. Venous stasis
 4. Hypercoagulability
 5. Abdominal surgery
 6. Malignant tumors
 7. Prolonged bed rest
 8. Obesity
 9. CVP line insertion

C. Pathophysiology
 1. Air, fat, or the tail of a thrombus that breaks off travels from the venous circulation to the right side of the heart and pulmonary artery

2. Blood flow is obstructed by the embolism, resulting in pulmonary hypertension and possible infarction

D. Possible assessment findings
   1. Dyspnea
   2. Tachycardia
   3. Elevated temperature
   4. Cough
   5. Hemoptysis
   6. Chest pain
   7. Tachypnea
   8. Anxiety
   9. Crackles
   10. Hypotension
   11. Arrhythmias

E. Possible diagnostic test findings
   1. Chest X-ray: dilated pulmonary arteries
   2. ABGs: respiratory alkalosis, hypoxemia
   3. Lung scan: decreased pulmonary circulation, blood flow obstruction
   4. Angiography: location of embolism, filling defect of pulmonary artery
   5. Blood chemistry: increased lactic dehydrogenase
   6. ECG: tachycardia, nonspecific ST changes

F. Medical management
   1. I.V. therapy: hydration, heparin lock
   2. Oxygen therapy
   3. Intubation and mechanical ventilation
   4. Position: high-Fowler's
   5. Activity: bed rest; active and passive ROM and isometric exercises
   6. Monitoring: VS, UO, CVP, ECG, I/O, and neurovascular checks
   7. Laboratory studies: ABGs, PT, and PTT
   8. Treatments: Indwelling urinary catheter, incentive spirometry
   9. Analgesic: meperidine hydrochloride (Demerol), oxycodone (Percocet, Tylox)
   10. Diuretics: furosemide (Lasix), ethacrynic acid (Edecin)
   11. Anticoagulants: heparin (Lipo-Hepin), warfarin sodium (Coumadin)
   12. Fibrinolytics: streptokinase, urokinase
   13. Pulse oximetry

G. Nursing interventions
   1. Administer I.V. fluids
   2. Administer oxygen
   3. Provide suction and TCDB
   4. Assess respiratory status

5. Keep the patient in high-Fowler's position

6. Monitor and record VS, UO, CVP, I/O, urine for blood, laboratory studies, and pulse oximetry

7. Administer medications, as prescribed

8. Allay the patient's anxiety

CLINICAL ALERT

9. Monitor and record color, consistency, and amount of sputum

10. Assess for positive Homans' sign

11. Monitor PT and PTT to maintain therapeutic level

12. Individualize home care instructions

CLINICAL ALERT

    a. Recognize the signs and symptoms of respiratory distress

    b. Avoid activities which promote venous stasis

      (1) Prolonged sitting and standing

      (2) Wearing constrictive clothing

      (3) Crossing legs when seated

      (4) Using oral contraceptives

    c. Recognize signs and symptoms of excessive anticoagulants

H. Possible complications: pulmonary infarction

I. Possible surgical interventions

1. Vein ligation

2. Plication of inferior vena cava (see page 65)

3. Embolectomy (see page 64)

◆ XVIII. Lung cancer

A. Definition—malignant tumor of the lung that may be primary or metastatic

B. Possible etiology

1. Cigarette smoking

2. Exposure to environmental pollutants

3. Exposure to occupational pollutants

C. Pathophysiology

1. Unregulated cell growth and uncontrolled cell division result in the development of a neoplasm

2. Four histologic types include epidermoid (squamous), adenocarcinoma, large cell anaplastic, small cell anaplastic

3. Lungs are a common target site for metastasis from other organs

D. Possible assessment findings

1. Cough

2. Dyspnea

3. Hemoptysis

4. Chest pain

5. Chills

6. Fever

      7. Weight loss

      8. Weakness

      9. Anorexia

    10. Wheezing

    11. Fatigue

E. Possible diagnostic test findings

    1. Chest X-ray: lesion or mass

    2. Bronchoscopy: positive biopsy

    3. Involvement of pulmonary artery or pulmonary veins

    4. Sputum studies: positive cytology for cancer cells

    5. Lung scan: mass

F. Medical management

    1. Diet: high-protein, high-calorie

    2. I.V. therapy: heparin lock

    3. Oxygen therapy

    4. Intubation and mechanical ventilation

    5. Position: semi-Fowler's

    6. Activity: active and passive ROM exercises, as tolerated

    7. Monitoring: VS, UO, and I/O

    8. Laboratory studies: ABGs

    9. Nutritional support: TPN

   10. Radiation therapy

   11. Antineoplastics: cyclophosphamide (Cytoxan), doxorubicin hydrochloride (Adriamycin)

   12. Treatment: incentive spirometry

   13. Isotope implant

   14. Laser photocoagulation

   15. Diuretics: furosemide (Lasix), ethacrynic acid (Edecrin)

   16. Chemotherapy: cisplatin (Platinol), vinblastine sulfate (Velban)

   17. Analgesics: meperidine hydrochloride (Demerol), morphine sulfate (Roxanol)

   18. Antiemetic: prochlorperazine (Compazine), ondansetron hydrochloride (Zofran)

   19. Pulse oximetry

G. Nursing interventions

    1. Maintain the patient's diet

    2. Encourage fluids

    3. Administer I.V. fluids

    4. Administer oxygen

    5. Provide suction, and TCDB

    6. Assess respiratory status

    7. Keep the patient in semi-Fowler's position

8. Monitor and record VS, UO, I/O, laboratory studies, and pulse oximetry
9. Administer TPN
10. Administer medications, as prescribed
11. Encourage the patient to express feelings about changes in body image and a fear of dying
12. Assess the patient's pain and administer analgesics, as prescribed
13. Provide postchemotherapeutic and postradiation nursing care
    a. Provide skin and mouth care
    b. Monitor dietary intake
    c. Administer antiemetics and antidiarrheals, as prescribed
    d. Monitor for bleeding, infection, and electrolyte imbalance
    e. Provide rest periods
14. Provide information about the American Cancer Society
15. Individualize home care instructions
    a. Demonstrate deep breathing and coughing exercises
    b. Alternate rest periods with activity
    c. Follow dietary recommendations and restrictions

H. Possible complications
   1. Respiratory insufficiency
   2. Pneumonia

I. Possible surgical interventions
   1. Lung resection (see page 63)
   2. Lobectomy (see page 63)
   3. Wedge resection (see page 63)
   4. Pneumonectomy (see page 63)

♦ XIX. Laryngeal cancer

A. Definition—benign or malignant tumor of the larynx

B. Possible etiology
   1. Cigarette smoking
   2. Alcohol abuse
   3. Exposure to environmental pollutants
   4. Exposure to radiation
   5. Voice strain

C. Pathophysiology
   1. Unregulated cell growth and uncontrolled cell division result in the development of a neoplasm through the growth of abnormal cells
   2. Most laryngeal cancers are squamous cell carcinomas
   3. Intrinsic cancer is cancer within the larynx
   4. Extrinsic cancer is cancer outside the larynx

D. Possible assessment findings
1. Throat pain
2. Burning sensation
3. Palpable lump in neck
4. Dysphagia
5. Dyspnea
6. Cough
7. Hemoptysis
8. Progressive hoarseness
9. Sore throat
10. Weakness
11. Weight loss
12. Foul breath

E. Possible diagnostic test findings
1. Laryngoscopy: lesions, ulcerations, positive biopsy
2. Biopsy: cytology positive for cancer cells
3. Computed tomography: laryngeal tumor
4. Magnetic resonance imaging: laryngeal tumor

F. Medical management
1. Diet: high-calorie, high-vitamin, high-protein
2. I.V. therapy: heparin lock
3. Oxygen therapy
4. Position: semi-Fowler's
5. Activity: as tolerated
6. Monitoring: VS, UO, and I/O
7. Laboratory studies: Hgb, HCT, and ABGs
8. Nutritional support: TPN, NG tube feedings, and gastrostomy feedings
9. Radiation therapy
10. Chemotherapy: experimental protocols
11. Treatment: incentive spirometry
12. Analgesic: oxycodone hydrochloride (Tylox)
13. Antineoplastics: methotrexate sodium (Mexate), vincristine sulfate (Oncovin), bleomycin sulfate (Blenoxane), cisplatin (Platinol)
14. Antiemetic: prochlorperazine (Compazine)

G. Nursing interventions
1. Maintain high-calorie, high-vitamin, high-protein diet
2. Administer I.V. fluids
3. Administer oxygen
4. Provide incentive spirometry, TCDB
5. Assess respiratory status
6. Maintain activity, as tolerated
7. Keep the patient in semi-Fowler's position

8. Monitor and record VS, UO, I/O, and laboratory studies
9. Administer TPN, NG tube feedings, and gastrostomy feedings
10. Administer medications, as prescribed
11. Encourage the patient to express feelings about potential loss of voice and changes in body image
12. Monitor and record the color, amount, and consistency of sputum
13. Provide postchemotherapeutic and postradiation nursing care
  a. Provide prophylactic skin and mouth care
  b. Monitor dietary intake
  c. Administer antiemetics and antidiarrheals, as prescribed
  d. Monitor for bleeding, infection, and electrolyte imbalance
  e. Provide rest periods
14. Provide information about the Lost Chord Club, New Voice Club, and International Association of Laryngectomies
15. Individualize home care instructions
  a. Recognize the signs and symptoms of respiratory distress
  b. Limit using voice
  c. Demonstrate tracheostomy care, suctioning, alternative communication

H. Possible complications
  1. Laryngeal obstruction
  2. Respiratory distress

I. Possible surgical interventions
  1. Partial laryngectomy (see page 60)
  2. Total laryngectomy (see page 60)
  3. Radical neck dissection (see page 61)

POINTS TO REMEMBER

Objective assessment findings in respiratory disorders include dyspnea, adventitious sounds, sputum, clubbing of fingers, fremitus, crepitus, and a change in patterns and character of respirations.

♦ After a bronchoscopy, food and fluids should be withheld until the patient's gag reflex returns.

♦ The stimulus for breathing in emphysema is low Po_2.

♦ The patient with ARDS, pneumothorax, or pulmonary embolism should be placed in high-Fowler's position.

♦ Lung cancer has been linked to cigarette smoking and environmental and occupational pollutants.

STUDY QUESTIONS

To evaluate your understanding of this chapter, answer the following questions in the space provided; then compare your responses with the correct answers in Appendix B, pages 382 and 383.

1. Which nursing interventions are a priority for the patient post bronchoscopy? _____

   _____

   _____

2. What is a key postoperative assessment for a patient with a radical neck dissection? _____

   _____

   _____

3. How should the nurse position the patient who has had a pneumonectomy?

   _____

   _____

4. What are the assessment findings in a patient with pneumonia? _____

   _____

   _____

5. What should the nurse teach the patient about how TB is spread? _____

   _____

   _____

6. What is the key assessment finding in a patient with a pneumothorax? _____

   _____

   _____

7. What are the most important home care instructions for a patient with a pulmonary embolism? _____

   _____

   _____

CRITICAL THINKING AND APPLICATION EXERCISES

1. Observe a pulmonary resection. Prepare an oral presentation for your fellow students, describing the procedure and patient care before, during, and after the procedure.

2. Develop a chart comparing the major bronchodilators.

3. Interview a patient with lung cancer. Evaluate the information for possible risk factors and identify ways to modify them.

4. Follow a patient with a respiratory disorder from admission through discharge. Develop a patient-specific plan of care, including any needs for follow-up and home care.

CHAPTER

3

Nervous System

CHAPTER OVERVIEW

Caring for the patient with a neurologic disorder requires a sound understanding of anatomy and physiology of the nervous system. A thorough assessment is essential to planning and implementing appropriate patient care. The assessment includes a complete history, physical examination, diagnostic testing, identification of modifiable and nonmodifiable risk factors, and information related to the psychosocial impact of the disorder on the patient. Nursing diagnoses focus primarily on self-care deficits, altered cerebral tissue perfusion, and decreased adaptive intracranial capacity. Nursing interventions are designed to increase the transmission of nerve impulses, thereby improving muscular function. Patient teaching, a crucial nursing activity, involves information about medical follow-up, medication regimens, providing a safe environment, signs and symptoms of possible complications, and reduction of modifiable risk factors through weight control, activity and diet restrictions, stress management, and smoking cessation. The impact of neurologic dysfunction on self-esteem also should be considered with self-care deficits.

◆ I. Anatomy and physiology review

A. Neuron
  1. The nerve cell, or neuron, is the basic functional unit of the nervous system
  2. The neuron consists of a cell body, dendrites, and an axon, surrounded by a myelin sheath (myelinated neuron)
  3. The neuron conducts impulses across a synapse to muscles, glands, and organs
  4. Neurotransmitters (acetylcholine, serotonin, dopamine, endorphins, gamma-aminobutyric acid, and norepinephrine) help conduct impulses across the synapse

B. Central nervous system (CNS)
  1. The CNS includes the brain and the spinal cord
    a. Brain
      (1) The *cerebrum* is divided into two hemispheres that contain four lobes each
        (a) The frontal lobe is the site of personality, intellectual functioning, and motor speech
        (b) The parietal lobe is the site of sensation, integration of sensory information, and spatial relationships
        (c) The temporal lobe is the site of hearing, taste, smell, and speech
        (d) The occipital lobe is the site of vision
      (2) The *diencephalon* consists of the thalamus and the hypothalamus
        (a) The thalamus relays sensory impulses of pain, temperature, and touch to the cortex
        (b) The hypothalamus controls temperature, respiration, blood pressure, and emotional states
      (3) The *brain stem* comprises the midbrain, pons, and medulla oblongata
        (a) The midbrain consists of the tectum and the cerebral peduncles
        (b) The pons consists of the pons dorsalis and pons ventralis

        (c) The medulla oblongata contains the vomiting, vasomo-tor, respiratory, and cardiac centers

        (d) Pyramidal tracts decussate at the medulla oblongata

    (4) The *cerebellum* coordinates muscle tone, movement, equilibrium, and posture

    (5) Blood is supplied to the brain via the internal carotid arteries, vertebral arteries, and circle of Willis

    (6) The *reticular activating system* coordinates sensory input and regulates level of arousal and response to stimuli

    (7) The *corpus callosum* consists of nerve fibers that transmit nerve impulses from one hemisphere of the brain to the other

    (8) *The blood-brain barrier* consists of endothelial cells within the capillaries of the brain that prevent substances in plasma from reaching the brain and cerebrospinal fluid (CSF)

    (9) The *limbic system* stores recent memories, stimulates "arousal-attention" responses, and provides semi-automatic responses to stimuli

  b. Spinal cord

    (1) The *spinal cord* consists of grey matter and white matter

        (a) Grey matter forms an H-shaped core in the spinal cord

        (b) White matter includes the spinal cord's ascending (sensory) and descending (motor) tracts

    (2) The spinal cord's reflex arc is an involuntary response to a stimulus

2. The CNS is covered and protected by the meninges, which comprise three membranous layers

  a. Dura mater

  b. Pia mater

  c. Arachnoid membrane

3. Four ventricles produce and circulate CSF

  a. CSF surrounds and protects the brain and spinal cord

  b. CSF exchanges nutrients and wastes at the cellular level

C. Peripheral nervous system (PNS)

1. The PNS and the CNS together constitute the nervous system

2. The PNS comprises 12 pairs of cranial nerves, 31 pairs of spinal nerves, and the autonomic nervous system

  a. The cranial nerves consist of the olfactory, optic, oculomotor, trochlear, trigeminal, abducent, facial, acoustic, glossopharyngeal, vagus, accessory, and hypoglossal nerves

  b. Spinal nerves carry mixed impulses (motor and sensory) to and from the spinal cord

    c. The autonomic nervous system regulates smooth muscle, cardiac muscle, and glands; it comprises the sympathetic and parasympathetic nervous systems

       (1) Sympathetic activity results in adrenergic responses

       (2) Parasympathetic activity results in cholinergic responses

♦ II. Assessment findings

A. History

1. Memory impairment
2. Numbness and tingling
3. Muscle weakness
4. Twitching and spasm
5. Ringing in the ears
6. Difficulty chewing, swallowing, talking, and walking
7. Headache
8. Dizziness
9. Fainting
10. Loss of balance and coordination
11. Nausea and vomiting
12. Pain
13. Mental confusion or excitement
14. Blurred or double vision
15. Change in bowel and bladder patterns
16. Sexual dysfunction
17. Tremors
18. Stiff neck
19. Drooping eyelids

B. Physical examination

CLINICAL
ALERT

1. Paresthesia
2. Change in level of consciousness (LOC)
3. Ataxic gait
4. Dyskinesia
5. Tinnitus
6. Dysphagia
7. Aphasia
8. Seizures
9. Diplopia
10. PAPILLEDEMA
11. Change in visual fields
12. Loss of vision
13. Abnormal temperature
14. Pulse changes
15. Abnormal respirations

16. Hypertension
17. Change in muscle reflexes
18. Abnormal pupil size and reaction
19. Positive Babinski's reflex
20. Loss of cough, gag, corneal, oculocephalic, and oculovestibular reflexes
21. PTOSIS

♦ **III. Diagnostic tests and procedures**

A. EEG
   1. Definition and purpose
     a. Noninvasive test of the brain
     b. Graphical representation of the brain's electrical activity
   2. Nursing interventions before the procedure
     a. Determine the patient's ability to lie still
     b. Reassure the patient that electrical shock will not occur
     c. Explain that the patient will be subjected to stimuli, such as lights and sounds
     d. Withhold medications and caffeine 8 hours before the procedure

B. Computerized tomography (CT) scan
   1. Definition and purpose
     a. Noninvasive scan after injection of a contrast dye
     b. Visualization of the brain and its structures
   2. Nursing interventions before the procedure
     a. Note the patient's allergies to iodine, seafood, and radiopaque dyes
     b. Allay the patient's anxiety
     c. Inform the patient about possible throat irritation and flushing of the face

C. Magnetic resonance imaging (MRI)
   1. Definition and purpose
     a. Noninvasive scan using magnetic and radio waves
     b. Visualization of the brain and its structures
   2. Nursing interventions before the procedure
     a. Be aware that patients with pacemakers, surgical and orthopedic clips, or shrapnel should not be scanned
     b. Remove jewelry and metal objects from the patient
     c. Determine the patient's ability to lie still
     d. Administer sedation, as prescribed

D. Cerebral angiogram
   1. Definition and purpose
     a. Fluoroscopic procedure using a radiopaque dye
     b. Examination of the cerebral arteries

CLINICAL ALERT

CLINICAL ALERT

2. Nursing interventions before the procedure
   a. Note the patient's allergies to iodine, seafood, or radiopaque dyes
   b. Inform the patient about possible throat irritation and flushing of the face
3. Nursing interventions after the procedure
   a. Monitor vital signs (VS)
   b. Allay the patient's anxiety
   c. Check the insertion site for bleeding
   d. Monitor NEUROVITAL SIGNS

E. Lumbar puncture (LP)
   1. Definition and purpose
      a. Invasive procedure
      b. Collection of CSF from the lumbar subarachnoid space and measurement of CSF pressure and injection of radiopaque dye for myelogram
   2. Nursing interventions before the procedure
      a. Determine the patient's ability to lie still in a flexed, lateral, recumbent position

      b. Explain the procedure to the patient
      c. Know that the presence of increased intracranial pressure (ICP) is a contraindication for having the test
   3. Nursing interventions after the procedure
      a. Keep the patient flat in bed for 24 hours
      b. Administer analgesics, as prescribed
      c. Check the puncture site for bleeding
      d. Monitor neurovital signs
      e. Force fluids

F. CSF analysis
   1. Definition and purpose
      a. Laboratory test of CSF obtained via LP
      b. Microscopic examination of CSF for blood, white blood cells (WBCs), immunoglobulins, bacteria, protein, glucose, and electrolytes
   2. Nursing interventions
      a. Label specimens properly and send to the laboratory immediately
      b. Adhere to nursing interventions after an LP

G. Electromyography (EMG)
   1. Definition and purpose
      a. Noninvasive test of muscles
      b. Graphical recording of the electrical activity of a muscle at rest and during contraction

2. Nursing interventions
   a. Explain that the patient must flex and relax the muscles during the procedure
   b. Explain that the patient will feel some discomfort but not pain
   c. Administer analgesics, as prescribed, after the procedure

H. Myelogram
   1. Definition and purpose
      a. Injection of radiopaque dye by LP
      b. Visualization of the subarachnoid space, spinal cord, and vertebrae under fluoroscopy

   2. Nursing interventions before the procedure
      a. Note the patient's allergies to iodine, seafood, and radiopaque dyes
      b. Inform the patient about possible throat irritation and flushing of the face
   3. Nursing interventions after the procedure
      a. Keep the patient flat in bed, as directed
      b. Check the puncture site for bleeding
      c. Monitor neurovital signs
      d. Force fluids

I. Brain scan
   1. Definition and purpose
      a. Procedure that involves injection of a radiopaque dye
      b. Visual imaging of blood flow and distribution and brain structures

   2. Nursing interventions before the procedure
      a. Note the patient's allergies to iodine, seafood, and radiopaque dyes
      b. Inform the patient about possible throat irritation and flushing of the face
      c. Determine the patient's ability to lie still during the procedure

J. Skull X-rays
   1. Definition and purpose
      a. Noninvasive examination
      b. Radiographic picture of head and neck bones
   2. Nursing interventions before the procedure
      a. Determine the patient's ability to lie still during the procedure
      b. Explain the events that will occur during the procedure

K. Positron emission tomography
   1. Definition and purpose
      a. Imaging that involves injection of a radioisotope
      b. Visualization of oxygen uptake, blood flow, and glucose metabolism
   2. Nursing interventions
      a. Determine the patient's ability to lie still during the procedure
      b. Withhold alcohol, tobacco, and caffeine for 24 hours before the procedure

      c. Withhold medications, as directed, before the procedure

      d. Check the injection site for bleeding after the procedure

L. Blood chemistry

  1. Definition and purpose

      a. Laboratory test of a blood sample

      b. Analysis for potassium, sodium, calcium, phosphorus, protein, albumin, osmolality, glucose, bicarbonate, blood urea nitrogen (BUN), and creatinine

  2. Nursing interventions

      a. Withhold food and fluids before the procedure

      b. Monitor the site for bleeding after the procedure

M. Hematologic studies

  1. Definition and purpose

      a. Laboratory test of a blood sample

      b. Analysis for WBCs, red blood cells (RBCs), erythrocyte sedimentation rate, prothrombin time (PT), partial thromboplastin time (PTT), platelets, hemoglobin (Hgb), and hematocrit (HCT)

  2. Nursing interventions

      a. Note current drug therapy before the procedure

      b. Check the venipuncture site for bleeding after the procedure

◆ IV. Psychosocial impact of nervous system disorders

A. Developmental impact

  1. Changes in body image

  2. Loss of control over body functions

  3. Fear of rejection

  4. Embarrassment from changes in body structure and function

  5. Decreased self-esteem

  6. Fear of dying

  7. Dependence

B. Economic impact

  1. Disruption or loss of employment

  2. Cost of hospitalizations

  3. Cost of home health care

  4. Cost of special equipment

C. Occupational and recreational impact

  1. Restrictions in work activity

  2. Changes in leisure activity

  3. Restrictions in physical activity

  4. Need for vocational retraining

   D. Social impact
   1. Changes in eating modes
   2. Changes in elimination patterns and modes
   3. Social isolation
   4. Changes in sexual function
   5. Changes in role performance

♦ **V. Risk factors for developing nervous system disorders**

   A. Modifiable risk factors
   1. Exposure to chemical or environmental pollutants
   2. Substance abuse
   3. Participation in contact sports
   4. Hypertension

   B. Nonmodifiable risk factors
   1. Aging
   2. Family history of neurologic disease
   3. History of cardiac disease
   4. History of head injury
   5. Exposure to viral or bacterial infection

♦ **VI. Nursing diagnostic categories for a patient with a nervous system disorder**

   A. Probable nursing diagnostic categories
   1. Impaired physical mobility
   2. Feeding self-care deficit
   3. Bathing/hygiene self-care deficit
   4. Dressing/grooming self-care deficit
   5. Toileting self-care deficit
   6. Sensory-perceptual alteration: visual
   7. Sensory-perceptual alteration: tactile
   8. Altered thought processes
   9. Social isolation
   10. Impaired home maintenance management
   11. Unilateral neglect
   12. Body image disturbance
   13. Self-esteem disturbance
   14. Dysreflexia

   B. Possible nursing diagnostic categories
   1. Sexual dysfunction
   2. Altered urinary elimination
   3. Impaired verbal communication
   4. Bowel incontinence

5. Altered nutrition: less than body requirements
6. Ineffective airway clearance
7. Ineffective individual coping
8. Risk for injury
9. Altered cerebral tissue perfusion
10. Powerlessness
11. Risk for violence
12. Sleep pattern disturbance
13. Risk for aspiration
14. Decreased adaptive capacity: intracranial

◆ VII. Craniotomy

A. Description
    1. Surgical opening in the skull to excise a tumor, evacuate a blood clot, relieve intracranial pressure, or repair an aneurysm
    2. Classified as supratentorial or infratentorial

B. Preoperative nursing interventions
    1. Complete patient and family preoperative teaching
        a. Determine the patient's understanding of the procedure
        b. Describe the operating room (OR), postanesthesia care unit (PACU), and preoperative and postoperative routines; demonstrate postoperative turning, coughing, and deep breathing (TCDB), splinting, leg exercises, and range-of-motion (ROM) exercises
        c. Explain the postoperative need for drainage tubes, surgical dressings, oxygen therapy, I.V. therapy, and pain control
    2. Complete a preoperative checklist
    3. Administer preoperative medications, as prescribed
    4. Allay the patient's and family's anxiety about surgery
    5. Document the patient's history and physical assessment data base
    6. Administer antibiotics, as prescribed
    7. Prepare the patient for preoperative shaving of the head

C. Postoperative nursing interventions
    1. Assess cardiac, respiratory, and neurologic status, including LOC
    2. Assess pain and administer postoperative analgesics, as prescribed
    3. Assess for return of peristalsis; give solid foods and liquids, as tolerated
    4. Administer I.V. fluids and total parenteral nutrition (TPN)
    5. Allay the patient's anxiety
    6. Inspect the surgical dressing and change, as directed
    7. Reinforce TCDB
    8. Keep the patient in semi-Fowler's position
    9. Provide incentive spirometry

10. Maintain active or passive ROM exercises, as tolerated

11. Administer oxygen and maintain endotracheal tube (ET) to ventilator

12. Monitor VS, urine output (UO), urine specific gravity, intake and output (I/O), central venous pressure (CVP), laboratory studies, electrocardiogram (ECG), neurovital signs, neurovascular checks, ICP, and pulse oximetry

13. Monitor and maintain the position and patency of drainage tubes: nasogastric (NG), indwelling urinary catheter, wound drainage

14. Assess cough and gag reflexes

15. Encourage the patient to express feelings about changes in body image or a fear of dying

16. Check for signs of diabetes insipidus

17. Provide eye care

18. Allow a rest period between each nursing activity

19. Observe for signs of increasing ICP

20. Administer corticosteroids, as prescribed

21. Administer anticonvulsants, as prescribed

22. Administer laxatives, as prescribed

23. Administer antacids, as prescribed

24. Administer osmotic diuretics, as prescribed

25. Maintain seizure precautions

26. Individualize home care instructions
   a. Recognize the signs and symptoms of infection
   b. Monitor for change in LOC
   c. Demonstrate safety measures during seizure activity

D. Possible surgical complications
   1. Increased ICP
   2. Seizures
   3. Respiratory distress
   4. Diabetes insipidus
   5. Motor and sensory deficits
   6. Infection
   7. Meningitis

♦ VIII. Endarterectomy

A. Description—surgical removal of atheromas from arteries and a patch graft repair of the vessel

B. Preoperative nursing interventions
   1. Complete patient and family preoperative teaching
      a. Determine the patient's understanding of the procedure
      b. Describe the OR, PACU, and preoperative and postoperative routines

       c. Demonstrate postoperative TCDB, splinting, and leg and ROM exercises

       d. Explain the postoperative need for drainage tubes, surgical dressings, oxygen therapy, I.V. therapy, and pain control

  2. Complete a preoperative checklist

  3. Administer preoperative medications, as prescribed

  4. Allay the patient's and family's anxiety about surgery

  5. Document the patient's history and physical assessment data base

  6. Administer antibiotics, as prescribed

  7. Protect the surgical site from trauma

  8. Obtain a preoperative vascular assessment

C. Postoperative nursing interventions

  1. Assess cardiac, respiratory, and neurologic status

  2. Assess pain and administer postoperative analgesics, as prescribed

  3. Assess for return of peristalsis; give solid foods and liquids, as tolerated

  4. Administer I.V. fluids

  5. Allay the patient's anxiety

  6. Inspect the surgical dressing and change, as directed

  7. Reinforce TCDB

  8. Keep the patient in semi-Fowler's position

  9. Provide incentive spirometry

 10. Maintain activity: active or passive ROM and isometric exercises, as tolerated

 11. Administer oxygen

 12. Monitor VS, UO, I/O, laboratory studies, neurovital signs, neurovascular checks, and pulse oximetry

 13. Monitor and maintain the position and patency of drainage tubes: NG, indwelling urinary catheter, and wound drainage

 14. Check the surgical site for bleeding

 15. Maintain a pressure dressing

CLINICAL ALERT

 16. Provide special care for carotid endarterectomy

       a. Check neck edema

       b. Assess ability to swallow

 17. Administer anticoagulants

 18. Individualize home care instructions

       a. Recognize the signs and symptoms of infection

       b. Monitor for motor and sensory deficits

D. Possible surgical complications

  1. Bleeding

  2. Embolism

  3. Thrombosis

4. Neurologic deficits

5. Infection

◆ IX. Parkinson's disease (paralysis agitans)

A. Definition—progressive degenerative disease of the extrapyramidal system associated with dopamine deficiency

B. Possible etiology

1. Unknown

2. Imbalance of dopamine and acetylcholine in basal ganglia

3. Cerebral vascular disease

4. Drug-induced: phentolamine (Regitine), reserpine (Serpasil), methyldopa (Aldomet)

5. Dopamine deficiency

C. Pathophysiology

1. Nerve cells in the basal ganglia are destroyed, resulting in impaired muscular function

2. Dopamine in the substantia nigra degenerates

3. Lack of dopamine results in decreased inhibition of the synaptic transmitter for muscle tone and coordination

D. Possible assessment findings

1. "Pill rolling" tremors

2. Shuffling gait

3. Stiff joints

4. Masklike facial expression

5. Dyskinesia

6. Dysphagia

7. Drooling

8. "Cogwheel" rigidity

9. Fatigue

10. Stooped posture

11. Tremors at rest

12. Small handwriting

13. Difficulty in initiating voluntary activity

E. Possible diagnostic test findings

1. EEG: minimal slowing

2. CT scan: normal

F. Medical management

1. Diet: high-residue, high-calorie, and high-protein; soft foods

2. Physical therapy

3. Activity: as tolerated

4. Monitoring: VS, UO, I/O, and neurovital signs

5. Anticholinergics: benztropine mesylate (Cogentin), trihexyphenidyl (Artane)
6. Antiparkinsonian agents: levodopa (Larodopa), carbidopa-levodopa (Sinemet), benztropine mesylate (Cogentin)
7. Antispasmodic: procyclidine (Kemadrin)
8. Antidepressant: amitriptyline (Elavil)
9. Antiviral: amantadine (Symmetrel)
10. MAO-B inhibitor: selegiline hydrochloride (Eldepryl)
11. Dopamine receptor agonists: pergolide mesylate (Permax), bromocriptine mesylate (Parlodel)

G. Nursing interventions
1. Maintain the patient's diet
2. Assess neurovascular and respiratory status
3. Position the patient to prevent contractures
4. Monitor and record VS, UO, and I/O
5. Administer medications, as prescribed
6. Encourage the patient to express feelings about changes in body image

CLINICAL ALERT

7. Promote daily ambulation
8. Maintain a patent airway
9. Provide active and passive ROM exercises
10. Provide skin care daily
11. Provide oral hygiene
12. Reinforce gait training
13. Reinforce independence in care
14. Provide information about the American Parkinson's Disease Association, Inc.; the Parkinson Disease Foundation; and the National Parkinson's Foundation
15. Individualize home care instructions (For more information about patient teaching, see *Patients with nervous system disorders,* page 100)
    a. Recognize the signs and symptoms of respiratory distress
    b. Alternate rest periods with activity
    c. Promote a safe environment
    d. Take measures to prevent choking
       (1) Cut food into small pieces
       (2) Suction the mouth frequently
       (3) Eat soft foods
    e. Increase intake of roughage and fluids to prevent constipation

H. Possible complications
1. Depression
2. Corneal ulceration
3. Injury
4. Aspiration
5. Constipation

TEACHING TIPS
Patients with nervous system disorders

Be sure to include the following topics in your teaching plan when caring for patients with neurologic disorders.
- Smoking cessation
- Optimal weight maintenance
- Regular exercise
- Medication therapy including action, adverse effects, and scheduling of medications
- Dietary recommendations and restrictions
- Stress reduction strategies
- Rest and activity patterns
- Frequent blood pressure monitoring
- Environmental safety
- Community resources
- Self-monitoring for infection
- Avoidance of alcohol
- Danger signs, including changes in mentation and level of consciousness
- Rehabilitation, including adaptive and assistive devices
- Coping mechanisms

   I. Possible surgical intervention: stereotaxic thalamotomy to relieve tremor and rigidity

◆ X. Multiple sclerosis

  A. Definition—progressive demyelinating disease of both motor and sensory neurons that has periods of remissions and exacerbation

  B. Possible etiology
    1. Unknown
    2. Autoimmune disease
    3. Viral

  C. Pathophysiology
    1. Scattered demyelinization occurs in the brain and spinal cord
    2. Degeneration of myelin sheath results in patches of sclerotic tissue and impaired conduction of motor nerve impulses

  D. Possible assessment findings
    1. Weakness
    2. Nystagmus
    3. Scanning speech
    4. ATAXIA
    5. Diplopia
    6. Paresthesia

7. Blurred vision

8. Impaired sensation

9. Feelings of euphoria

10. Paralysis

11. Urinary incontinence

12. Intention tremor

13. Inability to sense or gauge body position

14. Optic neuritis

15. Intolerance to heat

E. Possible diagnostic test findings

1. CSF analysis: increased immunoglobulin G (IgG), protein, WBCs

2. CT scan: normal except in chronic illness, when atrophy is found

3. MRI: normal except in chronic illness, when atrophy is found

4. Evoked potentials: slowing of nerve conduction

5. Oligoclonal banding: positive

6. EMG: abnormal

F. Medical management

1. Diet: high-calorie, high-protein, and high-vitamin; gluten-free; low-fat

2. Activity: as tolerated

3. Monitoring: VS, UO, I/O, and neurovital signs

4. Speech therapy

5. Plasmapheresis

6. Muscle relaxant: baclofen (Lioresal)

7. Physical therapy

8. Glucocorticoids: prednisone (Deltasone), dexamethasone (Decadron), corticotropin (ACTH)

9. Antacids: magnesium and aluminum hydroxide (Maalox), aluminum hydroxide gel (AlternaGEL)

10. Fluids: increased intake

11. Antineoplastic (immunosuppressant): cyclophosphamide (Cytoxan)

12. Skeletal muscle relaxant: quinine sulfate (Quinamm)

G. Nursing interventions

1. Maintain the patient's diet

2. Force fluids

3. Assess neurologic status

4. Monitor and record: VS, UO, I/O, and neurovital signs

5. Administer medications, as prescribed

6. Encourage the patient to express feelings about changes in body image

7. Maintain active and passive ROM exercises

8. Establish bowel and bladder program

9. Maintain activity, as tolerated

10. Protect the patient from falls
11. Maintain a stress-free environment
12. Provide information about the National Multiple Sclerosis Society
13. Individualize home care instructions
    a. Identify ways to reduce stress
    b. Recognize the signs and symptoms of exacerbation
    c. Avoid exposure to people with infections
    d. Alternate rest periods with activity
    e. Maintain a safe, quiet environment
    f. Use assistive devices in activities of daily living (ADLs), such as specialized eating utensils, and wheelchair ramps
    g. Reinforce independence
    h. Avoid temperature extremes

H. Possible complications
  1. Urinary tract infection
  2. Respiratory tract infection
  3. Contractures
  4. Depression
  5. Paraplegia
  6. Quadriplegia

I. Possible surgical intervention: contralateral thalamotomy

♦ XI. Myasthenia gravis

A. Definition—neuromuscular disorder that results in weakness of voluntary muscles

B. Possible etiology
  1. Insufficient acetylcholine
  2. Autoimmune disease
  3. Excessive cholinesterase

C. Pathophysiology
  1. Disturbance occurs in transmission of nerve impulses at the myoneural junction
  2. Transmission defect results from deficiency in release of acetylcholine or deficient number of acetylcholine receptor sites
  3. Thymus gland may remain active, triggering autoimmune reaction

D. Possible assessment findings
  1. Muscle weakness that increases with activity and decreases with rest
  2. Dysphagia
  3. Diplopia
  4. Dysarthria
  5. Ptosis

6. Strabismus
7. Impaired speech
8. Respiratory distress
9. Masklike expression
10. Drooling

E. Possible diagnostic test findings
  1. Neostigmine (Prostigmin) or edrophonium (Tensilon) test: relief of symptoms after medication administration
  2. EMG: decreased amplitude of evoked potentials
  3. Thymus scan: hyperplasia or thymoma

F. Medical management
  1. Diet: high-calorie; soft foods
  2. Activity: as tolerated
  3. Monitoring: VS, UO, I/O, and neurovital signs
  4. Glucocorticoids: prednisone (Deltasone), dexamethasone (Decadron), corticotropin (ACTH)
  5. Antacids: magnesium and aluminum hydroxide (Maalox), aluminum hydroxide gel (AlternaGEL)
  6. Anticholinesterases: neostigmine (Prostigmin), pyridostigmine bromide (Mestinon), ambenonium chloride (Mytelase)
  7. Plasmapheresis
  8. Immunosuppressant: azathioprine (Imuran)
  9. Antineoplastic: cyclophosphamide (Cytoxan)

G. Nursing interventions
  1. Maintain the patient's diet; encourage small, frequent meals

CLINICAL ALERT

  2. Assess neurologic and respiratory status
  3. Assess swallow and gag reflexes
  4. Monitor and record VS, UO, I/O, and neurovital signs
  5. Administer medications, as prescribed
  6. Encourage the patient to express feelings about changes in body image and about difficulty in communicating verbally
  7. Determine the patient's activity tolerance
  8. Provide rest periods
  9. Provide oral hygiene
  10. Protect the patient from falls
  11. Watch the patient for choking while eating
  12. Provide information about the Myasthenia Gravis Foundation
  13. Individualize home care instructions
    a. Identify ways to reduce stress
    b. Recognize the signs and symptoms of respiratory distress
    c. Recognize the signs and symptoms of myasthenic crisis
    d. Adhere to activity limitations
    e. Avoid hot foods and tonic preparations containing quinine

H. Possible complications
   1. Myasthenic crisis
      a. Increased symptoms of muscular weakness from under medication or stress
      b. Symptoms improve with edrophonium (Tensilon)

   2. Cholinergic crisis
      a. Increased symptoms of muscular weakness and adverse effects of anticholinesterase medications from overmedication with cholinergic drugs
      b. Symptoms worsen with edrophonium (Tensilon)

I. Possible surgical intervention: thymectomy

♦ XII. Guillain-Barré syndrome (polyradiculitis, acute infectious polyneuritis)

A. Definition—peripheral polyneuritis characterized by ascending paralysis

B. Possible etiology
   1. Unknown
   2. Virus
   3. Infection
   4. Autoimmune disease

C. Pathophysiology
   1. Preceding infection synthesizes lymphocytes, which attack the myelin sheath, causing demyelinization
   2. Demyelinization is followed by inflammation around nerve roots, veins, and capillaries
   3. Inflammatory process compresses nerve roots

D. Possible assessment findings
   1. Generalized weakness
   2. Paralysis that starts in the legs
   3. Ascending paralysis
   4. Respiratory paralysis
   5. Tachycardia
   6. Hypertension
   7. Increased temperature
   8. Ptosis
   9. Facial weakness
   10. Dysphagia
   11. Dysarthria

E. Possible diagnostic test findings
   1. CSF analysis: increased protein
   2. EMG: slowed nerve conduction

F. Medical management
   1. Diet: high-calorie, high-protein
   2. Position: semi-Fowler's
   3. Activity: bed rest, active and passive ROM and isometric exercises
   4. Monitoring: VS, UO, I/O, and neurovital signs
   5. Plasmapheresis
   6. Nutritional support: gastrostomy feedings, NG feedings
   7. Intubation and mechanical ventilation
   8. Physical therapy
   9. Indwelling urinary catheter, chest physiotherapy, postural drainage, and suction
   10. Antibiotics: amoxicillin (Amoxil), ampicillin (Omnipen), gentamicin (Garamycin)
   11. Glucocorticoids: prednisone (Deltasone), dexamethasone (Decadron), corticotropin (ACTH)
   12. Antacids: magnesium and aluminum hydroxide (Maalox), aluminum hydroxide gel (AlternaGEL)
   13. IgG antibody: immune globulin I.V. (Gammagard)
   14. Pulse oximetry

G. Nursing interventions
   1. Maintain the patient's diet
   2. Administer oxygen
   3. Provide suction and TCDB
   4. Assess respiratory and neurologic status
   5. Maintain the position and patency of NG and endotracheal tubes
   6. Keep the patient in semi-Fowler's position
   7. Monitor and record VS, UO, I/O, neurovital signs, and pulse oximetry
   8. Administer medications, as prescribed
   9. Encourage the patient to express feelings about powerlessness, changes in body image, and difficulty in communicating verbally

CLINICAL ALERT

   10. Assess muscle strength
   11. Assess gag and swallow reflexes
   12. Provide eye and mouth care
   13. Establish alternate means of communicating with the patient
   14. Protect the patient from falls
   15. Prevent skin breakdown
   16. Provide ROM exercises
   17. Assess for Homans' sign
   18. Establish a bowel and bladder program
   19. Apply antiembolism stockings
   20. Turn the patient every 2 hours
   21. Provide information about the Guillain-Barré Foundation

22. Individualize home care instructions
    a. Identify ways to reduce stress
    b. Maintain a safe, quiet environment
    c. Minimize environmental stress
    d. Exercise hands, arms, and legs regularly

H. Possible complications
    1. Respiratory failure
    2. Contractures
    3. Aspiration
    4. Pneumonia

I. Possible surgical interventions: none

◆ XIII. Seizure disorders

A. Definition
    1. Involuntary muscle contractions caused by abnormal discharge of electrical impulses from nerve cells
    2. Classification of seizures
        a. Generalized seizures
            (1) Generalized absence (petit mal)
            (2) Generalized tonic-clonic (grand mal)
            (3) Myoclonic
            (4) Atonic
        b. Partial seizures (focal seizures)
            (1) Simple partial
            (2) Complex partial
        c. Unclassified seizures

B. Possible etiology
    1. Idiopathic origin
    2. Head injury
    3. Hypoglycemia
    4. Brain tumor
    5. Infection
    6. Anoxia

C. Pathophysiology
    1. Many neurons fire in a synchronous pattern, resulting in a transient physiologic disturbance
    2. Physiologic disturbances include abnormal movements, abnormal sensations, and a change in the LOC

D. Possible assessment findings
    1. Aura
    2. Loss of consciousness
    3. Dyspnea

    4. Fixed and dilated pupils

    5. Incontinence

E. Possible diagnostic test findings

    1. EEG: abnormal wave patterns, focus of seizure activity

    2. CT scan: a space-occupying lesion

    3. MRI: pathologic changes

    4. Brain mapping: identification of seizure areas

F. Medical management

    1. Diet: ketogenic

    2. I.V. therapy: heparin lock

    3. Activity: bed rest

    4. Monitoring: VS, UO, I/O, and neurovital signs

    5. Laboratory studies: glucose, potassium, and phenytoin levels

    6. Special care: seizure precautions

    7. Anticonvulsants: phenytoin (Dilantin), ethosuximide (Zarontin), phenobarbital (Luminal), diazepam (Valium), carbamazepine (Tegretol), valproic acid (Depakote)

G. Nursing interventions

    1. Maintain the patient's diet

    2. Assess neurologic and respiratory status

    3. Monitor and record VS, UO, I/O, neurovital signs, and laboratory studies

    4. Administer medications, as prescribed

CLINICAL ALERT

    5. Encourage the patient to express feelings about powerlessness

    6. Maintain seizure precautions

    7. Protect the patient during seizure activity

    8. Observe and record seizure activity

        a. Initial movement

        b. Respiratory pattern

        c. Duration of seizure

        d. Loss of consciousness

        e. Aura

        f. Incontinence

        g. Pupillary changes

    9. Assess postictal state

  10. Maintain a patent airway

  11. Protect the patient from falls

  12. Provide information about the Epilepsy Foundation of America; the National Epilepsy League, Inc.; and the National Association to Control Epilepsy

  13. Individualize home care instructions

        a. Recognize the signs and symptoms of seizure activity

        b. Avoid drinking alcohol

c. Promote a safe environment
d. Wear a medical identification bracelet
e. Identify and time seizure activity
f. Prevent injury during seizure activity

H. Possible complications
1. Musculoskeletal injury
2. Hypoxia
3. Status epilepticus

I. Possible surgical intervention: excision of epileptogenic area (rare)

◆ XIV. Increased intracranial pressure

A. Definition—elevated ICP beyond the normal pressure exerted by blood, brain, and CSF within the skull

B. Possible etiology
1. Tumor
2. Abscess
3. Space-occupying lesion
4. Edema
5. Hemorrhage
6. Hydrocephalus
7. Head injury
8. Infection
9. Congenital abnormality

C. Pathophysiology
1. Because the skull cannot expand, an increase in brain tissue, CSF, or blood results in increased ICP
2. Increased ICP results in decreased cerebral circulation and anoxia, which can lead to permanent brain damage

D. Possible assessment findings
1. Restlessness
2. Hypertension
3. Bradycardia
4. Pupillary changes
   a. Sluggish reaction
   b. Dilation
5. Weakness
6. Decreased LOC
7. Widening pulse pressure
8. Abnormal posturing
   a. Decortication
   b. DECEREBRATION
9. Headache

10. Vomiting
11. Papilledema

E. Possible diagnostic test findings

    1. ICP measurement via ventriculostomy, epidural sensor, and subarachnoid screw: increased pressure
    2. LP: contraindicated

F. Medical management
    1. Diet: withhold food and fluids, as ordered
    2. I.V. therapy: electrolyte replacement, heparin lock
    3. Oxygen therapy
    4. Intubation and mechanical ventilation with hyperventilation
    5. GI decompression: NG tube
    6. Position: semi-Fowler's
    7. Activity: bed rest, passive ROM exercises
    8. Monitoring: VS, UO, I/O, ECG, ICP, neurovital signs, and arterial pressure
    9. Laboratory studies: potassium, sodium, glucose, osmolality, BUN, and creatinine levels
    10. Indwelling urinary catheter
    11. ICP monitoring: ventriculostomy, subarachnoid screw, epidural sensor
    12. Diuretics: mannitol (Osmitrol), furosemide (Lasix)
    13. Antacids: magnesium and aluminum hydroxide (Maalox)
    14. CSF drainage via ventriculostomy
    15. Anticonvulsant: phenytoin (Dilantin)
    16. Glucocorticoid: dexamethasone (Decadron)
    17. Histamine antagonists: cimetidine (Tagamet), ranitidine (Zantac)
    18. Barbiturate-induced coma
    19. Seizure precautions
    20. Pulse oximetry
    21. Mucosal barrier fortifier: sucralfate (Carafate)

G. Nursing interventions
    1. Maintain fluid restrictions
    2. Administer I.V. fluids
    3. Administer oxygen
    4. Provide suction, TCDB
    5. Assess neurologic and respiratory status
    6. Maintain the position and patency of the NG tube; provide low suctioning
    7. Maintain the position and patency of the ET tube and indwelling urinary catheter
    8. Keep the patient in semi-Fowler's position

9. Monitor and record VS, UO, I/O, ICP, neurovital signs, laboratory studies, and pulse oximetry

10. Administer medications, as prescribed

11. Allay the patient's anxiety

12. Maintain neutral alignment of the neck with the body

13. Turn the patient every 2 hours

14. Prevent jugular venous constriction

15. Allow a period of rest between each nursing activity

16. Maintain a quiet environment

17. Continue bed rest

18. Prevent Valsalva's maneuver

19. Provide mouth and skin care

20. Provide appropriate sensory input and stimuli with frequent reorientation

21. Assist with ADLs; make referrals to appropriate community agencies

22. Maintain seizure precautions

23. Individualize home care instructions
   a. Recognize the signs and symptoms of decreased LOC
   b. Recognize the signs and symptoms of seizures
   c. Minimize environmental stress
   d. Set limits for impulsive behavior
   e. Continue fluid restrictions

H. Possible complications
   1. Tentorial herniation
   2. Herniation through foramen magnum
   3. Coma
   4. Seizure
   5. Death

I. Possible surgical intervention: craniotomy for surgical decompression (see page 95)

◆ XV. Head injury

A. Definition—classified by the type of fracture, hemorrhage, or trauma to the brain
   1. Fractures
      a. Depressed
      b. Comminuted
      c. Linear
   2. Hemorrhages
      a. Epidural
      b. Subdural
      c. Intracerebral
      d. Subarachnoid

      3. Trauma
        a. Concussion
        b. Contusion

B. Possible etiology
      1. Auto accidents
      2. Falls
      3. Assaults
      4. Blunt trauma
      5. Penetrating trauma

C. Pathophysiology: brain injury or bleeding within the brain results in edema and hypoxia

D. Possible assessment findings
      1. Disorientation to time, place, or person
      2. Paresthesia
      3. Positive Babinski's reflex
      4. Decreased LOC
      5. Otorrhea
      6. Rhinorrhea
      7. Unequal pupil size
      8. Loss of pupil reaction

E. Possible diagnostic test findings
      1. Skull X-ray: skull fracture
      2. CT scan: hemorrhage, cerebral edema, or shift of midline structures
      3. MRI: hemorrhage, cerebral edema, or shift of midline structures
      4. Cerebral angiography: intracerebral, subdural, epidural hematoma
      5. Echoencephalogram: shift of midline structures

F. Medical management
      1. Diet: restricted fluids
      2. I.V. therapy: electrolyte replacement, heparin lock
      3. Oxygen therapy
      4. Intubation and mechanical ventilation with hyperventilation
      5. GI decompression: NG tube
      6. Position: semi-Fowler's
      7. Activity: bed rest, active and passive ROM exercises
      8. Monitoring: VS, UO, I/O, ECG, hemodynamic variables, ICP, CVP, neurovital signs, and arterial line
      9. Laboratory studies: potassium, sodium, osmolality, arterial blood gases (ABGs), Hgb, and HCT
    10. Indwelling urinary catheter
    11. Analgesic: codeine phosphate (Paveral)
    12. Diuretics: mannitol (Osmitrol), furosemide (Lasix)

13. Antacids: magnesium and aluminum hydroxide (Maalox), aluminum hydroxide gel (AlternaGEL)
14. Anticonvulsant: phenytoin (Dilantin)
15. Glucocorticoid: dexamethasone (Decadron)
16. Histamine antagonists: cimetidine (Tagamet), ranitidine (Zantac)
17. Antifibrinolytics: aminocaproic acid (Amicar)
18. Cervical collar
19. Reflex checks: oculocephalic, oculovestibular, corneal, cough, and gag
20. Mucosal barrier fortifier: sucralfate (Carafate)
21. Pulse oximetry

G. Nursing interventions
1. Restrict fluids
2. Administer I.V. fluids
3. Administer oxygen
4. Provide suction, TCDB
5. Assess neurologic and respiratory status
6. Maintain position, patency, and low suction of NG tube
7. Maintain position and patency of ET and indwelling urinary catheter
8. Keep the patient in semi-Fowler's position
9. Monitor and record VS, UO, I/O, hemodynamic variables, ICP, CVP, specific gravity, urine glucose and ketones, laboratory studies, and pulse oximetry
10. Maintain seizure precautions
11. Administer medications, as prescribed
12. Encourage the patient to express feelings about changes in body image
13. Assess for CSF leak: otorrhea, rhinorrhea
14. Assess pain
15. Check for signs of diabetes insipidus
16. Check cough and gag reflex
17. Provide appropriate sensory input and stimuli with frequent reorientation
18. Provide means of communication
19. Observe for signs of increasing ICP
20. Provide eye, skin, and mouth care
21. Turn the patient every 2 hours
22. Assist with ADLs
23. Provide information about the National Head Injury Foundation
24. Individualize home care instructions
    a. Recognize the signs and symptoms of decreased LOC
    b. Recognize the signs and symptoms of seizures

      c. Set limits for impulsive behavior

      d. Adhere to fluid restrictions

H. Possible complications

   1. Shock

   2. Meningitis

   3. Increased ICP

   4. Stress ulcer

   5. Diabetes insipidus

   6. Infection

I. Possible surgical intervention: craniotomy for evacuation of hematomas (see page 95)

◆ XVI. Cerebrovascular accident

A. Definition—disruption of cerebral circulation that results in motor and sensory deficits

B. Possible etiology

   1. Cerebral arteriosclerosis

   2. Syphilis

   3. Trauma

   4. Hypertension

   5. Thrombosis

   6. Embolism

   7. Hemorrhage

   8. Vasospasm

C. Pathophysiology

   1. Disruption of cerebral blood flow causes cerebral anoxia

   2. Cerebral anoxia results in cerebral infarction

   3. Infarction results in edema

D. Possible assessment findings

   1. Syncope

   2. Change in LOC

   3. Paresthesia

   4. Headache

   5. Aphasia

   6. Seizures

   7. Labile emotional responses

   8. Paralysis

E. Possible diagnostic test findings

   1. LP: increased pressure, bloody CSF

   2. CT scan: intracranial bleeding, infarct, or shift of midline structures

   3. EEG: focal slowing in area of lesion

   4. MRI: intracranial bleeding, infarct, or shift of midline structures

     5. Brain scan: decreased perfusion

     6. Digital subtraction angiography: occlusion or narrowing of vessels

F. Medical management

     1. Diet: low-sodium, increased potassium

     2. I.V. therapy: heparin lock

     3. Oxygen therapy

     4. Intubation and mechanical ventilation

     5. GI decompression: NG tube

     6. Position: semi-Fowler's

     7. Activity: bed rest, active and passive ROM and isometric exercises

     8. Monitoring: VS, UO, I/O, ECG, ICP, and neurovital signs

     9. Laboratory studies: sodium, potassium, glucose, ABGs, PT, and PTT

    10. Nutritional support: TPN

    11. Indwelling urinary catheter, incentive spirometry

    12. Seizure precautions

    13. Analgesic: codeine phosphate (Paveral)

    14. Diuretics: mannitol (Osmitrol), furosemide (Lasix)

    15. Antacids: magnesium and aluminum hydroxide (Maalox), aluminum hydroxide gel (AlternaGEL)

    16. Anticonvulsant: phenytoin (Dilantin)

    17. Glucocorticoid: dexamethasone (Decadron)

    18. Histamine antagonists: cimetidine (Tagamet), ranitidine (Zantac)

    19. Antihypertensive: diazoxide (Hyperstat)

    20. Anticoagulants: warfarin sodium (Coumadin), heparin

    21. Pulse oximetry

    22. Physical therapy

G. Nursing interventions

     1. Maintain the patient's diet

     2. Administer I.V. fluids

     3. Administer oxygen

     4. Provide suction, TCDB

     5. Assess neurovascular, cardiac, and respiratory status

     6. Maintain position, patency, and low suction of NG tube

     7. Keep the patient in semi-Fowler's position

     8. Monitor and record VS, UO, I/O, ICP, neurovital signs, laboratory studies, and pulse oximetry

     9. Administer TPN

    10. Administer medications, as prescribed

    11. Encourage the patient to express feelings about changes in body image and about difficulty in communicating verbally

    12. Maintain a quiet environment

    13. Assess for receptive and expressive aphasia

14. Assess for hemianopia
15. Protect the patient from falls and injury
16. Apply antiembolism stockings
17. Maintain seizure precautions
18. Provide passive ROM exercises
19. Turn and position the patient every 2 hours
20. Provide means of communication
21. Provide skin and mouth care
22. Provide information about the American Heart Association and the National Stroke Foundation
23. Individualize home care instructions
24. Identify ways to reduce stress
    a. Recognize the signs and symptoms of seizures
    b. Minimize environmental stress
    c. Reinforce established methods of communication (aphasic patient)
    d. Monitor blood pressure
    e. Use assistive devices in ADLs
    f. Teach scanning

H. Possible complications
   1. Cerebral edema
   2. Vasospasm
   3. Pneumonia
   4. Increased ICP
   5. Problems from immobility
      a. Thrombophlebitis
      b. Pulmonary embolism
      c. Osteoporosis
      d. Urinary stasis

I. Possible surgical interventions
   1. Carotid endarterectomy (see page 96)
   2. Craniotomy for evacuation of a clot (see page 95)
   3. Craniotomy for superior temporal artery—middle cerebral artery anastomosis (see page 95)

♦ **XVII. Cerebral aneurysm**

A. Definition
   1. Dilation or localized weakness of the middle layer of an artery
   2. Classified by aneurysm type
      a. Saccular (berry)
      b. Fusiform
      c. Mycotic

B. Possible etiology
1. Atherosclerosis
2. Trauma
3. Congenital weakness
4. Syphilis

C. Pathophysiology
1. Enlargement of aneurysm compresses nerves
2. Enlargement of the aneurysm finally results in dissolution of the wall and rupture of the aneurysm
3. Rupture of the aneurysm results in subarachnoid hemorrhage
4. Release of serotonin, prostaglandins, and catecholamines from blood precipitates vasospasm

D. Possible assessment findings
1. Diplopia
2. Ptosis
3. Headache
4. Hemiparesis
5. Nuchal rigidity
6. Decreased LOC
7. Seizure activity
8. Blurred vision

E. Possible diagnostic test findings
1. CT scan: shift of intracranial midline structures, blood in subarachnoid space
2. MRI: shift of intracranial midline structures, blood in subarachnoid space
3. Cerebral angiogram: identification of vasospasm and vasculature associated with aneurysm
4. LP (contraindicated with increased ICP): increased pressure, protein, WBC; bloody and xanthochromic CSF

F. Medical management
1. I.V. therapy: heparin lock
2. Oxygen therapy
3. Position: semi-Fowler's
4. Activity: bed rest, passive ROM exercises
5. Monitoring: VS, UO, I/O (fluid restrictions), ICP, neurovital signs, and arterial line
6. Precautions: aneurysm and seizure
7. Antacids: magnesium and aluminum hydroxide (Maalox), aluminum hydroxide gel (AlternaGEL)
8. Anticonvulsant: phenytoin (Dilantin)
9. Glucocorticoid: dexamethasone (Decadron)
10. Histamine antagonists: cimetidine (Tagamet), ranitidine (Zantac)

11. Stool softener: docusate sodium (Colace)
12. Antifibrinolytic: aminocaproic acid (Amicar)
13. Antihypertensives: methyldopa (Aldomet), hydralazine (Apresoline)
14. Ergot alkaloid: methysergide (Sansert)
15. Calcium channel blocker: nimodipine hydrochloride (Nimotop)
16. Intubation and mechanical ventilation
17. Pulse oximetry
18. Mucosal barrier fortifier: sucralfate (Carafate)

G. Nursing interventions
   1. Restrict fluids
   2. Administer oxygen
   3. Assess neurologic status
   4. Keep the patient in semi-Fowler's position
   5. Monitor and record VS, UO, I/O, ICP, and pulse oximetry
   6. Administer medication, as prescribed
   7. Encourage the patient to express feelings about a fear of dying
   8. Allay the patient's anxiety
   9. Maintain a quiet, darkened environment
   10. Assess pain
   11. Allow a rest period between nursing activities
   12. Maintain bed rest
   13. Prevent Valsalva's maneuver
   14. Assess for signs of increased ICP
   15. Maintain seizure and aneurysm precautions
   16. Provide passive ROM exercises
   17. Limit visitors
   18. Provide skin care
   19. Assist with ADLs
   20. Prevent constipation
   21. Assess for meningeal irritation
   22. Individualize home care instructions
      a. Recognize the signs and symptoms of decreasing LOC
      b. Minimize environmental stress
      c. Alter ADLs to compensate for neurologic deficits
      d. Prevent constipation

H. Possible complications
   1. Vasospasm
   2. Rebleeding of the aneurysm
   3. Increased ICP
   4. Rupture of the aneurysm
   5. Hydrocephalus
   6. Brain herniation

I. Possible surgical interventions
   1. Craniotomy for clipping or wrapping of an aneurysm (see page 95)
   2. Craniotomy for evacuation of hematomas (see page 95)

◆ XVIII. Brain tumor

A. Definition—malignant or benign tumor of the brain that may be primary or metastatic

B. Possible etiology
   1. Genetic
   2. Environmental

C. Pathophysiology
   1. Unregulated cell growth and uncontrolled cell division result in the development of a neoplasm
   2. Tumors are classified according to tissue of origin
      a. Gliomas
      b. Meningiomas
      c. Metastatic
   3. Tumors can be infiltrative and destroy surrounding tissue or be encapsulated and displace brain tissue
   4. Presence of lesion and compression of blood vessels produces ischemia, edema, and increased ICP

D. Possible assessment findings
   1. Tumor in any brain area
      a. Headache
      b. Vomiting
      c. Papilledema
   2. Tumor in the frontal lobe
      a. Personality changes
      b. Aphasia
      c. Memory loss
   3. Tumor in the temporal lobe
      a. Seizures
      b. Aphasia
   4. Tumor in the parietal lobe
      a. Motor seizures
      b. Sensory impairment
   5. Tumor in the occipital lobe
      a. Visual impairment
      b. Homonymous hemianopia
      c. Visual hallucinations

      6. Tumor in the cerebellum
        a. Impaired equilibrium
        b. Impaired coordination

E. Possible diagnostic test findings
    1. EEG: seizure activity
    2. CT scan: location and size of tumor
    3. Skull X-ray: location and size of tumor
    4. Angiography: location and size of tumor
    5. LP (contraindicated with increased ICP): increased protein

F. Medical management
    1. Diet: high-protein, high-calorie
    2. I.V. therapy: heparin lock
    3. Oxygen therapy
    4. Position: semi-Fowler's
    5. Activity: bed rest
    6. Monitoring: VS, UO, I/O, ICP, and neurovital signs
    7. Laboratory studies: sodium and potassium glucose levels
    8. Nutritional support: TPN
    9. Radiation therapy
    10. Antineoplastics: vincristine sulfate (Oncovin), lomustine (CeeNu), carmustine (BiCNU)
    11. Diuretics: mannitol (Osmitrol), furosemide (Lasix)
    12. Antacids: magnesium and aluminum hydroxide (Maalox), aluminum hydroxide gel (AlternaGEL)
    13. Anticonvulsant: phenytoin (Dilantin)
    14. Glucocorticoid: dexamethasone (Decadron)
    15. Histamine antagonists: cimetidine (Tagamet), ranitidine (Zantac)
    16. Seizure precautions
    17. Chemotherapy
    18. Stereotactic brachytherapy
    19. Stereotaxic radiosurgery (Roentgen knife)
    20. Mucosal barrier fortifier: sucralfate (Carafate)

G. Nursing interventions
    1. Maintain the patient's diet
    2. Encourage the patient to drink fluids
    3. Administer I.V. fluids
    4. Administer oxygen
    5. Assess neurologic and respiratory status
    6. Keep the patient in semi-Fowler's position
    7. Monitor and record VS, UO, I/O, ICP, neurovital signs, and laboratory studies
    8. Administer TPN
    9. Administer medications, as prescribed

10. Encourage the patient to express feelings about changes in body image and a fear of dying
11. Assess pain
12. Assess for increased ICP
13. Provide oral hygiene
14. Provide postchemotherapeutic and postradiation nursing care
   a. Provide prophylactic skin and mouth care
   b. Monitor dietary intake
   c. Administer antiemetics and antidiarrheals, as prescribed
   d. Monitor for bleeding, infection, and electrolyte imbalance
   e. Provide rest periods
15. Maintain seizure precautions
16. Provide information about the National Head Injury Foundation and the Association for Brain Tumor Research
17. Individualize home care instructions
   a. Recognize the signs and symptoms of change in LOC
   b. Maintain a safe, quiet environment
   c. Respect quality of life decisions
   d. Make referrals for hospice care

H. Possible complications
   1. Increased ICP
   2. Brain herniation
   3. Seizures

I. Possible surgical intervention: craniotomy for surgical excision of a tumor (see page 95)

◆ XIX. Spinal cord injury

A. Definition
   1. Traumatic injury to the spinal cord that results in sensory and motor deficits
   2. Two types of spinal cord injury
      a. Paraplegia, paralysis of the legs
      b. Quadriplegia, paralysis of all four extremities

B. Possible etiology
   1. Car accidents
   2. Falls
   3. Gunshot wounds
   4. Stab wounds
   5. Diving into shallow water
   6. Infections
   7. Tumors
   8. Congenital anomalies

C. Pathophysiology
   1. Injury may result in complete transection of the spinal cord
   2. Associated edema and hemorrhage from the injury cause ischemia
   3. Necrosis and scar tissue form in the area of the traumatized cord
   4. Injury may result in paraplegia or quadriplegia

D. Possible assessment findings
   1. Paralysis below the level of the injury
   2. Paresthesia below the level of the injury
   3. Neck pain
   4. Loss of bowel and bladder control
   5. Respiratory distress
   6. Numbness and tingling
   7. Flaccid muscle
   8. Absence of reflexes below the level of the injury

E. Possible diagnostic test findings
   1. Spinal X-rays: vertebral fracture
   2. CT scan: spinal cord edema, vertebral fracture, spinal cord compression
   3. MRI: spinal cord edema, vertebral fracture, spinal cord compression

F. Medical management
   1. Diet: low-calcium, high-protein
   2. I.V. therapy: heparin lock
   3. Oxygen therapy
   4. Intubation and mechanical ventilation
   5. GI decompression: NG tube

CLINICAL ALERT

   6. Position: flat, neck immobilized
   7. Activity: bed rest, passive ROM exercises
   8. Monitoring: VS, UO, I/O, ECG, ICP, and neurovital signs
   9. Laboratory studies: sodium, potassium, and glucose levels and WBC count
   10. Indwelling urinary catheter
   11. Antacids: magnesium and aluminum hydroxide (Maalox), aluminum hydroxide gel (AlternaGEL)
   12. Anticonvulsant: phenytoin (Dilantin)
   13. Glucocorticoid: dexamethasone (Decadron)
   14. Histamine antagonists: cimetidine (Tagamet), ranitidine (Zantac)
   15. Cervical collar
   16. Maintenance of vertebral alignment: Stryker turning frame, Crutchfield tongs, Halo brace

17. Laxative: bisacodyl (Dulcolax)
18. Antianxiety agent: diazepam (Valium)
19. Antihypertensives: diazoxide (Hyperstat), hydralazine (Apresoline)
20. Muscle relaxant: dantrolene sodium (Dantrium)
21. Pulse oximetry
22. Specialized bed: rotation (Rotorest, Tilt and Turn, Paragon)
23. Mucosal barrier fortifier: sucralfate (Carafate)

G. Nursing interventions
   1. Maintain the patient's diet
   2. Force fluids
   3. Administer I.V. fluids
   4. Administer oxygen
   5. Provide suction, TCDB
   6. Assess neurologic and respiratory status
   7. Keep the patient flat
   8. Monitor and record VS, UO, I/O, laboratory studies, and pulse oximetry
   9. Administer medications, as prescribed
  10. Encourage the patient to express feelings about changes in body image, changes in sexual expression and function, altered mobility
  11. Turn the patient every 2 hours using the logrolling technique
  12. Maintain body alignment
  13. Initiate bowel and bladder retraining
  14. Provide sexual counseling
  15. Provide passive ROM exercises
  16. Check for autonomic dysreflexia
  17. Assess for spinal shock
  18. Provide skin care
  19. Provide heel and elbow protectors and sheepskin
  20. Apply antiembolism stockings
  21. Provide information about the National Spinal Cord Injury Association
  22. Individualize home care instructions
    a. Exercise regularly to strengthen muscles
    b. Recognize the signs and symptoms of autonomic dysreflexia, urinary tract infection, and upper respiratory infection
    c. Continue bowel and bladder program
    d. Maintain acidic urine with cranberry juice
    e. Consume adequate fluids: 3,000 ml/day
    f. Use assistive devices for ADLs

CLINICAL ALERT

    g. Maintain skin integrity

    h. Stay mobile using a wheelchair

    i. Reinforce independence

H. Possible complications

    1. Spinal shock

    2. Autonomic dysreflexia

    3. Respiratory distress

I. Possible surgical interventions

    1. Laminectomy (see page 293)

    2. Spinal fusion (see page 294)

◆ XX. Amyotrophic lateral sclerosis (ALS)—Lou Gehrig's disease

A. Definition—Progressive degenerative neurologic disease resulting in decreased motor function in the upper and lower motor neuron systems

B. Possible etiology

    1. Unknown cause

    2. Genetic predisposition

    3. Viral infection

    4. Excess of glutamate

C. Pathophysiology

    1. Myelin sheaths are destroyed and replaced with scar tissue, resulting in distorted or blocked nerve impulses

    2. Nerve cells die and muscle fibers have atrophic changes

D. Possible assessment findings

    1. Fatigue

    2. Awkwardness of fine finger movements

    3. Dysphagia

    4. Muscle weakness of hands and arms

    5. Fasciculations of face

    6. Nasal quality of speech

    7. Spasticity

    8. Atrophy of tongue

E. Possible diagnostic test findings

    1. EMG: decreased amplitude of evoked potentials

    2. No one specific diagnostic test used

    3. Diagnosis based on assessment findings

F. Medical Management
   1. Focused on symptomatic relief

CLINICAL
ALERT

   2. Activity: as tolerated
   3. Monitoring: VS, UO, I/O, neurovital signs
   4. Mechanical ventilation: negative-pressure ventilators
   5. NG tube feedings
   6. Gastrostomy tube feedings
   7. Antispasmodics: baclofen (Lioresal), diazepam (Valium)
   8. Muscle cramps: Quinine therapy
   9. Investigational: thyrotropin-releasing hormone, interferon

G. Nursing interventions
   1. Maintain the patient's diet
   2. Assess neurologic and respiratory status
   3. Assess swallow and gag reflexes
   4. Monitor and record VS, UO, I/O, and neurovital signs
   5. Administer medications, as prescribed
   6. Encourage patient to complete advanced directives or a "living will"
   7. Monitor for choking while eating
   8. Suction oral pharynx, as necessary
   9. Provide information about the ALS Foundation
   10. Individualize home care instructions
      a. Teach patient to maintain tucked chin position while eating or drinking
      b. Teach patient to use tonsillar suction tip to clear oral pharynx
      c. Inform patient about prosthetic devices to assist with ADLs

H. Possible complications
   1. Respiratory failure
   2. Pneumonia
   3. Death

I. Possible surgical intervention: none

POINTS TO REMEMBER

♦ Nervous system disorders can affect the patient's body image, control over body functions, self-esteem, and fears of rejection, dependence, or dying.

♦ Before the patient has a myelogram, the nurse should check the patient for allergies to iodine, seafood, and radiopaque dyes.

♦ Typical nursing diagnoses for a patient with a nervous system disorder include powerlessness, changes in body image, and lowered self-esteem.

♦ Nursing assessment for a patient who has had a craniotomy should focus on changes in the LOC and on signs of increasing ICP.

♦ Alternate methods of communication need to be established for a patient with myasthenia gravis.

STUDY QUESTIONS

To evaluate your understanding of this chapter, answer the following questions in the space provided; then compare your responses with the correct answers in Appendix B, page 383.

1. Which nursing interventions are appropriate after an LP? _____

   _____

   _____

2. What are two key nursing interventions after a craniotomy? _____

   _____

   _____

3. When a patient has a seizure, which activities should the nurse observe and record? _____

   _____

   _____

4. Which assessment findings would be present in a patient with a cerebellar tumor? _____

   _____

   _____

5. What are two key nursing interventions for a patient with spinal cord injury? _____

   _____

   _____

CRITICAL THINKING AND APPLICATION EXERCISES

1. Observe a lumbar puncture. Prepare an oral presentation for your fellow students, describing the procedure and patient care before, during, and after the procedure.

2. Develop a chart comparing the major drug classes used for treating seizures.

3. Draw a diagram showing the physiology of increased ICP.

4. Interview a patient with a neurologic disorder. Evaluate the information for possible risk factors and identify ways to modify them.

5. Follow a patient with a neurologic disorder from admission through discharge. Develop a patient-specific plan of care, including any needs for follow-up and home care.

CHAPTER

Sensory System: Eyes and Ears

LEARNING OBJECTIVES

After studying this chapter, you should be able to:

♦ Describe the psychosocial impact of sensory disorders.

♦ Differentiate between the modifiable and non-modifiable risk factors in the development of a sensory disorder.

♦ List three probable and three possible nursing diagnoses for a patient with a sensory disorder.

♦ Identify nursing interventions for a patient with a sensory disorder.

♦ Identify three teaching topics for a patient with a sensory disorder.

CHAPTER OVERVIEW

Caring for the patient with a sensory disorder requires a sound understanding of the anatomy and physiology of the eye and ear, and the psychological impact of the loss of hearing and sight. A thorough assessment is essential to planning and implementing appropriate patient care. The assessment includes a complete history, physical examination, diagnostic testing, identification of modifiable and non-modifiable risk factors, and information related to the psychosocial impact of the disorder on the patient. Nursing diagnoses focus primarily on sensory/perceptual alteration, social isolation, and knowledge deficit. Nursing interventions are designed to improve patient safety and decrease the patient's anxiety about body image changes. Patient teaching, a crucial nursing activity, involves information about medical follow-up, medication regimens, signs and symptoms of possible complications, and the reduction of modifiable risk factors through the use of safety precautions to protect the eyes and ears.

◆ I. Anatomy and physiology review

A. Eyes
1. External structures
   a. Eyelids—two movable, musculofibrous folds that protect the eye by opening and closing
   b. Palpebral fissure—space between the open lids
   c. Conjunctiva—thin transparent mucous membrane that lines the lid
   d. Tears—produced by lacrimal glands and distributed by blink of lids; two types include lubricating and water-based tears
   e. Extraocular muscles—focus muscles abduct, adduct, elevate or depress; two muscles direct the eye laterally, inferiorly, or superiorly
   f. Eyeball—spherical organ surrounded by orbital fat and positioned in orbit; three layers include the sclera, uvea, and retina
2. Internal structures
   a. Sclera—dense, white fibrous protective coating of eye; optic nerve and central retinal vessel pass through posterior opening; anterior opening serves as refracting window; provides structural strength to front of eye
   b. Choroid—highly vascular posterior portion of uveal tract that nourishes retina
   c. Iris—thin, circular pigmented muscular structure in eye; gives color to eye; divides space between cornea and lens into anterior and posterior chamber; peripheral border attaches to ciliary body
   d. Ciliary body—muscular fibers in middle pigmented layer of eye that contract and relax the lens zonules; maintain INTRAOCULAR PRESSURE (IOP) by secreting AQUEOUS HUMOR
   e. Pupil—circulation aperture in iris that changes size as iris adapts to amount of light entering eye
   f. Lens—biconvex, avascular, colorless and transparent structure suspended behind the iris by the zonules
   g. Vitreous body—clear, transparent, avascular, gelatinous fluid that fills the space in the posterior portion of the eye; bounded by the lens, retina, and optic disk; maintains transparency and form of the eye

      h. Retina—thin, semitransparent layer of nerve tissue that lines the eye wall; rods and cones respond to light energy and initiate the neural response that is interpreted in the brain

      i. Lens zonules—suspends lens; contraction and relaxation of zonules changes shape of lens and allows it to focus light on the retina

      j. Retinal cones—responsible for visual acuity and color discrimination

      k. Retinal rod—responsible for peripheral vision under decreased light conditions

      l. Macula lutea—center of posterior retina with fovea centralis for acute vision, color vision, and resolution of image

      m. Optic nerve—convergence of nerve fibers of retina

      n. Optic disk—head of the optic nerve known as the blind spot

  3. Image formation

      a. Light rays enter the eye through the cornea and pass through the pupil, lens, and vitreous body to the retina

      b. Light rays stimulate the retinal sensory receptors to send impulses through the optic nerve to the occipital cortex, where the impulses are registered as visual sensations

  4. Aqueous humor formation

      a. Watery, transparent liquid which flows through anterior and posterior chambers and exits through Schlemm's canal

      b. Serves circulatory function for avascular tissues of eye

      c. Responsible for maintaining IOP

  5. Accommodation—the process of contraction and relaxation of the lens zonules that changes the shape of lens and allows it to focus light on the retina

B. Ears

  1. External ear

      a. Portion of ear that includes the pinna (auricle) and external auditory canal

      b. Separated from the middle ear by the tympanic membrane

  2. Middle ear

      a. Air filled cavity in the temporal bone

      b. Contains three small bones (malleus, incus, and stapes)

      c. Also known as the tympanum

  3. Inner ear

      a. Portion of the ear that consists of the cochlea, vestibule, and semicircular canals

      b. Also known as the labyrinth

  4. Sound transmission—airborne vibrations are transformed to sound through mechanical stimulation of the endolymphatic fluids

  5. Equilibrium—maintained by semicircular canals

♦ II. Assessment findings

A. History

   1. Eyes

      a. Blurred distance vision

      b. Difficulty watching television or reading

      c. Headaches

      d. Dizziness

      e. Eye or brow pain

      f. Eye weeping

      g. Scratchy or itchy eye

      h. Inflamed eye

      i. Watery eye

      j. Puffy eyelids

      k. Crossed eyes

      l. Unequal pupils

      m. Squinting

      n. Increased blinking

      o. Rubbing eye

      p. Encrusted eye

      q. Burning sensation in eye

      r. Double vision

      s. Spots before the eye

      t. Difficulty differentiating colors

      u. Difficulty driving at night

   2. Ears

      a. TINNITUS

      b. Increased inability to hear at group meetings

      c. Need to turn up volume on television and radio

      d. Social withdrawal

      e. Fatigue

      f. Indifference

      g. Insecurity

      h. Suspiciousness

B. Physical examination

   1. Eyes

      a. Visual acuity changes

      b. VERTIGO

      c. Discharge from eye

      d. Sty

      e. PRESBYOPIA

      f. PTOSIS

      g. NYSTAGMUS

      h. OPTIC ATROPHY

     i. MYOPIA
     j. HYPEROPIA
     k. ANISOMETROPIA
     l. ASTIGMATISM
  2. Ears
     a. Speech deterioration
     b. Ear pain
     c. Ear deformities
     d. Ear lesions
     e. Ear canal discharge
     f. Mastoid pain
     g. Pressure of CERUMEN
     h. Eye canal inflammation
     i. Foreign body in ear canal
     j. Change in position and color of tympanic membrane

◆ III. Diagnostic tests and procedures

A. Visual acuity
  1. Definition and purpose
     a. Tests clarity of vision using letter chart (Snellen's) placed 20′ (6 m) from the patient
     b. Expressed in a ratio that relates what a person with normal vision sees at 20′ to what the patient can see at 20′
  2. Nursing interventions
     a. Explain testing procedure to patient
     b. Answer patient questions
     c. Remind patient to bring eyeglasses or contact lenses, if presently prescribed
     d. Advise examiner if patient is unable to read alphabet letters
     e. Advise examiner if patient has difficulty hearing or following directions

B. Extraocular eye muscle testing
  1. Definition and purpose
     a. Tests parallel alignment of the eyes and integrity of nervous control of muscles of the eye
     b. Correlated action of the extraocular muscles results in parallel gaze
  2. Nursing interventions
     a. Explain the testing procedure to patient
     b. Answer patient questions
     c. Advise examiner if patient has difficulty hearing or following directions

C. Visual field
  1. Definition and purpose
      a. Tests degree of peripheral vision of each eye
      b. Examiner and patient sit directly facing each other at a distance of 2'; patient covers one eye while looking directly at examiner's nose; examiner covers one eye; examiner moves an object along a horizontal plane into central view from peripheral points about one half distance between them
  2. Nursing interventions
      a. Explain testing procedure to patient
      b. Answer patient questions
      c. Advise examiner if patient has difficulty hearing or following directions

D. Tonometry
  1. Definition and purpose
      a. Test to measure intraocular pressure
      b. Examiner uses applanation tonometer or pneumotonometer
  2. Nursing interventions
      a. Ask patient to remain still
      b. Depending on method of exam, advise patient that a puff of air or the instrument may be felt touching the eye

CLINICAL ALERT

E. Auditory acuity
  1. Definition and purpose
      a. General estimation for the patient's hearing
      b. Assesses the patient's ability to hear a whispered phrase or ticking watch
  2. Nursing interventions
      a. Explain testing procedure to patient
      b. Answer patient questions
      c. Advise examiner if patient has difficulty following directions

F. Endothelial cell counter
  1. Definition and purpose
      a. Test to observe high resolution details of endothelial cell morphology
      b. Photographic instrument is attached to a slit lamp
  2. Nursing interventions
      a. Explain testing procedure to patient
      b. Answer patient questions
      c. Advise patient to remain still

G. A-scan ultrasound
  1. Definition and purpose
      a. Test to detect tumors or lesions of the eye
      b. High frequency pulses of ultrasound are emitted from a small probe placed on the eye

2. Nursing interventions before the procedure
   a. Explain the procedure to the patient
   b. Answer patient questions
   c. Administer topical anesthetic eye drops
3. Nursing interventions after the procedure
   a. Advise patient not to rub eyes
   b. Place patient on eye rest

H. Otoscopic examination
   1. Definition and purpose
      a. Test used to visualize the tympanic membrane
      b. Examiner uses otoscope
   2. Nursing interventions
      a. Advise patient to hold still
      b. Explain that a gentle pull will be felt on the auricle and a slight pressure will be felt in the ear

I. Audiometry
   1. Definition and purpose
      a. Test to measure the degree of deafness
      b. Examiner uses pure-tone or speech methods
   2. Nursing interventions
      a. Explain that the patient will need to wear earphones for the procedure
      b. Explain that the patient will be asked to signal when a tone is heard while sitting in a soundproof room

♦ IV. Psychosocial impact of sensory disorders

A. Developmental impact
   1. Failing in school
   2. Changes in body image
   3. Fear of rejection
   4. Decreased self-esteem

B. Economic impact
   1. Cost of adaptive equipment
   2. Disruption or loss of job
   3. Cost of hospitalization and follow-up care
   4. Cost of medications

C. Occupational and recreational impact
   1. Limited job opportunities
   2. Changes in leisure activity
   3. Restrictions in physical activity

    D. Social impact
       1. Social isolation
       2. Changes in role performance

◆ V. Possible risk factors

    A. Modifiable risk factors
       1. Eyes
          a. Work setting
          b. Leisure activities
          c. Sports activities
          d. Exposure to airborne irritants
          e. Work activities
       2. Ears
          a. Exposure to loud noises
          b. Use of streptomycin, neomycin, or aspirin
    B. Non-modifiable risk factors
       1. Eyes
          a. Glaucoma
          b. Diabetes
          c. Hypertension
          d. Eye trauma
          e. Eye surgery
          f. Family history: glaucoma, blindness, hypertension, cataracts, diabetes, eye infections
          g. Cataracts
          h. Aging
       2. Ears
          a. Diabetes
          b. Aging

◆ VI. Nursing diagnostic categories

    A. Probable nursing diagnostic categories
       1. Eyes
          a. Sensory/perceptual alteration: visual
          b. Fear
          c. Anxiety
          d. Knowledge deficit
          e. Body image disturbance
       2. Ears
          a. Sensory/perceptual alteration: auditory
          b. Social isolation
          c. Knowledge deficit

       d. Anxiety

       e. Pain

B. Possible nursing diagnostic categories

  1. Eyes

     a. Self-care deficit

     b. Pain

     c. Social isolation

     d. Risk for injury

  2. Ears

     a. Risk for injury

     b. Risk for infection

◆ VII. Eye surgeries

A. Description

  1. Cataract surgery

     a. Intracapsular—removal of the entire intact lens as a unit using a cryoprobe

     b. Extracapsular—removal of the anterior capsule by expressing the lens nucleus and aspirating the remaining soft and cortical fragments with the use of a special irrigation aspiration machine

  2. Corneal transplantation—microsurgical, full thickness replacement of the cornea with tissue from a deceased donor

  3. Retinal reattachment— transscleral cryotherapy (scleral buckling) is applied around the retinal tear producing a chorioretinal adhesion that seals the break so that liquid vitreous can no longer pass through the subretinal space

B. Preoperative nursing interventions

  1. Complete patient and family preoperative teaching

     a. Determine the patient's understanding of the procedure

     b. Describe the operating room (OR), post anesthesia care unit (PACU), and preoperative and postoperative routines

     c. Demonstrate postoperative turning, coughing, and deep breathing (TCDB)

     d. Explain the postoperative need for: surgical eye bandages, oxygen therapy, I.V. therapy, and pain control

  2. Complete the preoperative checklist

  3. Administer the preoperative medications, as prescribed

  4. Allay the patient's and family's anxiety about surgery

  5. Document the patient's history and physical assessment data base

C. Postoperative nursing interventions

  1. Assess pain and administer postoperative analgesics, as prescribed

  2. Assess for return of peristalsis

  3. Administer I.V. fluids, as prescribed

4. Allay the patient's anxiety

5. Reinforce TCDB

6. Provide incentive spirometry

7. Maintain activity: active and passive range of motion (ROM) and isometric exercises for extremities, as tolerated

8. Monitor and record vital signs (VS), urinary output (UO), intake and output (I/O), laboratory studies, and pulse oximetry

9. Assess cardiac and respiratory status

CLINICAL ALERT

10. Inspect the surgical eye bandages and change, as directed

11. Keep the patient's head elevated in a supine position with a small pillow under and at each side of the head

12. Bed rest with bathroom privileges

13. Encourage the patient to express feelings about the loss of sight

14. Assess the patient's ability to complete self-care activities and activities of daily living (ADLs)

15. Raise side rails

16. Administer antibiotics, as prescribed

17. Give solid foods and liquids, as tolerated

18. Administer stool softeners, as prescribed

19. Orient to time, place, and surroundings

CLINICAL ALERT

20. Assess eye for drainage, redness, swelling, cloudy vision, halos around lights, and impaired vision

21. Do not administer morphine because it causes miosis

22. Individualize home care instructions

   a. Encourage eye rest

   b. Use eye shield or patch, as prescribed

   c. Use dark glasses in strong light

   d. No reading, smoking, or shaving until permitted

   e. Apply cold or warm compresses, as prescribed

   f. Do not rub or wipe eyes

   g. Label medication bottles with large letters

   h. Wash hands before instilling eye drops

   i. Assess home for safety to prevent falls

   j. Adapt lighting to patient's needs

   k. Listen to radio for diversion

   l. Administer eye medications, as prescribed

   m. Avoid coughing, sneezing, lifting, squeezing eyes shut, and fast head movements

D. Possible surgical complications

   1. Cataract surgery: corneal endothelial damage, pupillary block, glaucoma, hemorrhage, wound fistula, choroidal detachment, uveitis

   2. Corneal transplant: hemorrhage, epithelial defects, wound leaks, glaucoma, graft rejection

3. Retinal reattachment: increased IOP, glaucoma, infection, choroidal detachment, diplopia

◆ **VIII. Ear surgeries**

A. Description
   1. Tympanoplasty—reconstruction of the middle ear bone to restore function to the middle ear structures that have become diseased or are deformed at birth
   2. Cochlear implant
      a. Placement of auditory prothesis for people who are profoundly deaf and designated as untreatable by other methods
      b. Helps patient detect environmental sounds, but does not restore normal hearing

B. Preoperative nursing interventions
   1. Complete patient and family preoperative teaching
      a. Determine the patient's understanding of the procedure
      b. Describe the OR, PACU, and preoperative and postoperative routines
      c. Demonstrate postoperative TCDB
      d. Explain the postoperative need for: drainage tubes, surgical dressings, oxygen therapy, I.V. therapy, and pain control
   2. Complete the preoperative checklist
   3. Administer the preoperative medications, as prescribed
   4. Allay the patient's and family's anxiety about surgery
   5. Document the patient's history and physical assessment data base

C. Postoperative nursing interventions
   1. Assess pain and administer postoperative analgesics, as prescribed
   2. Assess for return of peristalsis
   3. Administer I.V. fluids, as prescribed
   4. Allay the patient's anxiety
   5. Reinforce TCDB
   6. Provide incentive spirometry
   7. Maintain activity: active and passive ROM and isometric exercises for extremities, as tolerated
   8. Monitor and record VS, UO, I/O, laboratory studies, and pulse oximetry
   9. Assess cardiac and respiratory status

CLINICAL ALERT

   10. Inspect the surgical dressing and change, as directed
   11. Keep the patient in a supine position with head of bed elevated; maintain bed rest for first 24 hours, then ambulate with assistance
   12. Monitor and maintain the position and patency of wound drainage tubes
   13. Encourage the patient to express feelings about loss of hearing

14. Assess patient for dizziness and nystagmus
15. Administer antibiotics, as prescribed
16. Administer antivertigo agent, as prescribed
17. Administer antiemetic, as prescribed
18. Give solid foods and liquids, as tolerated
19. Individualize home care instructions
    a. Avoid blowing nose, sneezing, or coughing
    b. Avoid shampooing hair or showering
    c. Monitor self for mouth dryness, altered taste, facial paralysis, and ear pressure
    d. Avoid sudden head movements
    e. Decrease environmental noise
    f. Have people face patient directly while speaking slowly and loudly
    g. Use nonverbal clues when communicating
    h. Avoid people with colds
    i. Cover ears when outside
    j. Change dressing, as directed
    k. Do not fly, lift, bend, or swim
    l. Elevate head of bed

D. Possible surgical complications
   1. Infections
   2. Tissue rejection of graft or prothesis

♦ IX. Cataract

A. Definition—opacification of the normally clear, transparent crystalline lens

B. Possible etiology
   1. Aging
   2. Blunt or penetrating trauma
   3. Long-term steroid treatment
   4. Diabetes mellitus
   5. Hypoparathyroidism
   6. Radiation exposure
   7. Anterior uveitis
   8. Ultraviolet light exposure

C. Pathophysiology
   1. The nucleus of the lens takes on a yellowish-brown hue
   2. Surrounding opacities are spoke-like, white densities anterior and posterior to the nucleus

D. Possible assessment findings
   1. Disabling glare
   2. Dimmed or blurred vision

TEACHING TIPS
Patients with a sensory disorder

Be sure to include the following topics in your teaching plan for the patient with a sensory disorder.
- Follow-up appointments
- Medication therapy, including the action, adverse effects, and scheduling of medications
- Feelings about changes in lifestyle and activities of daily living (ADLs)
- Signs and symptoms of infection, hearing loss, and decreased vision
- Activity limitations
- Activities that prevent social isolation
- Safe, stress-free environment
- Independence with ADLs and any modifications and assistive devices needed to compensate for limited sensory input
- Community agencies and resources for supportive services
- Preventive care
- Eye: protection from injury, bright sun, and chemicals; need for eye rest; working in well-lighted areas
- Ear: wearing protective devices during work, leisure, and sports; avoiding exposure to high-frequency sounds

    3. Distorted images

    4. Poor night vision

    5. Yellow, gray, or white pupil

  E. Possible diagnostic test findings

    1. Endothelial cell counter: 2000 cells/μl

    2. A-scan ultrasound: areas of increased density around the nucleus of the lens

  F. Medical management

    1. No specific medical treatment

    2. Laboratory studies: IOP, endothelial cell counter, A-scan ultrasound

  G. Nursing interventions

    1. Assess vision status

    2. Allay the patient's anxiety

    3. Encourage the patient to express feelings about changes in body image and effect on ADLs

    4. Provide information about cataracts and cataract surgery

    5. Individualize home care instructions (For more information about teaching, see *Patients with a sensory disorder*)

      a. Wear dark glasses in bright light

      b. Arrange furniture to avoid sitting in direct sunlight

      c. Wear wide brimmed hat

      d. Lower visor while driving

H. Possible medical complications: glaucoma, blindness, severe visual loss

I. Possible surgical intervention: cataract extraction

♦ X. Glaucoma

A. Definition

  1. A group of diseases that differ in pathophysiology, clinical presentation, and treatment

  2. Characterized by visual field loss due to damage to the optic nerve caused by increased IOP

  3. The increased IOP results from pathologic changes that prevent normal circulation of aqueous humor

B. Possible etiology

  1. Diabetes mellitus

  2. African-American race

  3. Family history of glaucoma

  4. Previous eye trauma or surgery

  5. Long-term steroid treatment

  6. Uveitis

C. Pathophysiology

  1. Primary glaucoma

    a. Not associated with any known ocular or systemic condition that contributes to abnormal level of IOP

    b. Usually bilateral and may be inherited

  2. Secondary glaucoma

    a. Associated with ocular or systemic disorders that are responsible for increased IOP

    b. Often unilateral

  3. Open-angle glaucoma: increased IOP is caused by increased resistance to aqueous humor outflow

  4. Angle-closure glaucoma: increased resistance to aqueous humor flow caused by blockage of trabecular meshwork by peripheral iris

  5. Combined mechanism glaucoma: two or more forms of glaucoma

  6. Open-angle complicated by angle-closure is most common

D. Possible assessment findings

  1. Primary open-angle glaucoma

    a. Initially asymptomatic

    b. May have asymmetric involvement

    c. Narrowed field of vision

    d. Atrophy and cupping of optic nerve head
    e. Increased IOP
  2. Acute closed-angle glaucoma
    a. Acute ocular pain
    b. Halo vision
    c. Blurred vision
    d. Redness in eye
    e. Increased IOP
    f. Atrophy and cupping of optic nerve head
    g. Dilated pupil

E. Possible diagnostic test findings
  1. Tonometry: increased IOP
  2. Perimetry: decreased field of vision
  3. Gonioscopy: angle open or closed
  4. Ophthalmoscopy: atrophy and cupping of optic nerve head

F. Medical management
  1. Dietary restrictions: sodium and fluid
  2. Activity: as tolerated
  3. Monitoring: VS, UO, I/O
  4. Laboratory studies: tonometry, perimetry, opthalmascopy
  5. Primary open-angle glaucoma
    a. Beta-adrenergic antagonist: timolol (Timoptic)
    b. Adrenergic agonist: epinephrine (Epitrin)
    c. Carbonic anhydrase inhibitor: acetazolamide (Diamox)
  6. Acute closed-angle glaucoma
    a. Cholinergic agent: pilocarpine hydrochloride (Iopidine)
    b. Carbonic anhydrase inhibitor: acetazolamide (Diamox)

G. Nursing interventions
  1. Maintain the patient's diet restrictions
  2. Limit fluid intake
  3. Assess vision status
  4. Monitor and record VS, UO, I/O, and laboratory studies
  5. Administer medications, as prescribed
  6. Allay the patient's anxiety
  7. Encourage the patient to express feelings about changes in body image
  8. Assess eye pain
  9. Individualize home care instructions
    a. Avoid rubbing eye
    b. Use hypoallergenic cosmetics
    c. Wear goggles while swimming
    d. Wear protective glasses while playing sports and working

e. Monitor eye for redness, discharge, watering, blurred or cloudy vision, halos, flashes of light, and floaters

H. Possible medical complications: blindness

I. Possible surgical interventions

1. Primary open-angle glaucoma
   a. Laser or incisional trabeculoplasty with continued medication
   b. Laser or incisional trabeculectomy with continued medication
   c. Laser or incisional peripheral iridectomy
2. Acute closed-angle glaucoma
   a. Laser or incisional iridectomy

♦ XI. Meniere's disease

A. Definition—condition of the inner ear that is characterized by recurrent and usually progressive symptoms including vertigo, tinnitus, a sensation of pressure in the ears, and neurosensory hearing loss

B. Possible etiology

1. Exact mechanism unknown
2. Possible etiologies
   a. Abnormal hormones influence on the blood flow to the labyrinth
   b. Electrolyte disturbance in the labyrinth fluids
   c. Allergic reaction
   d. Autoimmune disorder
   e. Abnormal metabolites

C. Pathophysiology—the labyrinth does not function normally

D. Possible assessment findings

1. Paroxysmal whirling vertigo with nausea and vomiting
2. Tinnitus
3. Fluctuating unilateral neurosensory hearing loss of low tones
4. Sense of pressure in the ear
5. Nystagmus
6. Ataxia

E. Possible diagnostic test findings

1. Audiogram: hearing loss
2. Magnetic resonance imaging: negative
3. Electronystagmography: labyrinth dysfunction
4. Auditory dehydration test: positive audiometric fluctuation

F. Medical management

1. Dietary restrictions: fluid, sodium, caffeine
2. Activity: as tolerated
3. Monitoring: VS, UO, I/O
4. Glucocorticoid: dexamethasone (Decadron)

      5. Benzodiazipine: oxazepam (Serax)

      6. Anticholinergic: atropine sulfate (Atropine)

      7. Antihistamine: diphenhydramine hydrochloride (Benadryl)

      8. Diuretic: spironolactone (Aldactone)

      9. Antiemetic: prochlorperazine (Compazine)

     10. Vasodilators: nicotinic acid (Nicobid), tolazoline hydrochloride (Priscoline), methantheline (Banthine)

G. Nursing interventions

      1. Maintain the patient's diet

      2. Limit fluid

      3. Assess hearing status

      4. Monitor and record VS, UO, I/O, and laboratory studies

      5. Administer medications, as prescribed

      6. Allay the patient's anxiety

      7. Raise side rails of bed

      8. Individualize home care instructions

         a. Have patient lie down to relieve dizziness

         b. Learn to read lips

         c. Use hearing aid

         d. Use sign language and gestures to communicate

H. Possible medical complications: deafness

I. Possible surgical interventions

      1. Endolymphatic subarachnoid shunt

      2. Endolymphatic system-mastoid shunt

      3. Ultrasonic surgery

      4. Total labyrinthectomy

POINTS TO REMEMBER

♦ Eyes should be protected from injury, bright sun, and chemicals throughout life.

♦ Eye rest and well-lighted work areas prevent eyestrain.

♦ Ear protection should be worn during work, leisure, and sports activities that pose a danger from loud and high frequency sounds.

♦ Impaired vision or hearing may cause changes in personality, difficulties with communication, decreased awareness of surroundings, and increased exposure to injury.

STUDY QUESTIONS

To evaluate your understanding of this chapter, answer the following questions in the space provided; then compare your responses with the correct answer in Appendix B, page 383.

1. What is the primary complication of glaucoma?_____

_____

_____

2. List the principles of safe eye care. _____

_____

_____

3. Describe the patient positioning that should be used following eye surgery.

_____

_____

4. Which nursing behaviors improve communication with a patient who has a hearing loss?_____

_____

_____

CRITICAL THINKING AND APPLICATION EXERCISES

1. Observe cataract surgery. Prepare an oral presentation for your fellow students, describing the procedure and patient care before, during, and after the procedure.

2. Develop a chart comparing the major drug classes used for treating glaucoma.

3. Interview a patient with a hearing disorder. Evaluate the information for any possible risk factors and identify ways to modify them.

4. Follow a patient with a sensory disorder from admission through discharge. Develop a patient-specific plan of care, including any needs for follow-up and home care.

CHAPTER

5

Gastrointestinal System

LEARNING OBJECTIVES

After studying this chapter, you should be able to:

♦ Describe the psychosocial impact of gastrointestinal (GI) disorders.

♦ Differentiate between modifiable and nonmodifiable risk factors in the development of a GI disorder.

♦ List three probable and three possible nursing diagnoses for a patient with any GI disorder.

♦ Identify the nursing interventions for a patient with a GI disorder.

♦ Write three goals for teaching a patient with a GI disorder.

CHAPTER OVERVIEW

Caring for the patient with a gastrointestinal (GI) disorder requires a sound understanding of GI anatomy, physiology, and function. A thorough assessment is essential to planning and implementing appropriate patient care. The assessment includes a complete history, physical examination, diagnostic testing, identification of modifiable and nonmodifiable risk factors, and information related to the psychosocial impact of GI dysfunction on the patient. Nursing diagnoses focus primarily on a change in bowel habits and altered nutrition (constipation, diarrhea). Patient teaching, a crucial nursing activity, involves information about medical follow-up, medication regimens, signs and symptoms of possible complications, and reduction of modifiable risk factors through decreased alcohol consumption, diet restrictions, stress management, and smoking cessation. The psychosocial impact of changes in body image and decreased self-esteem is also an important focus for nursing care.

◆ I. Anatomy and physiology review

A. Mouth
   1. Mechanical and chemical digestion originate here
   2. Tongue and teeth are accessory organs of digestion
   3. Salivary glands secrete saliva, which combines with food during mastication

B. Esophagus
   1. This organ provides for the transfer of food from the oropharynx to the stomach
   2. Closure of the epiglottis prevents food from entering the trachea
   3. Closure of the cardiac sphincter prevents reflux of gastric contents

C. Stomach
   1. A hollow, 1-liter muscular pouch
   2. Secretes pepsin, renin, lipase, mucus, and hydrochloric (HCl) acid for digestion
   3. Mixes and stores chyme
   4. Secretes intrinsic factor necessary for absorption of cyanocobalamin (vitamin B_{12})

D. Small intestine
   1. Consists of duodenum, jejunum, and ileum
      a. Chyme, in liquid or semiliquid form, enters the duodenum through the pyloric sphincter
      b. Bile and pancreatic secretions enter the duodenum through the common bile duct at the ampulla of Vater
   2. Small intestine digests food
   3. Small intestine absorbs nutrients
   4. Small intestine is lined with villi that contain capillaries and lymphatics
   5. Motor activity of the small intestine includes mixing and peristalsis

E. Large intestine
   1. Consists of the cecum, colon, rectum, and anus
   2. Segments of the colon are the cecum, ascending colon, transverse colon, descending colon, and sigmoid colon
   3. Chyme enters the cecum through the ileocecal valve
   4. Large intestine has several functions
      a. Absorption of fluid and electrolytes
      b. Synthesis of vitamin K by intestinal bacteria
      c. Storage of fecal material

     5. Chyme becomes more solid as water is absorbed through the intestinal wall of the colon

     6. Defecation is the movement of feces from the rectum through the anal sphincter

F. Liver

     1. Largest organ in the body

     2. Produces bile (main function) which emulsifies fats and stimulates peristalsis

     3. Conveys bile from the gallbladder where it is stored until it enters the duodenum at Oddi's sphincter through the common bile duct

     4. Metabolizes carbohydrates, fats, and proteins

     5. Synthesizes coagulation factors VII, IX, X, and prothrombin

     6. Stores vitamins A, D, E, K, B_{12}, copper, and iron

     7. Detoxifies chemicals

     8. Excretes bilirubin

     9. Obtains dual blood supply from portal vein and hepatic artery

    10. Produces and stores glycogen

    11. Promotes erythropoiesis when bone marrow production is insufficient

G. Gallbladder

     1. Hollow, pear-shaped organ that stores bile

     2. Secretes bile via the cystic duct to the common bile duct

H. Pancreas

     1. Accessory gland of digestion

     2. Exocrine function: secretes three digestive enzymes

       a. Amylase

       b. Lipase

       c. Trypsin

     3. Endocrine function: secretes hormones from the islets of Langerhans

       a. Insulin

       b. Glucagon

       c. Somatostatin

     4. Main pancreatic duct joins the common bile duct and empties into the duodenum at the ampulla of Vater

     5. Responsible for secreting large amounts of sodium bicarbonate, which neutralizes acid chyme

◆ II. Assessment findings

A. History

CLINICAL ALERT

     1. Inadequate diet

     2. Change in bowel habits

       a. Constipation

       b. Diarrhea

       c. Flatus

DECISION TREE
Abdominal pain: Determining the possible causes

This flowchart highlights the decision-making process used to determine the possible causes of a patient's abdominal pain.

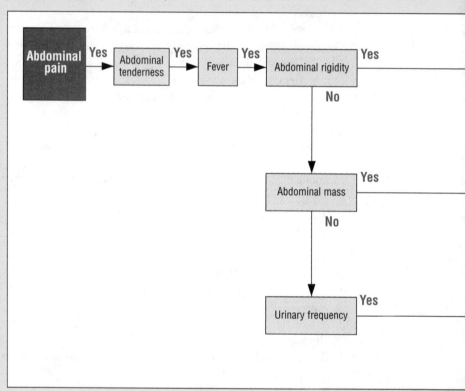

3. Complaints of indigestion
4. Nausea and vomiting
5. Abdominal pain (For more information, see *Abdominal pain: Determining the possible causes*)
6. DYSPHAGIA
7. Loss of appetite

B. Objective data associated with GI disorders

   1. Weight changes
   2. Abnormal color and consistency of stool
      a. MELENA
      b. Clay-colored stools

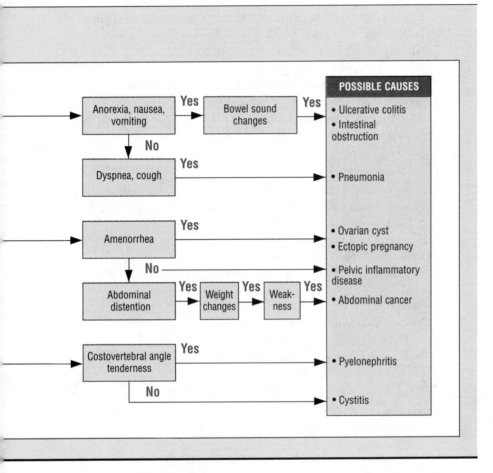

c. Frothy stools
d. STEATORRHEA
e. Occult blood in stool
3. Abnormal bowel sounds
4. Abdominal distention
5. Rectal bleeding
6. Jaundice
7. Edema
8. HEMATEMESIS
9. Anorexia

♦ III. Diagnostic tests and procedures

A. Upper GI series
  1. Definition and purpose
     a. Fluoroscopic procedure using barium as a contrast medium
     b. Examination of the esophagus, stomach, duodenum, and other portions of the small bowel after swallowing barium
  2. Nursing interventions before the procedure
     a. Withhold food and fluids
     b. Administer fluids, cathartics, and enemas, as prescribed
  3. Nursing interventions after the procedure
     a. Inform the patient that stool will be light-colored for several days
     b. Administer cathartics, fluids, and enemas, as prescribed

B. Lower GI series (barium enema)
  1. Definition and purpose
     a. Fluoroscopic procedure using barium as a contrast medium
     b. Examination of the large intestine after administration of barium via an enema
  2. Nursing interventions before the procedure
     a. Withhold food and fluids
     b. Encourage the patient to discuss feelings of embarrassment
     c. Administer bowel preparation (laxatives and enemas), as prescribed
  3. Nursing interventions after the procedure
     a. Determine if the patient is constipated
     b. Force fluids unless contraindicated
     c. Administer enemas and laxatives, as prescribed
     d. Monitor color and consistency of stool

C. Endoscopy
  1. Definition and purpose
     a. Procedure using an endoscope
     b. Direct visualization of the esophagus and stomach
  2. Nursing interventions before the procedure
     a. Withhold food and fluids
     b. Obtain written, informed consent
     c. Obtain baseline vital signs (VS)
     d. Administer sedatives, as prescribed
  3. Nursing interventions after the procedure

CLINICAL ALERT

     a. Withhold food and fluids until the gag reflex returns
     b. Assess gag and cough reflexes
     c. Assess vasovagal response

D. Fecal occult blood test
  1. Definition and purpose
     a. Laboratory test using a reagent
     b. Analysis of stool for blood

  2. Nursing interventions before the procedure
     a. Advise the patient to avoid red meat, iron, and high fiber for 1 to 3 days
     b. Document the administration of aspirin, vitamin C, and anti-inflammatory drugs

E. Fecal fat
  1. Definition and purpose
     a. Laboratory test using a stain
     b. Analysis of stool for fat
  2. Nursing interventions before the procedure
     a. Advise the patient to restrict alcohol intake and maintain a high-fat diet 72 hours before the examination
     b. Refrigerate specimen
     c. Document current medications

F. Proctosigmoidoscopy
  1. Definition and purpose
     a. Procedure using a lighted scope
     b. Direct visualization of the sigmoid colon, rectum, and anal canal
  2. Nursing interventions before the procedure
     a. Encourage the patient to discuss feelings of embarrassment
     b. Inform the patient that the procedure requires a knee-chest position
     c. Administer bowel preparation, as prescribed
     d. Obtain written, informed consent
     e. Document iron intake
  3. Nursing interventions after the procedure
     a. Check the patient for bleeding
     b. Monitor the patient's VS

G. Barium swallow
  1. Definition and purpose
     a. Procedure using barium as a contrast medium
     b. Fluoroscopic examination of the pharynx and esophagus after administration of barium
  2. Nursing interventions before the procedure
     a. Withhold food and fluids
     b. Explain the procedure to the patient
  3. Nursing interventions after the procedure
     a. Determine if the patient is constipated
     b. Force fluids unless contraindicated
     c. Administer laxatives, as prescribed

H. Cholangiography
   1. Definition and purpose
      a. Procedure using an injection of a radiopaque dye through a catheter
      b. Radiographic examination of the biliary duct system
   2. Nursing interventions before the procedure
      a. Encourage a low-residue, high-simple fat diet 1 day before the exam

      b. Withhold food and fluids after midnight
      c. Note the patient's allergies to iodine, seafood, and radiopaque dyes
      d. Inform the patient about possible throat irritation and flushing of the face
   3. Nursing interventions after the procedure
      a. Check the injection site for bleeding
      b. Monitor VS

I. Liver scan
   1. Definition and purpose
      a. Procedure using an I.V. injection of a radioisotope
      b. Visual imaging of the distribution of blood flow in the liver
   2. Nursing interventions before the procedure
      a. Determine the patient's ability to lie still during the procedure
      b. Check the patient for possible allergies
   3. Nursing interventions after the procedure
      a. Assess the I.V. insertion site for bleeding, bruising, or hematoma
      b. Assess the patient for signs of delayed allergic reaction to the radioisotope, such as itching and hives

J. Gastric analysis
   1. Definition and purpose
      a. Procedure that aspirates the contents of the stomach through a nasogastric (NG) tube
      b. Fasting analysis to measure the acidity of gastric secretions
   2. Nursing interventions before the procedure
      a. Withhold food and fluids after midnight
      b. Instruct the patient not to smoke for 8 to 12 hours before the test
      c. Withhold medications that can affect gastric secretions for 24 hours before the procedure
   3. Nursing interventions after the procedure
      a. Obtain VS
      b. Note reactions to gastric acid stimulant, if used

K. Ultrasonography
   1. Definition and purpose
      a. Noninvasive procedure examination that uses echoes from sound waves
      b. Visualization of body organs

CLINICAL ALERT

CLINICAL ALERT

CLINICAL ALERT

2. Nursing interventions before the procedure
   a. Withhold food and fluids for 8 to 12 hours
   b. Determine the patient's ability to lie still during the procedure
   c. Ask the patient not to smoke or chew gum for 8 to 12 hours before the test
   d. Administer enemas, as prescribed
   e. Remove abdominal dressings

L. Blood chemistry
   1. Definition and purpose
      a. Laboratory test of a blood sample
      b. Analysis for potassium, sodium, calcium, phosphorus, glucose, bicarbonate, blood urea nitrogen (BUN), creatinine, protein, albumin, osmolality, amylase, lipase, alkaline phosphatase, ammonia, bilirubin, lactic dehydrogenase (LDH), Bromsulphalein (BSP) test, aspartate aminotransferase (AST), serum alanine aminotransferase (ALT), hepatitis-associated antigens, carcinoembryonic antigen (CEA), and alpha-fetoprotein
   2. Nursing interventions
      a. Withhold food and fluid, as directed, before the procedure
      b. Check the site for bleeding after the procedure

M. Hematologic studies
   1. Definition and purpose
      a. Laboratory test of a blood sample
      b. Analysis for red blood cells (RBCs), white blood cells (WBCs), platelets, prothrombin time (PT), partial thromboplastin time (PTT), hemoglobin (Hgb), hematocrit (HCT)
   2. Nursing interventions
      a. Note current drug therapy before the procedure
      b. Check the site for bleeding after the procedure

N. Liver biopsy
   1. Definition and purpose
      a. Procedure using a needle for the percutaneous removal of a small amount of liver tissue
      b. Histologic evaluation of liver tissue
   2. Nursing interventions before the procedure
      a. Withhold food and fluids after midnight
      b. Obtain written, informed consent
      c. Assess baseline clotting studies and VS
      d. Instruct patient to exhale and hold breath during insertion of the needle

CLINICAL
ALERT

3. Nursing interventions after the procedure
   a. Check the insertion site for bleeding

   b. Monitor VS
   c. Observe the patient for signs of shock and pneumothorax
   d. Position patient on right lateral side for hemostasis

O. Colonoscopy
   1. Definition and purpose
      a. Procedure using flexible, lighted scope
      b. Direct visualization of large intestine; biopsies can be obtained
   2. Nursing interventions before the procedure
      a. Provide clear liquid diet 48 hours before test
      b. Administer bowel preparation 1 to 3 days before test
      c. Explain that the patient will feel cramping and the sensation of needing to have a bowel movement
      d. Explain use of air to distend bowel lumen

   3. Nursing interventions after the procedure
      a. Monitor for gross bleeding
      b. Withhold food and fluids for 2 hours
      c. Check for blood in stool if polyps removed

P. Endoscopic retrograde cholangiopancreatography (ERCP)
   1. Definition and purpose
      a. Radiographic examination of the hepatobiliary tree and pancreatic ducts using contrast medium and a lighted scope
      b. Used to evaluate the cause of obstructive jaundice
   2. Nursing interventions before the procedure

      a. Withhold food and fluid after midnight
      b. Check for allergies to iodine or seafood
      c. Remove dentures
      d. Explain that local anesthetic will be used

   3. Nursing interventions after the procedure
      a. Check for signs of respiratory depression
      b. Check for signs of urine retention

      c. Provide comfort measures for throat irritation
      d. Withhold food until gag reflex returns

Q. Percutaneous transhepatic cholangiography
   1. Definition and purpose
      a. Fluoroscopic examination of the biliary ducts through use of contrast medium
      b. Used to evaluate cause of severe jaundice and diagnose obstruction

2. Nursing interventions before the procedure
   a. Inform patient that the X-ray table will be tilted and rotated during the procedure
   b. Explain that transient pain will be felt with the injection of the anesthetic

   c. Check for allergies to iodine or seafood
   d. Check PT and PTT
   e. Withhold food and fluid after midnight
3. Nursing interventions after the procedure
   a. Rest for at least 6 hours in right sidelying position
   b. Check for bleeding at injection site
   c. Monitor vital signs
   d. Withhold food and fluids for 2 hours

◆ IV. Psychosocial impact of GI disorders

A. Developmental impact
   1. Changes in body image
   2. Feeling of lack of control over body function
   3. Fear of rejection
   4. Embarrassment from changes in body function and structure
   5. Decreased self-esteem

B. Economic impact
   1. Disruption of employment
   2. Cost of special diet
   3. Cost of special diversion appliances
   4. Cost of medications

C. Occupational and recreational impact
   1. Change of occupation
   2. Changes in leisure activity
   3. Restrictions in physical activity

D. Social impact
   1. Changes in eating patterns and modes
   2. Changes in elimination patterns and modes
   3. Social withdrawal and isolation
   4. Changes in sexual function

◆ V. Risk factors for developing GI disorders

A. Modifiable risk factors
   1. Diet: low-fiber
   2. Smoking
   3. Alcohol consumption
   4. Inactivity

     5. Stress

     6. Contaminated water and food

     7. Anger, fear, or anxiety

     8. Culturally based reluctance to discuss personal hygiene and health habits

B. Nonmodifiable risk factors

     1. Family history of GI disorders

     2. History of previous GI dysfunction

♦ VI. Nursing diagnostic categories for a patient with a GI disorder

A. Probable nursing diagnostic categories

     1. Constipation

     2. Diarrhea

     3. Pain

     4. Altered nutrition: less than body requirements

     5. Fluid volume deficit

B. Possible nursing diagnostic categories

     1. Body image disturbance

     2. Self-esteem disturbance

     3. Impaired skin integrity

     4. Noncompliance

     5. Knowledge deficit

     6. Anxiety

     7. Sexual dysfunction

     8. Impaired swallowing

     9. Incontinence, bowel

    10. Self-care deficit, toileting

♦ VII. Gallbladder and pancreatic surgeries

A. Description

     1. Cholecystostomy: surgical incision into the gallbladder to drain bile

     2. Choledochotomy: surgical incision into the common bile duct to remove stones

     3. Cholecystotomy: surgical incision into the gallbladder to remove gallstones

     4. Choledochostomy: surgical opening of the common bile duct to insert a T tube or catheter for drainage

     5. Cholecystectomy: surgical removal of the gallbladder

     6. Pancreatectomy: surgical removal of part or all of the pancreas

7. Extracorporeal shock-wave lithotripsy: use of shock waves to fragment gallstones into small pieces to either be removed by endoscopy or dissolved with solvents

8. Laparoscopic cholecystectomy: removal of gallbladder via small incision in abdomen and use of a fiberoptic endoscope

B. Preoperative nursing interventions

1. Complete patient and family preoperative teaching

   a. Determine the patient's understanding of the procedure

   b. Describe the operating room (OR), postanesthesia care unit (PACU), and preoperative and postoperative routines

   c. Demonstrate postoperative turning, coughing, and deep breathing (TCDB), splinting, leg exercises, and range-of-motion (ROM) exercises

   d. Explain the postoperative need for drainage tubes, surgical dressings, oxygen therapy, I.V. therapy, and pain control

2. Complete a preoperative checklist

3. Administer preoperative medications, as prescribed

4. Allay the patient's and family's anxiety about surgery

5. Document the patient's history and physical assessment data base

C. Postoperative nursing interventions

1. Check respiratory status and fluid balance

2. Assess pain and administer postoperative analgesics, as prescribed

3. Assess for return of peristalsis; give solid foods and liquids, as tolerated

4. Administer I.V. fluids and transfusion therapy, as prescribed

5. Allay the patient's anxiety

6. Inspect the surgical dressing and change, as directed

7. Reinforce TCDB and splinting of incision

8. Keep the patient in semi-Fowler's position

9. Provide incentive spirometry

10. Maintain activity, as tolerated

11. Monitor VS, urine output (UO), intake and output (I/O), and laboratory studies

12. Monitor and maintain position and patency of drainage tubes: NG, wound drainage, T tube

13. Administer antibiotics, as prescribed

14. Provide care for pancreatic surgery

   a. Use accuchecks to monitor glucose

   b. Monitor for signs of hyperglycemia

15. Individualize home care instructions

   a. Avoid lifting for 6 weeks

   b. Complete incision care daily

   c. Continue care of the T tube

   d. Adhere to a low-fat diet for 6 weeks

D. Possible surgical complications
   1. Pneumonia
   2. Atelectasis
   3. Peritonitis
   4. Hemorrhage

◆ **VIII. Portal-systemic shunts**

A. Definition
   1. Portacaval shunt: surgical anastomosis of the portal vein to the inferior vena cava to divert blood from the portal system to decrease pressure
   2. Splenorenal shunt: surgical anastomosis of the splenic vein to the left renal vein to divert blood from the portal system to decrease pressure
   3. Mesocaval shunt: surgical anastomosis of the inferior vena cava to the side of the superior mesenteric vein to divert blood from the portal system to decrease pressure
   4. Transjugular intrahepatic portosystemic shunt (TIPS): shunt between the portal and systemic venous circulation using the right internal jugular vein and placement of a stent

B. Preoperative nursing interventions
   1. Complete patient and family preoperative teaching
      a. Determine the patient's understanding of the procedure
      b. Describe the OR, PACU, and preoperative and postoperative routines; demonstrate postoperative TCDB, splinting, and leg and ROM exercises
      c. Explain the postoperative need for drainage tubes, surgical dressings, oxygen therapy, I.V. therapy, and pain control
   2. Complete a preoperative checklist
   3. Administer preoperative medications, as prescribed
   4. Allay the patient's and family's anxiety about surgery
   5. Document the patient's history and physical assessment data base

   6. Administer antibiotics, as prescribed (neomycin sulfate)
   7. Administer vitamin K, as prescribed
   8. Administer I.V. and transfusion therapy, as prescribed
   9. Administer lactulose, as prescribed
   10. Maintain patency of NG tube
   11. Monitor central venous pressure (CVP)
   12. Manage bleeding
      a. Administer Pitressin (vasopressin)
      b. Maintain Sengstaken-Blakemore tube

C. Postoperative nursing interventions
   1. Assess cardiac, respiratory, and neurologic status and fluid balance

2. Assess pain and administer postoperative analgesics, as prescribed
3. Administer I.V. fluids, total parental nutrition (TPN), and transfusion therapy, as prescribed
4. Allay the patient's anxiety
5. Inspect the surgical dressing
6. Reinforce TCDB and splinting of the incision
7. Keep the patient in semi-Fowler's position
8. Assess for return of peristalsis
9. Provide suction
10. Maintain activity: bed rest, active and passive ROM and isometric exercises
11. Administer oxygen and maintain endotracheal tube to ventilator
12. Monitor VS, UO, I/O, CVP, laboratory studies, electrocardiogram (ECG), neurovital signs, and pulse oximetry
13. Monitor and maintain position and patency of drainage tubes: NG, indwelling urinary catheter, wound drainage

CLINICAL ALERT

14. Allay the patient's anxiety
15. Measure and record the patient's abdominal girth
16. Monitor stool and NG drainage for occult blood
17. Monitor for hemorrhage
18. Check for peripheral edema
19. Provide skin, nares, and mouth care
20. Reorient frequently
21. Administer antibiotics, as prescribed (neomycin sulfate)
22. Administer vitamin K, as prescribed
23. Elevate extremities
24. Individualize home care instructions
    a. Adhere to activity limitations
    b. Complete incision care daily
    c. Avoid using alcohol
    d. Adhere indefinitely to a protein-restricted diet
    e. Avoid using over-the-counter medications
    f. Observe for symptoms of encephalopathy

D. Possible surgical complications
   1. Acute hepatic failure
   2. Chronic portal systemic encephalopathy
   3. Coagulopathy
   4. Shunt malfunction

◆ IX. Gastric surgery

A. Description
   1. Vagotomy: surgical ligation of the vagus nerve to decrease the secretion of gastric acid

2. Antrectomy: surgical removal of the antrum of the stomach
3. Pyloroplasty: surgical dilatation of the pyloric sphincter to increase the rate of gastric emptying
4. Gastroduodenostomy (Billroth I): surgical removal of the lower portion of the stomach with anastomosis of the remaining portion of the stomach to the duodenum
5. Gastrojejunostomy (Billroth II): surgical removal of the antrum and distal portion of the stomach and duodenum with anastomosis of the stomach to the jejunum
6. Subtotal gastrectomy: surgical removal of 60% to 80% of the stomach
7. Esophagojejunostomy (total gastrectomy): surgical removal of the entire stomach with a loop of the jejunum anastomosed to the esophagus

B. Preoperative nursing interventions
　1. Complete patient and family preoperative teaching
　　a. Determine the patient's understanding of the procedure
　　b. Describe the OR, PACU, and preoperative and postoperative routines
　　c. Demonstrate postoperative TCDB, splinting, and leg and ROM exercises
　　d. Explain the postoperative need for drainage tubes, surgical dressings, oxygen therapy, I.V. therapy, and pain control
　2. Complete a preoperative checklist
　3. Administer preoperative medications, as prescribed
　4. Allay the patient's and family's anxiety about surgery
　5. Document the patient's history and physical assessment data base
　6. Administer bowel preparation, as prescribed

C. Postoperative nursing interventions
　1. Assess respiratory status and fluid balance
　2. Assess pain and administer postoperative analgesics, as prescribed
　3. Administer I.V. fluids, NG tube feedings, and transfusion therapy, as prescribed
　4. Allay the patient's anxiety
　5. Inspect the surgical dressing and change, as directed
　6. Reinforce TCDB and splinting of incision
　7. Keep the patient in semi-Fowler's position
　8. Apply antiembolism or pneumatic stockings
　9. Assess for return of peristalsis
　10. Provide incentive spirometry
　11. Maintain activity, as tolerated
　12. Administer oxygen
　13. Monitor VS, UO, I/O, laboratory studies, and pulse oximetry

14. Monitor and maintain position and patency of drainage tubes: NG, indwelling urinary catheter, wound drainage

CLINICAL ALERT

15. Monitor NG drainage for overt bleeding
16. Irrigate NG tube gently; do not reposition NG tube
17. Weigh the patient daily
18. Monitor gastric pH
19. Individualize home care instructions
    a. Identify ways to reduce stress
    b. Increase food intake gradually
    c. Eat six small meals a day
    d. Limit fluids with meals

CLINICAL ALERT

D. Possible surgical complications
   1. Dumping syndrome after a partial gastrectomy
   2. Hemorrhage
   3. Dehydration
   4. Infection
   5. Dehiscence

◆ X. Hemorrhoidectomy

A. Description—surgical removal of hemorrhoids by clamp, excision, or cautery

B. Preoperative nursing interventions
   1. Complete patient and family preoperative teaching
      a. Determine the patient's understanding of the procedure
      b. Describe the OR, PACU, and preoperative and postoperative routines
      c. Demonstrate postoperative TCDB, splinting, and leg and ROM exercises
      d. Explain the postoperative need for drainage tubes, surgical dressings, oxygen therapy, I.V. therapy, and pain control
   2. Complete a preoperative checklist
   3. Administer preoperative medications, as prescribed
   4. Allay the patient's and family's anxiety about surgery
   5. Document the patient's history and physical assessment data base
   6. Administer bowel preparation, as prescribed
      a. Cleansing enemas
      b. Laxatives

C. Postoperative nursing interventions
   1. Assess pain and administer postoperative analgesics, as prescribed
   2. Assess for return of peristalsis; give solid foods and liquids, as tolerated
   3. Administer I.V. fluids
   4. Allay the patient's anxiety

5. Inspect the surgical dressing and remove anal packing, as directed
6. Reinforce TCDB
7. Keep the patient prone or on the side
8. Provide incentive spirometry
9. Maintain activity, as tolerated
10. Monitor VS, UO, I/O, and laboratory studies
11. Encourage the patient to discuss feelings of embarrassment and fear of defecation

CLINICAL ALERT

12. Administer analgesics, as prescribed, before the first bowel movement
13. Provide sitz baths
14. Provide a flotation pad when sitting
15. Administer stool softeners, as prescribed
16. Individualize home care instructions
    a. Avoid heavy lifting and prolonged standing or sitting
    b. Avoid constipation
    c. Defecate when urge is felt

CLINICAL ALERT

    d. Provide perineal care daily
    e. Anticipate a small amount of bleeding postoperatively with bowel movements
    f. Avoid Valsalva's maneuver
    g. Increase fluid intake

D. Possible surgical complications
   1. Rectal hemorrhage
   2. Urine retention

♦ XI. Bowel surgery

A. Description
   1. Abdominoperineal resection: removal of distal sigmoid colon, rectum, and anus with the creation of a permanent colostomy
   2. Colectomy: surgical excision of the right colon (right hemicolectomy) or left colon (left hemicolectomy)
   3. Ileostomy: surgical opening of the ileum to the abdominal surface to form a stoma
   4. Continent ileostomy (Koch's pouch): surgical creation of an intraabdominal reservoir for stool
   5. Bowel resection: surgical excision of a portion of the bowel
   6. Permanent colostomy: surgical opening of the colon to the abdominal surface to form a single stoma after the distal portion of the bowel is removed
   7. Double-barrel colostomy: surgical opening of the colon to the abdominal surface to form two stomas to prevent passage of stool into the distal bowel

  B. Preoperative nursing interventions
    1. Complete patient and family preoperative teaching
      a. Determine the patient's understanding of the procedure
      b. Describe the OR, PACU, and preoperative and postoperative routines
      c. Demonstrate postoperative TCDB, splinting, and leg and ROM exercises
      d. Explain the postoperative need for drainage tubes, gastrostomy feeding tube, surgical dressings, oxygen therapy, I.V. therapy, and pain control
    2. Complete a preoperative checklist
    3. Administer preoperative medications, as prescribed
    4. Allay the patient's and family's anxiety about surgery
    5. Document the patient's history and physical assessment data base
    6. Administer bowel preparation, as prescribed
      a. Antibiotics
      b. Cleansing enemas
    7. Arrange a preoperative visit with an enterostomal therapist
    8. Encourage the patient to express feelings about changes in body image

  C. Postoperative nursing interventions
    1. Assess cardiac status and fluid balance
    2. Assess pain and administer postoperative analgesics, as prescribed
    3. Assess for return of peristalsis; give solid foods and liquids, as tolerated
    4. Administer I.V. fluids, TPN, and transfusion therapy, as prescribed
    5. Allay the patient's anxiety
    6. Inspect the surgical dressing and change, as directed
    7. Reinforce TCDB and splinting of incision
    8. Keep the patient in semi-Fowler's position
    9. Provide incentive spirometry
   10. Maintain activity, as tolerated
   11. Apply antiembolism or pneumatic stockings
   12. Monitor VS, UO, I/O, laboratory studies, and pulse oximetry
   13. Monitor and maintain position and patency of drainage tubes: NG, indwelling urinary catheter, wound drainage
   14. Encourage the patient to express feelings about changes in body image
   15. Monitor and record the color, consistency, and amount of the patient's stool
   16. Provide routine colostomy care
      a. Prevent skin breakdown by thorough cleaning of skin around the stoma
      b. Check stoma

   c. Control odor
   d. Change ostomy bag, as needed
17. Increase fluid intake to 3,000 ml/day
18. Individualize home care instructions
   a. Recognize the signs and symptoms of intestinal obstruction
   b. Complete incision care daily

   c. Use ostomy bags
   d. Check the condition of the stoma daily and report bleeding and changes
   e. Report changes in consistency and color of stool
   f. Perform colostomy care daily
   g. Identify foods that cause flatus and irritability of the colon
   h. Teach the patient to catheterize a Koch's pouch
   i. Provide skin care around the stoma
   j. Discuss concerns about sexual activities

D. Possible surgical complications
1. Infection
2. Hemorrhage
3. Dehiscence
4. Evisceration
5. Paralytic ileus
6. Prolapsed stoma
7. Abscess

♦ XII. Hiatal hernia (esophageal hernia)

A. Definition—protrusion of the stomach through the diaphragm into the thoracic cavity

B. Possible etiology
1. Congenital weakness
2. Obesity
3. Pregnancy
4. Trauma
5. Increased abdominal pressure
6. Aging

C. Pathophysiology
1. The opening (hiatus) in the diaphragm where the esophagus enters the stomach becomes enlarged and weakened
2. The upper portion of the stomach enters the lower thorax
3. Sliding of the esophagus and stomach into the chest results in reflux of gastric acid

D. Possible assessment findings
1. Pyrosis

CLINICAL
ALERT

2. Dysphagia
3. Regurgitation
4. Sternal pain after eating
5. Vomiting
6. Feeling of fullness
7. Dyspnea
8. Cough
9. Tachycardia

E. Possible diagnostic test findings
1. Esophagoscopy: incompetent cardiac sphincter
2. Barium swallow: protrusion of the hernia
3. Chest X-ray: protrusion of abdominal organs into thorax
4. Gastric analysis: increased pH

F. Medical management
1. Diet: bland diet with decreased intake of caffeine and spicy foods
2. Oxygen therapy
3. GI decompression: NG tube
4. Position: semi-Fowler's
5. Activity: as tolerated
6. Monitoring: VS, UO, and I/O
7. Anticholinergic: propantheline bromide (Pro-Banthine)
8. Antacids: magnesium and aluminum hydroxide (Maalox), aluminum hydroxide gel (AlternaGEL)
9. Histamine antagonists: cimetidine (Tagamet), ranitidine (Zantac), famotidine (Pepcid), nizatidine (Axid)
10. Weight loss

G. Nursing interventions
1. Maintain the patient's diet
2. Administer oxygen
3. Assess respiratory status
4. Maintain position, patency, and low suction of NG tube
5. Keep the patient in semi-Fowler's position
6. Monitor and record VS, UO, I/O, and daily weight
7. Administer medications, as prescribed
8. Allay the patient's anxiety
9. Avoid flexion at the waist in positioning the patient
10. Individualize home care instructions (For more information about teaching, see *Patients with GI disorders,* page 166)
   a. Eat small, frequent meals
   b. Stop drinking carbonated beverages and alcohol
   c. Stay upright for 2 hours after eating
   d. Avoid wearing constrictive clothing
   e. Avoid lifting, bending, straining, and coughing

TEACHING TIPS
Patients with GI disorders

Be sure to include the following topics in your teaching plan for patients with GI disorders.
- Smoking cessation
- Stool monitoring, including color, amount, and consistency of stool
- Glucose level monitoring
- Signs of hyperglycemia
- Weight maintenance program
- Medication therapy, including the action, adverse effects, and scheduling of medications
- Dietary recommendations and restrictions
- Rest and activity patterns
- Signs and symptoms of GI bleeding
- Self-monitoring for infection

    H. Possible complications
        1. Hemorrhage
        2. Ulceration
        3. Aspiration
        4. Incarceration of stomach in chest

    I. Possible surgical interventions
        1. Reduction of hiatal hernia
        2. Fundoplication

◆ XIII. Gastric ulcer (peptic ulcer)

    A. Definition—erosion of mucosal lining of the stomach

    B. Possible etiology
        1. Alcohol abuse
        2. Stress
        3. Drug-induced: salicylates, steroids, indomethacin, reserpine
        4. Smoking
        5. Gastritis
        6. Zollinger-Ellison syndrome
        7. Infection: *Helicobacter pylori*

    C. Pathophysiology
        1. Increased emptying time of gastric acid from the gastric lumen into the small intestine causes an inflammatory reaction with tissue breakdown
        2. Bile refluxes into the stomach if the pyloric valve is involved
        3. Combination of HCl acid and pepsin destroys gastric mucosa

    4. Decreased resistance of gastric mucosa to action of HCl acid

D. Possible assessment findings

    1. Left epigastric pain 1 to 2 hours after eating

    2. Weight loss

    3. Nausea and vomiting

    4. Hematemesis

    5. Melena

    6. Anorexia

    7. Relief of pain after administration of antacids

E. Possible diagnostic test findings

    1. Hematology: decreased Hgb, HCT, PT, PTT

    2. Blood chemistry: increased sodium

    3. Gastric analysis: normal for gastric ulcer

    4. Upper GI: location of ulcer

    5. Barium swallow: ulceration of gastric mucosa

    6. Fecal occult blood: positive

    7. Serum gastrin: normal or increased

F. Medical management

    1. Diet: low-fiber in small, frequent feedings

    2. GI decompression: NG tube

    3. Position: semi-Fowler's

    4. Activity: bed rest

    5. Monitoring: VS, UO, and I/O

    6. Laboratory studies: Hgb, HCT

    7. Treatment: saline lavage by NG tube

    8. Transfusion therapy: packed RBCs

    9. Anticholinergics: propantheline bromide (Pro-Banthine), dicyclomine hydrochloride (Bentyl)

    10. Antacids: magnesium and aluminum hydroxide (Maalox), aluminum hydroxide gel (AlternaGEL)

    11. Histamine antagonists: cimetidine (Tagamet), ranitidine (Zantac), nizatidine (Axid), Famotidine (Pepcid)

    12. Prostaglandin: misoprostol (Cytotec)

    13. Mucosal barrier fortifier: sucralfate (Carafate)

    14. Endoscopic laser

    15. Photocoagulation

    16. Hormone: vasopressin (Pitressin) for management of bleeding

    17. Antibiotics

CLINICAL ALERT

G. Nursing interventions

    1. Maintain the patient's diet with small, frequent feedings

    2. Assess respiratory and cardiovascular status

    3. Maintain position, patency, and low suction of NG tube if gastric decompression is ordered

4. Keep the patient in semi-Fowler's position

5. Monitor and record VS, UO, I/O, laboratory studies, fecal occult blood, and gastric pH

6. Administer medications, as prescribed

7. Allay the patient's anxiety

8. Provide nares and mouth care

9. Minimize environmental stress

10. Maintain a quiet environment

11. Irrigate the NG tube with normal saline to maintain patency; do not use water, which may interfere with fluid and electrolyte balance

12. Monitor the consistency, color, amount, and frequency of stools

13. Individualize home care instructions

    a. Identify ways to reduce stress

    b. Follow dietary recommendations and restrictions; avoid caffeine, alcohol, and spicy and fried foods

    c. Maintain a quiet environment

H. Possible complications

  1. Hemorrhage

  2. Perforation

  3. Chemical peritonitis

  4. Intestinal obstruction

I. Possible surgical interventions

  1. Billroth I (see page 160)

  2. Billroth II (see page 160)

  3. Vagotomy and pyloroplasty (see pages 159 and 160)

♦ XIV. Gastric cancer

A. Definition—malignant stomach tumor that is primary or metastatic

B. Possible etiology

  1. High intake of salted and smoked foods

  2. Low intake of vegetables and fruits

  3. Chronic gastritis

  4. Achlorhydria

  5. Pernicious anemia

  6. Gastric ulcer

C. Pathophysiology

  1. Unregulated cell growth and uncontrolled cell division result in the development of a neoplasm

  2. Tumor usually develops in the distal third of stomach and metastasizes to the abdominal organs, lungs, and bones

  3. Most common neoplasm is adenocarcinoma

D. Possible assessment findings
1. Fatigue
2. Weakness
3. Syncope
4. Shortness of breath
5. Nausea and vomiting
6. Weight loss
7. Hematemesis
8. Indigestion
9. Epigastric fullness and pain
10. Malaise
11. Melena
12. Regurgitation
13. Anorexia

E. Possible diagnostic test findings
1. Fecal occult blood: positive
2. CEA: positive
3. Hematology: decreased Hgb, HCT
4. Blood chemistry: increased AST, LDH, and amylase
5. Gastric analysis: positive cancer cells, achlorhydria
6. GI series: gastric mass
7. Gastroscopy: biopsy positive for cancer cells

F. Medical management
1. Diet: high-protein, high-calorie, high-fat, and low-carbohydrate
2. I.V. therapy: heparin lock
3. GI decompression: NG tube
4. Position: semi-Fowler's
5. Activity: as tolerated
6. Monitoring: VS, UO, and I/O
7. Laboratory studies: Hgb, HCT, and fecal occult blood
8. Nutritional support: TPN
9. Radiation therapy
10. Antineoplastics: carmustine (BiCNU), 5-fluorouracil (Adrucil)
11. Vitamin supplements: folic acid (Folvite), cyanocobalamin (vitamin B_{12})
12. Chemotherapy
13. Analgesics: meperidine (Demerol), morphine sulfate (Roxanol)
14. Antiemetic: prochlorperazine (Compazine)

G. Nursing interventions
1. Maintain the patient's diet
2. Assess GI status
3. Maintain position, patency, and low suction of NG tube
4. Keep the patient in semi-Fowler's position

5. Monitor and record VS, UO, I/O, laboratory studies, and daily weight
6. Administer TPN
7. Administer medications, as prescribed
8. Encourage the patient to express feelings about a fear of dying
9. Provide skin and mouth care
10. Provide rest periods
11. Monitor the consistency, amount, and frequency of stool
12. Monitor the color of stool for blood
13. Provide postchemotherapeutic and postradiation nursing care
    a. Provide prophylactic skin and mouth care
    b. Monitor dietary intake
    c. Administer antiemetics and antidiarrheals, as prescribed
    d. Monitor for bleeding, infection, and electrolyte imbalance
    e. Provide rest periods
14. Provide information about the American Cancer Society
15. Individualize home care instructions
    a. Avoid exposure to people with infections
    b. Alternate rest periods with activity
    c. Monitor self for infection by taking temperature frequently
    d. Recognize the signs and symptoms of ulceration
    e. Complete skin care daily

H. Possible complications
   1. Obstruction
   2. Ulceration
   3. Metastasis

I. Possible surgical interventions
   1. Subtotal gastrectomy (see page 160)
   2. Total gastrectomy (see page 160)
   3. Billroth I (see page 160)
   4. Billroth II (see page 160)

◆ XV. Ulcerative colitis

A. Definition—inflammatory disorder of the large bowel
B. Possible etiology
   1. Emotional stress
   2. Autoimmune disease
   3. Genetics
   4. Idiopathic cause
   5. Allergies
   6. Viral and bacterial infections

C. Pathophysiology
   1. Inflammatory edema of the mucous membrane of the colon and rectum leads to bleeding and shallow ulcerations
   2. Abscess formation causes bowel-wall shortening, thinning, fragility, hypermotility, and decreased absorption
   3. Mucosal ulcerations begin in the distal end of the colon and ascend the large intestine

D. Possible assessment findings
   1. Abdominal tenderness
   2. Weakness
   3. Debilitation
   4. Anorexia
   5. Nausea and vomiting
   6. Dehydration
   7. Bloody, purulent, mucoid, watery stools (15 to 20/day)
   8. Elevated temperature
   9. Cachexia
   10. Weight loss
   11. Abdominal cramping
   12. Tenesmus
   13. Hyperactive bowel sounds
   14. Abdominal distention

E. Possible diagnostic test findings
   1. Sigmoidoscopy: ulceration and hyperemia
   2. Barium enema: ulcerations
   3. Blood chemistry: decreased potassium; increased osmolality
   4. Hematology: decreased Hgb, HCT
   5. Urine chemistry: increased specific gravity
   6. Stool specimen: positive for blood and mucus

F. Medical management
   1. Diet: two types
      a. High-protein, high-calorie, low-residue; bland foods in small, frequent feedings with restricted intake of milk and gas-forming foods
      b. No food and fluids
   2. I.V. therapy: hydration, electrolyte replacement, and heparin lock
   3. GI decompression: NG tube
   4. Position: semi-Fowler's
   5. Activity: bed rest with bedside commode
   6. Monitoring: VS, UO, I/O, daily weight, specific gravity, calorie count, and stools for occult blood
   7. Laboratory studies: potassium, Hgb, HCT, and osmolality
   8. Nutritional support: TPN

CLINICAL ALERT

CLINICAL ALERT

9. Treatments: indwelling urinary catheter, sitz baths
10. Antibiotic: sulfasalazine (Azulfidine)
11. Analgesic: meperidine hydrochloride (Demerol)
12. Sedative: phenobarbital (Luminal)
13. Anticholinergics: propantheline bromide (Pro-Banthine), dicyclomine hydrochloride (Bentyl)
14. Antacids: magnesium and aluminum hydroxide (Maalox), aluminum hydroxide gel (AlternaGEL)
15. Corticosteroid: hydrocortisone (Solu-Cortef)
16. Antiemetic: prochlorperazine (Compazine)
17. Antidiarrheals: diphenoxylate (Lomotil), loperamide (Imodium)
18. Transfusion therapy: packed RBCs
19. Antianemics: ferrous sulfate (Feosol), ferrous gluconate (Fergon)
20. Immunosuppressive agents: azathioprine (Imuran), cyclophosphamide (Cytoxan)
21. Vitamins and minerals
22. Tranquilizer: diazepam (Valium)
23. Potassium supplements: potassium chloride (K-Lor), potassium gluconate (Kaon)
24. Anti-inflammatory: olsalazine sodium (Dipentum)

G. Nursing interventions
1. Maintain the patient's diet; withhold food and fluids as necessary
2. Administer I.V. fluids
3. Assess GI status and fluid balance
4. Maintain position, patency, and low suction of NG tube
5. Keep the patient in semi-Fowler's position
6. Monitor and record VS, UO, I/O, laboratory studies, daily weight, specific gravity, calorie count, and fecal occult blood
7. Administer TPN and transfusion therapy
8. Administer medications, as prescribed
9. Allay the patient's anxiety
10. Provide skin, mouth, nares, and perianal care
11. Maintain bed rest with bedside commode
12. Turn the patient every 2 hours
13. Minimize environmental stress
14. Provide rest periods
15. Maintain a quiet environment
16. Promote independence in activities of daily living (ADLs)
17. Assess bowel sounds
18. Administer sitz baths
19. Monitor the number, amount, and character of stools
20. Assess perineal excoriation
21. Provide information about the United Ostomy Association and the National Foundation of Ileitis and Colitis

22. Individualize home care instructions
   a. Maintain a normal weight
   b. Identify ways to reduce stress
   c. Recognize the signs and symptoms of rectal hemorrhage and intestinal obstruction
   d. Complete sitz baths and perianal care daily

H. Possible complications
   1. Anemia
   2. Malnutrition
   3. GI perforation
   4. Megacolon
   5. Dehydration
   6. GI obstruction
   7. Hypokalemia
   8. Massive rectal hemorrhage
   9. Amyloidosis

I. Possible surgical interventions
   1. Ileostomy (see page 162)
   2. Colectomy (see page 162)

♦ XVI. Regional enteritis (Crohn's disease)

A. Definition
   1. Chronic inflammatory disease mostly of the small intestine, usually affecting the terminal ileum and sometimes affecting the large intestine, usually the ascending colon
   2. Slowly progressive with exacerbations and remissions

B. Possible etiology
   1. Unknown
   2. Emotional upsets
   3. Milk and milk products
   4. Fried foods

C. Pathophysiology
   1. Ulcerations of intestinal mucosa are accompanied by congestion, thickening of the small bowel, and fissure formations
   2. Enlarged regional mesenteric lymph nodes accompany fibrosis and narrowing of intestinal wall

D. Possible assessment findings
   1. Pain in lower right quadrant
   2. Mesenteric lymphadenitis
   3. Abdominal cramps and spasms after meals
   4. Nausea
   5. Flatulence

6. Weight loss
7. Elevated temperature
8. Chronic diarrhea with blood
9. Borborygmus

E. Possible diagnostic test findings
1. Abdominal X-ray: congested, thickened, fibrosed, and narrowed intestinal wall
2. Proctosigmoidoscopy: ulceration
3. Fecal occult blood: positive
4. Fecal fat test: increased
5. Upper GI: classic "string sign" at terminal ileum
6. Barium enema: lesions in terminal ileum

F. Medical management
1. Diet: two types
    a. High-protein, high-calorie, low-residue, low-fat, low-fiber, high-carbohydrate; bland foods in small, frequent feedings with restricted intake of milk and gas-forming foods
    b. No food and fluids
2. I.V. therapy: heparin lock
3. Activity: as tolerated
4. Monitoring: VS, I/O, daily weights, stools for occult blood, and specific gravity
5. Laboratory studies: potassium, Hgb, HCT, and osmolality
6. Nutritional support: TPN
7. Antibiotic: sulfasalazine (Azulfidine)
8. Analgesic: meperidine hydrochloride (Demerol)
9. Anticholinergics: propantheline bromide (Pro-Banthine), dicyclomine hydrochloride (Bentyl)
10. Antacids: magnesium and aluminum hydroxide (Maalox), aluminum hydroxide gel (AlternaGEL)
11. Corticosteroid: prednisone (Deltasone)
12. Antiemetic: prochlorperazine (Compazine)
13. Antidiarrheal: diphenoxylate (Lomotil)
14. Antianemics: ferrous sulfate (Feosol), ferrous gluconate (Fergon)
15. Vitamins and minerals
16. Potassium supplements: potassium chloride (K-Lor), potassium gluconate (Kaon)
17. Anti-inflammatory: olsalazine sodium (Dipentum)
18. Antibacterial: metronidazole (Flagyl)
19. Immunosuppressants: mercaptopurine (Purinethol), azathioprine (Imuran)

G. Nursing interventions
1. Maintain the patient's diet; withhold food and fluids as necessary

    2. Assess GI status and fluid balance

    3. Monitor and record VS, I/O, laboratory studies, daily weight, specific gravity, and fecal occult blood

    4. Administer TPN

    5. Administer medications, as prescribed

    6. Allay the patient's anxiety

    7. Provide skin and perianal care

    8. Minimize environmental stress

    9. Maintain a quiet environment

    10. Promote independence in ADLs

    11. Monitor the number, amount, and character of stools

    12. Assess abdominal distention

    13. Individualize home care instructions

       a. Avoid laxatives and aspirin

       b. Complete perianal care daily

       c. Identify ways to reduce stress

       d. Recognize the signs and symptoms of rectal hemorrhage and intestinal obstruction

H. Possible complications

    1. Intestinal obstruction

    2. Intestinal fistulas

    3. Intestinal perforation

    4. Hemorrhage

    5. Malnutrition

    6. Anemia

I. Possible surgical interventions

    1. Bowel resection with anastomosis (see page 162)

    2. Gastrojejunostomy with vagotomy (see page 160)

    3. Ileoanal reservoir

◆ XVII. Diverticulosis and diverticulitis

A. Definition

    1. Diverticulum: outpouching of intestinal mucosa through the muscular wall of the intestine

    2. Diverticulosis: multiple diverticula

    3. Diverticulitis: inflammation of diverticula

B. Possible etiology

    1. Stress

    2. Congenital weakening of the intestinal wall

    3. Low intake of roughage and fiber

    4. Straining at the stool

    5. Chronic constipation

CLINICAL ALERT

CLINICAL ALERT

C. Pathophysiology
   1. Muscle tone is weakened in the intestinal wall, resulting in a saclike outpouching (diverticulum)
   2. Inflammation (diverticulitis) is caused by bacteria and fecal material trapped in the diverticula
   3. Intestinal wall thickens and narrows
   4. Common site is sigmoid colon

D. Possible assessment findings
   1. Left lower quadrant pain
   2. Constipation and diarrhea
   3. Bloody stools
   4. Elevated temperature
   5. Rectal bleeding
   6. Change in bowel habits
   7. Flatulence
   8. Nausea

CLINICAL ALERT

E. Possible diagnostic test findings
   1. Sigmoidoscopy: diverticula, thickened wall
   2. Barium enema (contraindicated in acute diverticulitis): inflammation, narrow lumen of the bowel, diverticula
   3. Hematology: increased WBCs, erythrocyte sedimentation rate (ESR)

F. Medical management
   1. Diet: high-fiber, high-residue
   2. I.V. therapy: hydration, heparin lock
   3. GI decompression: NG tube
   4. Position: semi-Fowler's
   5. Activity: bed rest; active ROM and isometric exercises
   6. Monitoring: VS, UO, and I/O
   7. Laboratory studies: Hgb, HCT, and WBCs
   8. Nutritional support: TPN
   9. Antibiotics: gentamicin (Garamycin), tobramycin sulfate (Nebcin), clindamycin (Cleocin)
   10. Anticholinergic: propantheline bromide (Pro-Banthine)
   11. Stool softener: docusate sodium (Colace)

G. Nursing interventions
   1. Maintain the patient's diet
   2. Assess abdominal distention
   3. Maintain position, patency, and low suction of NG tube
   4. Keep the patient in semi-Fowler's position
   5. Monitor and record VS, UO, I/O, and laboratory studies
   6. Administer TPN
   7. Administer medications, as prescribed

8. Allay the patient's anxiety
9. Provide nares and mouth care
10. Provide rest periods
11. Administer cleansing enemas
12. Monitor stools for occult blood
13. Assess bowel sounds
14. Individualize home care instructions
    a. Identify ways to decrease constipation
    b. Follow dietary recommendations and restrictions; avoid corn, nuts, and fruits and vegetables with seeds
    c. Monitor stools for bleeding

H. Possible complications
   1. Bowel perforation
   2. Peritonitis
   3. Abscess
   4. Fistula
   5. Hemorrhage

I. Possible surgical intervention: bowel resection (see page 162)

♦ XVIII. Intestinal obstruction

A. Definition—blockage of intestinal lumen

B. Possible etiology
   1. Adhesions
   2. Hernias
   3. Tumors
   4. Fecal impaction
   5. Mesenteric thrombosis
   6. Paralytic ileus
   7. Diverticulitis
   8. Inflammation (Crohn's disease)
   9. Volvulus

C. Pathophysiology
   1. Gas, fluid, and digested substances accumulate proximal to the obstruction
   2. Fluids and gases cause bowel distention
   3. Peristalsis increases proximal to the obstruction
   4. Water and electrolytes are secreted into the blocked bowel
   5. Bowel inflammation increases and absorption by bowel mucosa is inhibited
   6. Fluid loss results in dehydration

D. Possible assessment findings
1. Cramping pain
2. Nausea
3. Abdominal distention
4. Vomiting fecal material
5. Constipation
6. Singultus
7. Elevated temperature
8. Diminished or absent bowel sounds
9. Weight loss

E. Possible diagnostic test findings
1. Blood chemistry: decreased sodium, potassium
2. Hematology: increased WBCs
3. Barium enema: stops at obstruction
4. Abdominal X-rays: increased amount of gas in bowel

F. Medical management
1. Diet: withhold food and fluids
2. I.V. therapy: hydration, electrolyte replacement, heparin lock
3. GI decompression: NG tube, Miller-Abbott tube, Cantor tube
4. Position: semi-Fowler's
5. Activity: bed rest
6. Monitoring: VS, UO, and I/O
7. Laboratory studies: sodium, potassium, and WBCs
8. Treatments: indwelling urinary catheter, NG irrigation
9. Antibiotic: gentamicin (Garamycin)
10. Analgesic: meperidine hydrochloride (Demerol)

G. Nursing interventions
1. Withhold food and fluids
2. Administer I.V. fluids
3. Assess bowel sounds
4. Measure and record the patient's abdominal girth
5. Monitor and record the frequency, color, and amount of stools
6. Maintain position, patency, and low suction of NG tube and Miller-Abbott tube
7. Keep the patient in semi-Fowler's position
8. Monitor and record VS, UO, I/O, and laboratory studies
9. Administer medications, as prescribed
10. Allay the patient's anxiety
11. Provide nares and mouth care
12. Provide information about the American Ostomy Association
13. Individualize home care instructions
   a. Avoid constipating foods
   b. Monitor the frequency and color of stools

     c. Recognize the signs and symptoms of diverticulitis

H. Possible complications
1. Peritonitis
2. Strangulation of bowel
3. Infection
4. Sepsis
5. Bowel necrosis

I. Possible surgical interventions
1. Bowel resection (see page 162)
2. Colostomy (see page 162)

◆ XIX. Peritonitis

A. Definition—localized or generalized inflammation of peritoneal cavity

B. Possible etiology
1. Bacterial infection
2. Pancreatitis
3. Blunt or penetrating trauma
4. Inflammation of colon or kidneys
5. Volvulus
6. Intestinal ischemia
7. Intestinal obstruction
8. Peptic ulceration
9. Biliary tract disease
10. Neoplasms
11. Nephrosis
12. Cirrhosis
13. Intestinal perforation

C. Pathophysiology
1. Peritoneal irritants cause inflammatory edema, vascular congestion, and hypermotility of the bowel
2. Movement of extracellular fluid into the peritoneal cavity leads to hypovolemia and decreased urine output

D. Possible assessment findings

CLINICAL ALERT

CLINICAL ALERT

1. Constant, diffuse, and intense abdominal pain
2. Rebound tenderness
3. Malaise
4. Nausea
5. Elevated temperature
6. Abdominal rigidity and distention
7. Anorexia
8. Decreased urine output
9. Shallow respirations

      10. Weak, rapid pulse

      11. Decreased peristalsis

      12. Decreased or absent bowel sounds

      13. Abdominal resonance and tympany on percussion

E. Possible diagnostic test findings

      1. Hematology: increased WBCs, HCT

      2. Peritoneal aspiration: positive for blood, pus, bile, bacteria, or amylase

      3. Abdominal X-ray: free air in abdomen under diaphragm

F. Medical management

      1. Diet: withhold food or fluid

      2. I.V. therapy: hydration, electrolyte replacement, heparin lock

      3. GI decompression: NG tube

      4. Position: semi-Fowler's

      5. Activity: bed rest

      6. Monitoring: VS, UO, I/O, CVP, and specific gravity

      7. Laboratory studies: Hgb, HCT, potassium, sodium, calcium, osmolality, and WBCs

      8. Nutritional support: TPN

      9. Treatments: indwelling urinary catheter, incentive spirometry

      10. Antibiotics: gentamicin (Garamycin), clindamycin (Cleocin), cephalothin (Keflin), ampicillin sodium/sulbactam sodium (Unasyn)

      11. Analgesic: meperidine hydrochloride (Demerol)

G. Nursing interventions

      1. Withhold food and fluids

      2. Administer I.V. fluids

      3. Provide TCDB

      4. Assess respiratory status and fluid balance

      5. Maintain position, patency, and low suction of NG tube

      6. Keep the patient in semi-Fowler's position

      7. Monitor and record VS, UO, I/O, laboratory studies, CVP, daily weight, and specific gravity

      8. Administer TPN

      9. Administer medications, as prescribed

      10. Allay the patient's anxiety

      11. Provide nares and mouth care

      12. Turn the patient every 2 hours

      13. Maintain bed rest

      14. Assess pain

      15. Assess bowel sounds

      16. Measure and record the patient's abdominal girth

      17. Avoid giving the patient laxatives

      18. Do not apply heat to the patient's abdomen

19. Individualize home care instructions
    a. Recognize the signs and symptoms of infection
    b. Monitor temperature daily
    c. Recognize the signs and symptoms of GI obstruction

H. Possible complications
   1. Adhesions
   2. Abscesses
   3. Obstructions
   4. Septic shock
   5. Paralytic ileus

I. Possible surgical interventions
   1. Exploratory laparotomy
   2. Bowel resection (see page 162)
   3. Incision and drainage of abscess
   4. Closure of perforation

◆ XX. Hemorrhoids

A. Definition—congested and dilated internal or external vessels of the rectum and anus

B. Possible etiology
   1. Chronic constipation
   2. Prolonged sitting or standing
   3. Straining at the stool
   4. Pregnancy
   5. Heavy lifting
   6. Portal hypertension
   7. Heredity
   8. Obesity
   9. Anal infection

C. Pathophysiology
   1. Increased abdominal pressure impairs the flow of blood through the hemorrhoidal venous plexus
   2. Decreased blood flow causes dilation and congestion of the vessels of the rectum and anus

D. Possible assessment findings
   1. Anal pain with defecation, sitting, or walking
   2. Anal pruritus
   3. Protrusion of hemorrhoids
   4. Rectal bleeding
   5. Rectal mucus discharge
   6. Bleeding during defecation
   7. Sensation of incomplete fecal evacuation

E. Possible diagnostic test findings
   1. Digital exam: hemorrhoids
   2. Barium enema: hemorrhoids
   3. Proctoscopy: internal hemorrhoids
   4. Hematology: decreased Hgb, HCT

F. Medical management
   1. Diet: high-fiber, low-roughage with increased fluid intake
   2. Position: side-lying or prone
   3. Activity: as tolerated
   4. Monitoring: VS, frequency of stools
   5. Laboratory studies: Hgb, HCT
   6. Treatments: witch hazel compresses, sitz baths
   7. Corticosteroid: hydrocortisone (Hydrocortisone Cream)
   8. Analgesic: acetaminophen (Tylenol)
   9. Antipruritic: diphenhydramine (Benadryl)
   10. Stool softener: docusate sodium (Colace)
   11. Anesthetic: lidocaine hydrochloride (Xylocaine)
   12. Laxative: magnesium hydroxide (milk of magnesia)
   13. Cryodestruction

G. Nursing interventions
   1. Maintain the patient's diet with increased fluids
   2. Assess bowel elimination and rectal bleeding
   3. Keep the patient on the side or prone
   4. Monitor and record VS, I/O, and laboratory studies
   5. Administer medications, as prescribed
   6. Allay the patient's anxiety
   7. Provide perineal care
   8. Administer sitz baths and witch hazel compresses
   9. Provide privacy and time for defecation
   10. Individualize home care instructions
       a. Use sitz baths and witch hazel compresses
       b. Defecate when urge is felt
       c. Avoid constipation
       d. Complete perineal care daily
       e. Avoid prolonged sitting or standing
       f. Avoid heavy lifting
       g. Recognize the signs and symptoms of rectal bleeding

H. Possible complications
   1. Megacolon
   2. Diverticulitis
   3. Hemorrhage

I. Possible surgical interventions
   1. Hemorrhoidectomy (see page 161)
   2. Barron rubber-band ligation

♦ **XXI. Colorectal cancer**

A. Definition—malignant tumor of the colon or rectum that is primary or metastatic

B. Possible etiology
   1. Diverticulosis
   2. Chronic ulcerative colitis
   3. Familial polyposis
   4. Aging
   5. Low-fiber, high-carbohydrate diet
   6. Chronic constipation

C. Pathophysiology
   1. Unregulated cell growth and uncontrolled cell division result in the development of a neoplasm
   2. Metastasis often occurs in the liver
   3. Adenocarcinomas occur in the colon, rectum, jejunum, and duodenum
   4. Adenocarcinomas infiltrate and cause obstruction, ulcerations, and hemorrhage

D. Possible assessment findings
   1. Abdominal cramps
   2. Abdominal distention
   3. Diarrhea and constipation
   4. Weakness
   5. Pallor
   6. Weight loss
   7. Anorexia
   8. Change in shape of stool
   9. Rectal bleeding
   10. Change in bowel habits
   11. Fecal oozing
   12. Palpable mass
   13. Melena
   14. Vomiting

CLINICAL ALERT

E. Possible diagnostic test findings
   1. Fecal occult blood: positive
   2. Hematology: decreased Hgb, HCT
   3. Sigmoidoscopy: identification and location of mass
   4. Barium enema: location of mass

     5. Biopsy: cytology positive for cancer cells

     6. CEA: positive

     7. GI series: location of mass

F. Medical management

     1. Diet: high-fiber, low-fat, low-refined carbohydrate

     2. I.V. therapy: heparin lock

     3. Position: semi-Fowler's

     4. Activity: as tolerated

     5. Monitoring: VS, U/O, and I/O

     6. Laboratory studies: Hgb, HCT

     7. Nutritional support: TPN

     8. Radiation therapy

     9. Antineoplastics: doxorubicin hydrochloride (Adriamycin), 5-fluorouracil (Adrucil)

     10. Chemotherapy

     11. Immunomodulator: levamisole hydrochloride (Ergamisol)

     12. Folic acid derivative: leucovorin (citrovorum factor)

     13. Antiemetics: prochlorperazine (Compazine), ondansetron hydrochloride (Zofran)

G. Nursing interventions

     1. Maintain the patient's diet

     2. Keep the patient in semi-Fowler's position

     3. Monitor and record VS, UO, I/O, laboratory studies, and daily weight

     4. Administer TPN

     5. Administer medications, as prescribed

     6. Encourage the patient to express feelings about changes in body image and a fear of dying

     7. Provide skin and mouth care

     8. Provide rest periods

CLINICAL ALERT

     9. Monitor and record the color, consistency, amount, and frequency of stools

     10. Assess for signs of intestinal obstruction and rectal bleeding

     11. Provide postchemotherapeutic and postradiation nursing care

        a. Provide prophylactic skin and mouth care

        b. Monitor dietary intake

        c. Administer antiemetics and antidiarrheals, as prescribed

        d. Monitor for bleeding, infection, and electrolyte imbalance

        e. Provide rest periods

     12. Provide information about the United Ostomy Association and the American Cancer Society

     13. Individualize home care instructions

        a. Monitor changes in bowel elimination

  b. Monitor self for infection

  c. Alternate rest periods with activity

H. Possible complications

 1. Anemia

 2. Hemorrhage

 3. Intestinal obstruction

I. Possible surgical interventions

 1. Abdominoperineal resection (see page 162)

 2. Colostomy (see page 162)

♦ XXII. Cholecystitis

A. Definition—acute or chronic inflammation of the gallbladder; most commonly associated with cholelithiasis

B. Possible etiology

 1. Cholelithiasis: cholesterol, bile pigment, calcium stones

 2. Obesity

 3. Infection of the gallbladder

 4. Estrogen therapy

C. Pathophysiology

 1. Inflamed gallbladder cannot contract in response to fatty foods entering the duodenum because of obstruction by calculi or edema

 2. Inability to constrict causes pain

 3. Accumulated bile is absorbed into the blood

**CLINICAL
ALERT**

D. Possible assessment findings

 1. Indigestion or chest pain after eating fatty or fried foods

 2. Episodic colicky pain in epigastric area, which radiates to back and shoulder

 3. Jaundice

 4. Nausea and vomiting

 5. Elevated temperature

 6. Flatulence

 7. Belching

 8. Clay-colored stools

 9. Dark amber urine

 10. Pruritus

 11. Ecchymosis

 12. Steatorrhea

E. Possible diagnostic test findings

 1. Cholangiogram: stones in biliary tree

 2. Gallbladder series: stones in biliary tree

 3. Ultrasound: bile duct distention and calculi

 4. Liver scan: obstruction of biliary tree

     5. Blood chemistry: increased alkaline phosphatase, bilirubin, direct bilirubin transaminase, amylase, lipase, AST, and LDH

     6. Hematology: increased WBCs

F. Medical management

     1. Diet: two types

       a. Low-fat, high-carbohydrate, high-protein, high-fiber, low-calorie in small, frequent feedings with restricted intake of gas-forming foods

       b. No foods and fluids, as directed

     2. I.V. therapy: hydration, electrolyte replacement, heparin lock

     3. GI decompression: NG tube, Miller-Abbott tube

     4. Position: semi-Fowler's

     5. Activity: bed rest

     6. Monitoring: VS, U/O, I/O, and specific gravity

     7. Laboratory studies: amylase, lipase, bilirubin, alkaline phosphatase, and WBCs

     8. Treatments: incentive spirometry, tepid baths without soap

     9. Antilithic: chenodiol (Chenix)

     10. Antibiotic: cephalothin (Keflin)

     11. Analgesic: meperidine hydrochloride (Demerol)

     12. Anticholinergics: propantheline bromide (Pro-Banthine), dicyclomine hydrochloride (Bentyl)

     13. Antiemetic: prochlorperazine (Compazine)

     14. Antipruritic: diphenhydramine (Benadryl)

     15. Vitamins: phytonadione (AquaMEPHYTON), cyanocobalamin (vitamin B_{12})

     16. Extracorporeal shock wave lithotripsy

     17. Endoscopic sphincterotomy

G. Nursing interventions

     1. Maintain the patient's diet; withhold food and fluids

     2. Administer I.V. fluids

     3. Provide TCDB

     4. Assess pain

     5. Maintain position, patency, and low suction of NG tube

     6. Keep the patient in semi-Fowler's position

     7. Monitor and record VS, U/O, I/O, laboratory studies, and specific gravity

     8. Administer medications, as prescribed

     9. Allay the patient's anxiety

     10. Provide skin, nares, and mouth care

     11. Maintain bed rest

     12. Maintain a quiet environment

     13. Administer tepid baths without soap

14. Prevent scratching if pruritus occurs
15. Individualize home care instructions
    a. Complete skin care daily
    b. Recognize the signs and symptoms of renal colic

H. Possible complications
1. Hemorrhage
2. Cirrhosis
3. Intestinal perforation
4. Peritonitis
5. Pancreatitis

I. Possible surgical interventions
1. Cholecystectomy (see page 156)
2. Choledochostomy (see page 156)
3. Cholecystostomy (see page 156)
4. Laparoscopic laser cholecystectomy (see page 157)

◆ XXIII. Pancreatitis

A. Definition—acute or chronic inflammation of the pancreas with vary-ing degrees of pancreatic edema, fat necrosis, and hemorrhage

B. Possible etiology
1. Biliary tract disease
2. Alcoholism
3. Hyperparathyroidism
4. Hyperlipidemia
5. Blunt trauma to pancreas or abdomen
6. Bacterial or viral infection
7. Duodenal ulcer
8. Drug induced: steroids, thiazide diuretics, oral contraceptives

C. Pathophysiology
1. Acute: pancreatic enzymes are activated in the pancreas rather than the duodenum, resulting in tissue damage and autodigestion of the pancreas
2. Chronic: chronic inflammation results in fibrosis and calcification of the pancreas, obstruction of the ducts, and destruction of the se-creting acinar cells

D. Possible assessment findings
1. Nausea and vomiting

CLINICAL
ALERT

2. Tachycardia
3. Abrupt onset of pain in epigastric area that radiates to the shoulder, substernal area, back, and flank
4. Aching, burning, stabbing, pressing pain
5. Abdominal tenderness and distention

6. Elevated temperature
7. Steatorrhea
8. Weight loss
9. Jaundice
10. Hypotension
11. Pain upon eating
12. Dyspnea
13. Decreased or absent bowel sounds
14. Positioning knee-chest, fetal, or leaning forward for comfort

E. Possible diagnostic test findings
1. CT scan: enlarged pancreas
2. Blood chemistry: increased amylase, lipase, lactic dehydrogenase, glucose, aspartate aminotransferase (AST), lipids; decreased calcium and potassium
3. Hematology: increased WBCs, RBCs
4. Grey Turner's sign: positive
5. Ultrasonography: cysts, bile duct inflammation and dilation
6. Cullen's sign: positive
7. Urine chemistry: increased amylase
8. Fecal fat: positive
9. Arteriography: fibrous tissue and calcification of pancreas
10. Glucose tolerance test: increased
11. ERCP: biliary obstruction

F. Medical management
1. Diet: low-fat, low-protein, high-carbohydrate in small, frequent feedings with restricted intake of caffeine, alcohol, and gas-forming foods
2. I.V. therapy: hydration, electrolyte replacement, heparin lock
3. GI decompression: NG tube
4. Position: semi-Fowler's
5. Activity: bed rest
6. Monitoring: VS, UO, I/O, CVP, specific gravity, and urine glucose and ketones
7. Laboratory studies: glucose, potassium, amylase, lipase, calcium, and lipids
8. Nutritional support: TPN
9. Transfusion therapy: packed RBCs
10. Antibiotic: cephalothin (Keflin)
11. Analgesic: meperidine hydrochloride (Demerol)
12. Anticholinergics: propantheline bromide (Pro-Banthine), dicyclomine hydrochloride (Bentyl)
13. Antacids: magnesium and aluminum hydroxide (Maalox), aluminum hydroxide gel (AlternaGEL)

14. Corticosteroid: hydrocortisone (Solu-Cortef)
15. Antiemetic: prochlorperazine (Compazine)
16. Histamine antagonists: cimetidine (Tagamet), ranitidine (Zantac)
17. Vitamins and minerals
18. Tranquilizers: lorazepam (Ativan), alprazolam (Xanax)
19. Digestants: pancrelipase (Viokase, Cotazym)
20. Potassium supplements: potassium chloride (K-Lor), potassium gluconate (Kaon)
21. Peritoneal lavage
22. Dialysis
23. Calcium supplements: calcium gluconate (Kalcinate), calcium carbonate (Os-Cal)
24. Antidiabetic agent: insulin
25. Mucosal barrier fortifier: sucralfate (Carafate)

G. Nursing interventions
1. Maintain the patient's diet; withhold food and fluids, as necessary
2. Administer I.V. fluids
3. Assess fluid balance
4. Maintain position, patency, and low suction of NG tube
5. Keep the patient in semi-Fowler's position
6. Monitor and record VS, UO, I/O, laboratory studies, CVP, daily weight, specific gravity, and urine glucose and ketones
7. Administer TPN
8. Administer medications, as prescribed
9. Allay the patient's anxiety
10. Provide skin, nares, and mouth care
11. Keep the patient in bed and turn every 2 hours
12. Provide a quiet, restful environment
13. Monitor urine and stool for color, character, and amount
14. Individualize home care instructions
    a. Monitor accuchecks for glucose levels
    b. Monitor stool for steatorrhea
    c. Monitor self for infection
    d. Recognize the signs and symptoms of increased blood glucose
    e. Adhere to activity limitations
    f. Alternate rest periods with activity

H. Possible complications
1. Ileus
2. Hypovolemic shock
3. Diabetes mellitus
4. Infection
5. Jaundice
6. Pancreatic fistula

7. Pancreatic abscess
8. Hypocalcemia
9. Septic shock

I. Possible surgical intervention: pancreatectomy (see page 156)

◆ XXIV. Hepatic cirrhosis

A. Definition
   1. Chronic, progressive disease characterized by inflammation, fibrosis, and degeneration of liver parenchymal cells
   2. Three types of hepatic cirrhosis
      a. Laënnec's (micronodular)
      b. Postnecrotic (macronodular)
      c. Biliary

B. Possible etiology
   1. Alcohol use or abuse
   2. Malnutrition
   3. Viral hepatitis
   4. Cholecystitis
   5. Obstructions from neoplasms, strictures, or gallstones

C. Pathophysiology
   1. Inflammation causes liver parenchymal cell destruction, with subsequent fibrosis
   2. Fibrotic changes cause obstruction of hepatic blood flow and normal liver function
   3. Obstruction causes portal hypertension
   4. Decreased liver function results in changes in body chemistry
      a. Decreased absorption and utilization of fat-soluble vitamins (A, D, E, and K)
      b. Increased secretion of aldosterone
      c. Ineffective detoxification of protein wastes

D. Possible assessment findings
   1. Nausea and vomiting
   2. Weakness and fatigue
   3. Anorexia and weight loss
   4. Jaundice
   5. Ecchymosis
   6. Palmar erythema
   7. Indigestion
   8. Pruritus
   9. Irregular bowel habits
   10. Pain in right upper quadrant
   11. Peripheral edema

12. Petechiae
13. Epistaxis
14. Hematemesis
15. Telangiectasis
16. Gynecomastia and impotence
17. Amenorrhea
18. Hemorrhoids
19. Hepatomegaly
20. Melena
21. Esophageal varices

E. Possible diagnostic test findings
   1. Blood chemistry: increased AST, ALT, LDH, alkaline phosphatase, ammonia, bilirubin, BSP; decreased albumin, total protein
   2. Hematology: decreased Hgb, HCT, WBCs; increased PT
   3. Liver scan: fibrotic liver, increased uptake
   4. Liver biopsy: destruction of parenchymal cells
   5. Esophagoscopy: esophageal varices
   6. Arterial blood gases (ABGs): metabolic acidosis, respiratory acidosis, respiratory alkalosis
   7. Urine chemistry: proteinuria
   8. CT scan: ASCITES

F. Medical management
   1. Diet: high-calorie, high-carbohydrate, low-fat, low-sodium in small, frequent feedings with restricted intake of alcohol and fluids
   2. I.V. therapy: hydration, electrolyte replacement, heparin lock
   3. Oxygen therapy
   4. GI decompression: NG tube
   5. Position: semi-Fowler's
   6. Activity: bed rest
   7. Monitoring: VS, U/O, I/O, neurovital signs, ECG, hemodynamic variables, and stools for occult blood
   8. Laboratory studies: AST, ALT, LDH, PT, amylase, lipase, Hgb, HCT, bilirubin, albumin, WBCs, and ABGs
   9. Nutritional support: TPN, NG feedings
   10. Treatments: indwelling urinary catheter; incentive spirometry; tepid bath; cool, moist compresses

CLINICAL ALERT

   11. Precautions: standard
   12. Transfusion therapy: platelets, packed RBCs, fresh frozen plasma (FFP)
   13. Antibiotic: neomycin sulfate (Neobiotic)
   14. Diuretics: spironolactone (Aldactone), furosemide (Lasix)
   15. Sedative: phenobarbital (Luminal)
   16. Stool softener: docusate sodium (Colace)

17. Ammonia detoxicant: lactulose (Cephulac)
18. Vitamins: phytonadione (AquaMEPHYTON), cyanocobalamin (vitamin B_{12})
19. Antacids: magnesium and aluminum hydroxide (Maalox), aluminum hydroxide gel (AlternaGEL)
20 Analgesic: oxycodone hydrochloride (Tylox)
21. Enzyme replacement: pancrelipase (Viokase)
22. Endoscopy sclerotherapy: ethanolamine oleate (Ethamolin)
23. Abdominal paracentesis
24. Balloon tamponade of varices: Sengstaken-Blakemore tube

G. Nursing interventions
1. Maintain the patient's diet; withhold food and fluids, as necessary
2. Administer I.V. fluids
3. Administer oxygen
4. Provide TCDB, incentive spirometry
5. Assess respiratory status, GI bleeding, and fluid balance
6. Maintain position, patency, and low suction of NG tube
7. Keep the patient in semi-Fowler's position
8. Monitor and record VS, UO, I/O, laboratory studies, hemodynamic variables, daily weight, specific gravity, fecal occult blood, and neurovital signs
9. Measure and record the patient's abdominal girth
10. Monitor for infection
11. Administer TPN
12. Administer medications, as prescribed
13. Allay the patient's anxiety
14. Provide skin, nares, and mouth care
15. Maintain universal precautions
16. Maintain bed rest
17. Maintain a quiet environment
18. Administer tepid baths without soap; apply cool, moist compresses

19. Prevent scratching
20. Use small-gauge needles to decrease risk of bleeding; avoid I.M. injections where possible
21. Apply prolonged pressure after venipuncture
22. Monitor stool for color, consistency, and amount
23. Provide information on Alcoholics Anonymous (AA)
24. Individualize home care instructions
    a. Avoid using over-the-counter medications
    b. Avoid using alcohol
    c. Avoid exposure to people with infections
    d. Know the action, adverse effects, and scheduling of medications
    e. Complete skin care daily

   f. Avoid straining while defecating, vigorously blowing nose, cough-
      ing, and using a hard toothbrush

H. Possible complications
   1. Ascites
   2. Esophageal varices
   3. Hemorrhoids
   4. Hemorrhage
   5. Estrogen and androgen imbalance
   6. Portal hypertension
   7. Hepatic coma
   8. Pancytopenia

I. Possible surgical interventions
   1. Portacaval shunt (see page 158)
   2. LeVeen peritoneovenous shunt
   3. TIPS (see page 158)

◆ **XXV. Hepatitis**

A. Definition
   1. Inflammation of the liver
   2. Five types of hepatitis
      a. Hepatitis A (formerly infectious)
      b. Hepatitis B (formerly serum)
      c. Hepatitis C (post-transfusion hepatitis)
      d. Hepatitis D
      e. Hepatitis E

B. Possible etiology, transmission
   1. Hepatitis A: Contaminated food, milk, water, feces (food-borne
      most common)
   2. Hepatitis B: Parenteral, sexual, oral
   3. Hepatitis C: blood or serum (blood transfusions, exposure to con-
      taminated blood)
   4. Hepatitis D: Similar to type B virus (HBV)
   5. Hepatitis E: Fecal, oral route

C. Pathophysiology
   1. Inflammation of liver tissue causes inflammation of hepatic cells, hy-
      pertrophy, and proliferation of Kupffer's cells and bile stasis
   2. Type A virus (HAV) is transmitted by fecal or oral route and causes
      hepatitis A
   3. HBV is transmitted by blood and body fluids and causes hepatitis B

D. Possible assessment findings
   1. Preicteric
      a. Anorexia
      b. Nausea and vomiting
      c. Fatigue
      d. Constipation and diarrhea
      e. Weight loss
      f. Right upper quadrant pain
      g. Hepatomegaly
      h. Splenomegaly
      i. Malaise
      j. Elevated temperature
      k. Pharyngitis
      l. Nasal discharge
      m. Headache
      n. Pruritus
   2. Icteric
      a. Fatigue
      b. Weight loss
      c. Clay-colored stools
      d. Dark urine
      e. Hepatomegaly
      f. Jaundice
      g. Splenomegaly
      h. Pruritus
   3. Posticteric
      a. Fatigue
      b. Decreasing hepatomegaly
      c. Decreasing jaundice
      d. Improved appetite

CLINICAL ALERT

E. Possible diagnostic test findings
   1. Blood chemistry: increased ALT, AST, alkaline phosphatase, LDH, bilirubin, ESR, positive anti-HAV (IgM) or positive hepatitis B surface (antigen)
   2. Hematology: increased PT
   3. BSP: increased
   4. Urine chemistry: increased urobilinogen
   5. Stool: hepatitis A virus

F. Medical management
   1. Diet: high-calorie, moderate-protein, high-carbohydrate, and low-fat
   2. Activity: bed rest
   3. Monitoring: VS, UO, and I/O

4. Laboratory studies: ALT, AST, LDH, bilirubin, PT, and PTT

5. Precautions: standard

6. Antiemetic: prochlorperazine (Compazine)

7. Vitamins and minerals: vitamin K (AquaMEPHYTON), Vitamin C, B-complex

G. Nursing interventions

1. Maintain the patient's diet

2. Monitor and record VS, UO, I/O, and laboratory studies

3. Administer medications, as prescribed

4. Allay the patient's anxiety

5. Maintain standard precautions

6. Provide rest periods

7. Encourage small, frequent meals

8. Avoid skin irritation

9. Prevent complications of bleeding

10. Individualize home care instructions

   a. Administer gammaglobulin to individuals exposed to hepatitis

   b. Avoid exposure to people with infections

   c. Avoid alcohol

   d. Maintain good personal hygiene

   e. Refrain from donating blood

   f. Increase fluid intake to 3,000 ml/day

   g. Abstain from sexual intercourse until serum liver studies are within normal limits

H. Possible complications

1. Pancreatitis

2. Aplastic anemia

3. Glomerulonephritis

4. Vasculitis

5. Cirrhosis

I. Possible surgical interventions: none

◆ **XXVI. Esophageal varices**

A. Definition—dilation of esophageal veins in the lower part of the esophagus

B. Possible etiology

1. Portal hypertension

2. Increased intra-abdominal pressure

3. Alcohol abuse

4. Cirrhosis

C. Pathophysiology
1. Venous drainage from the liver into the portal vein is decreased
2. Drainage obstruction results in portal hypertension
3. Return of venous blood from the intestinal tract and spleen to the right atrium via the collateral circulation is obstructed
4. The increased pressure dilates the esophageal veins, which then protrude into the esophageal lumen

D. Possible assessment findings
1. Anorexia
2. Nausea and vomiting
3. Hematemesis
4. Fatigue and weakness
5. Splenomegaly
6. Ascites
7. Peripheral edema
8. Melena
9. Dysphagia
10. Pallor

E. Possible diagnostic test findings
1. Hematology: increased PT; decreased RBCs, Hgb, HCT
2. Blood chemistry: increased BUN, LDH, AST; decreased albumin
3. Barium swallow: narrowed and irregular esophagus
4. Esophagoscopy: varices

F. Medical management
1. Diet: soft; withhold food and fluids with active bleeding
2. I.V. therapy: hydration, heparin lock
3. Oxygen therapy
4. GI decompression: NG tube
5. Position: semi-Fowler's
6. Activity: bed rest
7. Monitoring: VS, UO, and I/O
8. Laboratory studies: Hgb, HCT, PT, and PTT
9. Treatments: indwelling urinary catheter
10. Transfusion therapy: packed RBCs, FFP
11. Esophageal balloon tamponade: Sengstaken-Blakemore or Minnesota tube
12. Paracentesis
13. Endoscopy sclerotherapy: ethanolamine oleate (Ethamolin)
14. Diuretic: furosemide (Lasix)
15. Hormone: I.V. vasopressin (Pitressin) with nitroglycerin therapy
16. Antacids: magnesium and aluminum hydroxide (Maalox), aluminum hydroxide gel (AlternaGEL)
17. Histamine antagonists: cimetidine (Tagamet), ranitidine (Zantac)

18. Vitamins: vitamin K (AquaMEPHYTON)
19. Iced saline lavage by NG tube
20. Stool softener: docusate sodium (Colace)
21. Mucosal barrier fortifier: sucralfate (Carafate)

G. Nursing interventions
  1. Withhold food and fluids
  2. Administer I.V. fluids
  3. Administer oxygen
  4. Assess cardiovascular and respiratory status
  5. Maintain position, patency, and low suction of NG tube and Sengstaken-Blakemore tube

CLINICAL ALERT

  a. Maintain emergency measures for gastric balloon rupture
  b. Have suction, scissors to cut tube available
  6. Keep the patient in semi-Fowler's position
  7. Monitor and record VS, UO, I/O, laboratory studies, CVP, and daily weight
  8. Administer medications, as prescribed
  9. Allay the patient's anxiety
  10. Provide nares and mouth care

CLINICAL ALERT

  11. Minimize environmental stress
  12. Check for signs of bleeding
  13. Avoid activities that increase intra-abdominal pressure
  14. Monitor and record amount, color, frequency, and consistency of stools

CLINICAL ALERT

  15. Assess level of consciousness and impending encephalopathy
  16. Provide information about AA
  17. Individualize home care instructions
    a. Monitor stools for occult blood
    b. Avoid lifting and straining
    c. Avoid using alcohol

H. Possible complications
  1. Hemorrhage
  2. Shock
  3. Metabolic imbalance

I. Possible surgical interventions
  1. Ligation of varices
  2. Portacaval shunt (see page 158)
  3. Splenorenal shunt (see page 158)
  4. Mesocaval shunt (see page 158)
  5. TIPS (see page 158)

POINTS TO REMEMBER

♦ Occult blood in stool and emesis is a common finding in GI disorders.

♦ Imposed changes in eating and bowel habits may result in social isolation.

♦ Peritonitis, pneumonia, atelectasis, and hemorrhage are potential complications of gallbladder surgeries.

STUDY QUESTIONS

To evaluate your understanding of this chapter, answer the following questions in the space provided; then compare your responses with the correct answers in Appendix B, pages 383 and 384.

1. What are the nursing interventions before and after an endoscopy? _____
   _____
   _____

2. What are the key teaching goals for a patient after pancreatic surgery? _____
   _____
   _____

3. What are the home care instructions for a patient with a hiatal hernia? _____
   _____
   _____

4. Which foods should the patient with a gastric ulcer avoid? _____
   _____
   _____

5. What are the assessment findings in a patient with intestinal obstruction?__
   _____
   _____

6. How are type A and type B hepatitis transmitted? _____
   _____
   _____

CRITICAL THINKING AND APPLICATION EXERCISES

1. Observe a colonoscopy. Prepare an oral presentation for your fellow students, describing the procedure and patient care before, during, and after the procedure.

2. Develop a chart comparing the major drug classes used for treating gastric ulcers.

3. Interview a patient with colorectal cancer. Evaluate the information for possible risk factors and identify ways to modify them.

4. Follow a patient with a GI disorder from admission through discharge. Develop a patient-specific plan of care, including any needs for follow-up and home care.

CHAPTER

6

Endocrine System

CHAPTER OVERVIEW

Caring for the patient with an endocrine disorder requires a sound understanding of endocrine anatomy and physiology and fluid and electrolyte balance. A thorough assessment is essential to planning and implementing appropriate patient care. The assessment includes a complete history, physical examination, diagnostic testing, identification of modifiable and nonmodifiable risk factors, and information related to the psychosocial impact of the disorder on the patient. Nursing diagnoses focus primarily on altered nutrition, fluid volume excess or deficit, and body image disturbance. Nursing interventions are designed to assess patient hydration and nutritional status, teach the patient and family about long-term use of medications, and assist the patient in adjusting to changes in body image and the effects of chronic illness. Patient teaching — a crucial nursing activity — involves information about medical follow-up, medication regimens, signs and symptoms of possible complications, and reduction of modifiable risk factors through adherence to dietary and medication recommendations and restrictions.

◆ I. Anatomy and physiology review

A. Hypothalamus
1. Controls temperature, respiration, and blood pressure
2. Affects the emotional states of fear, anxiety, anger, rage, pleasure, and pain
3. Produces hypothalamic-stimulating hormones, which affect the inhibition and release of pituitary hormones

B. Pituitary gland
1. Considered the "master gland"
2. Composed of anterior and posterior lobes
   a. Posterior lobe (neurohypophysis) secretes VASOPRESSIN (antidiuretic hormone: ADH) and oxytocin
   b. Anterior lobe (adenohypophysis) secretes follicle-stimulating hormone (FSH), luteinizing hormone (LH), prolactin, adrenocorticotropic hormone (ACTH), thyroid-stimulating hormone (TSH), and growth hormone (GH)
3. Affects all hormonal activity; factors altering pituitary gland function affect all hormonal activity

C. Thyroid gland
1. Accelerates cellular reactions, including basal metabolic rate (BMR) and growth
2. Controlled by secretion of TSH
3. Produces thyroxine (T4), tri-iodothyronine (T3), and thyrocalcitonin

D. Parathyroid glands
1. Secrete parathyroid hormone (parathormone: PTH), which regulates calcium and phosphorus metabolism
2. Require active form of vitamin D for PTH function

E. Adrenal glands
1. Adrenal cortex secretes three major hormones
   a. Glucocorticoids (cortisol)
   b. MINERALOCORTICOIDS (aldosterone)
   c. Sex hormones (androgens, estrogens, and progesterone)
2. Adrenal medulla secretes two hormones
   a. Norepinephrine
   b. Epinephrine

F. Pancreas
  1. Accessory gland of digestion
     a. Exocrine function: secretion of digestive enzymes
        (1) Amylase
        (2) Lipase
        (3) Trypsin
     b. Endocrine function: secretion of hormones from islets of Langerhans
        (1) Insulin
        (2) Glucagon
        (3) Somatostatin
  2. Main pancreatic duct joins the common bile duct and empties into the duodenum at the ampulla of Vater

♦ II. Assessment findings

A. History
  1. Changes in weight; hair quality and distribution; body proportions, muscle mass, and fat distribution
  2. Fatigue and weakness
  3. Change in mood or behavior
  4. Anorexia
  5. Constipation, diarrhea, urinary frequency
  6. Change in menses and libido
  7. History of infections
  8. Intolerance of heat or cold

B. Physical examination
  1. Vital sign (VS) changes
  2. Skin color and temperature changes
  3. Change in level of consciousness
  4. Pattern and character of respirations
  5. Change in urinary patterns
  6. Change in thirst
  7. Abnormalities of nails
  8. Change in visual acuity

♦ III. Diagnostic tests and procedures

A. Hematologic studies
  1. Definition and purpose
     a. Laboratory test of a blood sample
     b. Analysis for white blood cells (WBCs), red blood cells (RBCs), erythrocyte sedimentation rate (ESR), platelets, prothrombin time (PT), partial thromboplastin time (PTT), hemoglobin (Hgb), and hematocrit (HCT)

      2. Nursing interventions
         a. Note current drug therapy that might alter test results
         b. Check the venipuncture site for bleeding after the procedure

B. Blood chemistry
      1. Definition and purpose
         a. Laboratory test of a blood sample
         b. Analysis for potassium, sodium, calcium, phosphorus, ketones, glucose, osmolality, chloride, blood urea nitrogen (BUN), creatinine, T_3, T_4, protein-bound iodine (PBI), cortisol
      2. Nursing interventions
         a. Withhold food and fluids, as directed, before the procedure
         b. Check for recent studies using radiopaque dyes that may alter test results
         c. Note pregnancy
         d. List current medications that contain iodine
         e. Check the venipuncture site for bleeding after the procedure

C. Fasting serum glucose and two-hour postprandial glucose test
      1. Definition and purpose
         a. Laboratory test of a blood sample
         b. Analysis to measure the body's use and disposal of glucose
      2. Nursing interventions
         a. Withhold food and fluids for 8 hours before fasting sample is drawn
         b. Withhold insulin until the test is completed
         c. Administer 100 g of glucose orally, and request the laboratory to draw blood 2 hours later

CLINICAL ALERT

         d. Assess the patient for hypoglycemia or hyperglycemia

D. Glucose tolerance test (GTT)
      1. Definition and purpose
         a. Laboratory test of blood and urine
         b. Analysis to measure absorption of carbohydrates
      2. Nursing interventions
         a. List any medications that might interfere with the test
         b. Note pregnancy, trauma, or infectious disease
         c. Provide the patient with a high-carbohydrate diet 2 days before the test; then have the patient fast for 12 hours before the test
         d. Instruct the patient to avoid smoking, caffeine, alcohol, and exercise for 8 hours before the procedure
         e. Withhold all medications after midnight
         f. Obtain fasting serum glucose and urine specimen
         g. Administer test load oral glucose, and record time
         h. Request laboratory collection of serum glucose and urine specimens at 30, 60, 120, and 180 minutes

      i. Refrigerate samples

      j. Assess the patient for hyperglycemia or hypoglycemia

E. Adrenocorticotropic hormone (ACTH) stimulation test

  1. Definition and purpose

    a. Laboratory test of a blood sample

    b. Analysis for cortisol

  2. Nursing interventions

    a. List any medications that might interfere with the test

    b. Monitor 24-hour I.V. infusion of ACTH after baseline serum sample is drawn

    c. Check the venipuncture site for bleeding

F. Dexamethasone suppression test

  1. Definition and purpose

    a. Laboratory test of urine samples

    b. Analysis of serum cortisol and urinary 17-hydroxycorticosteroids (17-OHCS) after administration of dexamethasone

  2. Nursing interventions

    a. Administer dexamethasone and an antacid, as prescribed

    b. Obtain single urine and 24-hour urine samples, as directed

    c. List any medications that might interfere with the test

G. 24-hour urine test for 17-ketosteroids (17-KS) and 17-OHCS

  1. Definition and purpose

    a. Laboratory test of urine samples

    b. Quantitative laboratory analysis of urine collected over 24 hours to determine hormone precursors

  2. Nursing interventions

    a. Withhold all medications for 48 hours before the test

    b. Instruct the patient to void and note the time (collection of urine starts with the next voiding)

    c. Place urine container on ice

    d. Measure each voided urine

    e. Instruct the patient to void at the end of the 24-hour period

    f. List any medications that might interfere with the test

H. Urine vanillylmandelic acid (VMA) test

  1. Definition and purpose

    a. Laboratory test of urine samples

    b. Quantitative analysis of urine collected over 24 hours to determine the end products of catecholamine metabolism (epinephrine and norepinephrine)

2. Nursing interventions

   a. List any medications, previous tests, and medical conditions that might interfere with the test

   b. Restrict foods that contain vanilla, coffee, tea, citrus fruits, bananas, nuts, and chocolate for 3 days before 24-hour urine collection

   c. Instruct the patient to void and note the time (collection of urine starts with the next voiding)

   d. Place urine container on ice

   e. Measure each voided urine

   f. Instruct the patient to void at the end of the 24-hour period

I. BMR

  1. Definition and purpose

   a. Noninvasive test

   b. Indirect measurement of oxygen consumed by the body during a given time

  2. Nursing interventions

   a. List medications taken before the procedure

   b. Note environmental and emotional stressors

J. Visual acuity and field testing

  1. Definition and purpose

   a. Noninvasive test

   b. Measurement of central and peripheral vision

  2. Nursing interventions

   a. Ask the patient to wear or bring corrective lenses for the test

   b. Determine the patient's hearing and ability to follow directions

K. Computerized tomography (CT)

  1. Definition and purpose

   a. Noninvasive scan that may use I.V. injection of contrast dye

   b. Visualization of the sella turcica and abdomen

  2. Nursing interventions

   a. Explain the procedure

   b. Note the patient's allergies to iodine, seafood, and radiopaque dyes

   c. Allay the patient's anxiety

   d. Inform the patient about possible throat irritation and flushing of the face

L. Ultrasonography

  1. Definition and purpose

   a. Noninvasive procedure using echoes from sound waves

   b. Visualization of the thyroid, pelvis, and abdomen

2. Nursing interventions
    a Withhold food and fluids 8 to 12 hours before the test
    b. Determine the patient's ability to lie still
    c. Ask the patient not to smoke or chew gum for 8 to 12 hours be-
       fore the test
    d. Administer an enema before the procedure, as directed
    e. Remove abdominal dressing before the procedure

M. Closed percutaneous thyroid biopsy
  1. Definition and purpose
    a. Procedure involving a percutaneous, sterile aspiration of a small
       amount of thyroid tissue
    b. Histologic evaluation
  2. Nursing interventions before the procedure
    a. Withhold food and fluids after midnight
    b. Place obtained written, informed consent in patient's chart
  3. Nursing interventions after the procedure
    a. Maintain bed rest for 24 hours
    b. Monitor VS

CLINICAL ALERT

    c. Check the biopsy site for bleeding
    d. Assess the patient for esophageal or tracheal puncture

N. Thyroid uptake (radioactive iodine uptake: RAIU)
  1. Definition and purpose
    a. Procedure using oral or I.V. radioactive iodine
    b. Measurement of the amount of radioactive iodine taken up by
       the thyroid gland in 24 hours
  2. Nursing interventions before the procedure
    a. Advise the patient not to eat iodine-rich foods, such as iodized
       salt or shellfish, for 24 hours before the test
    b. Discontinue all thyroid and cough medications 7 to 10 days be-
       fore the test
    c. Schedule a thyroid scan before tests using iodine-based dyes

O. Thyroid scan
  1. Definition and purpose
    a. Procedure using an oral or I.V. radioactive isotope
    b. Visual imaging of radioactivity distribution in the thyroid gland
  2. Nursing interventions before the procedure
    a. Advise the patient not to eat iodine-rich foods, such as iodized
       salt or shellfish, for 24 hours before the test
    b. Discontinue all thyroid and cough medications 7 to 10 days be-
       fore the test
    c. Schedule the scan before other tests using iodine-based dyes or ra-
       dioactive iodine

P. Arteriography
  1. Definition and purpose
    a. Procedure using an injection of a radiopaque dye through a catheter
    b. Fluoroscopic examination of the arterial blood supply to the parathyroid, adrenal, or pancreatic glands
  2. Nursing interventions before the procedure

CLINICAL ALERT

    a. Obtain written, informed consent
    b. Note the patient's allergies to iodine, seafood, and radiopaque dyes
    c. Inform the patient about possible throat irritation and flushing of the face after the dye injection
    d. Withhold food and fluids after midnight
  3. Nursing interventions after the procedure
    a. Monitor VS
    b. Check the insertion site for bleeding

Q. Sulkowitch's test
  1. Definition and purpose
    a. Laboratory test of urine
    b. Analysis to measure the amount of calcium being excreted
  2. Nursing interventions
    a. If hypercalcemia is indicated, collect a single urine sample before a meal
    b. If hypocalcemia is indicated, collect a single urine sample after a meal

♦ **IV. Psychosocial impact of endocrine disorders**

A. Developmental impact
  1. Decreased self-esteem
  2. Changes in body image
  3. Embarrassment from the changes in body function and structure, such as changes in secondary sex characteristics and sexual functioning

B. Economic impact
  1. Disruption of employment
  2. Cost of vocational retraining
  3. Cost of medications
  4. Cost of special diet
  5. Cost of hospitalizations and follow-up care

C. Occupational and recreational impact
  1. Physical activity restrictions
  2. Adjustment to change in occupation

    D. Social impact

       1. Social withdrawal and isolation

       2. Changes in eating patterns

       3. Changes in role performance

       4. Changes in sexual function

◆ V. Possible risk factors

    A. Modifiable risk factors

       1. Medication

       2. Stress

       3. Diet

       4. Obesity

    B. Nonmodifiable risk factors

       1. Family history of endocrine illness

       2. History of trauma

       3. Aging

◆ VI. Nursing diagnostic categories

    A. Probable nursing diagnostic categories

       1. Fluid volume excess

       2. Risk for fluid volume deficit

       3. Altered nutrition: potential for more than body requirements

       4. Body image disturbance

       5. Altered urinary elimination

       6. Altered nutrition: less than body requirements

    B. Possible nursing diagnostic categories

       1. Risk for injury

       2. Social isolation

       3. Knowledge deficit

       4. Noncompliance

       5. Sensory/perceptual alteration: visual

       6. Sensory/perceptual alteration: tactile

       7. Risk for impaired skin integrity

       8. Altered thought processes

◆ VII. Adrenalectomy

    A. Description—surgical removal of one or both adrenal glands

    B. Preoperative nursing interventions

       1. Complete patient and family preoperative teaching

          a. Determine the patient's understanding of the procedure

          b. Describe the operating room (OR), postanesthesia care unit (PACU), and preoperative and postoperative routines

    c. Demonstrate postoperative turning, coughing, and deep breathing (TCDB); splinting; leg exercises; and range-of-motion (ROM) exercises

    d. Explain the postoperative need for drainage tubes, surgical dressings, oxygen therapy, I.V. therapy, and pain control

2. Complete a preoperative checklist
3. Administer preoperative medications, as prescribed
4. Allay the patient's and family's anxiety about surgery
5. Document the patient's history and physical assessment data base
6. Administer steroids, as prescribed
7. Administer vasopressors, as prescribed

C. Postoperative nursing interventions

1. Assess cardiac, respiratory, and neurologic status and fluid balance

    a. Monitor fluid intake and output and serum electrolyte levels

    b. Keep in mind that adrenalectomy disturbs mineralocorticoid and glucocorticoid secretion, resulting in altered fluid and electrolyte balance

CLINICAL ALERT

2. Assess pain and administer postoperative analgesics, as prescribed
3. Assess for return of peristalsis; provide solid foods and liquids, as tolerated
4. Administer I.V. fluids
5. Allay the patient's anxiety
6. Inspect the surgical dressing and change, as directed
7. Reinforce TCDB and splinting of incision
8. Keep the patient in semi-Fowler's position
9. Provide incentive spirometry
10. Maintain activity, as tolerated
11. Monitor VS, urinary output (UO), intake and output (I/O), central venous pressure (CVP), laboratory studies, electrocardiogram (ECG), neurovital signs, daily weight, specific gravity, urine for glucose and ketones, and pulse oximetry
12. Monitor and maintain position and patency of drainage tubes: nasogastric (NG), indwelling urinary catheter, and wound drainage
13. Encourage the patient to express feelings about changes in body image and the need for lifelong medication replacement
14. Administer antacids, as prescribed
15. Maintain a quiet environment
16. Administer hormone replacements, as prescribed
17. Administer vasopressors, as prescribed
18. Individualize home care instructions

    a. Recognize the signs and symptoms of infection, hypovolemia, and hypoglycemia

    b. Avoid exposure to people with infections

    c. Complete incision care daily, as directed

    d. Comply with lifelong hormone replacement
    e. Monitor blood pressure daily
    f. Explore methods to reduce insomnia
    g. Avoid extreme temperatures

D. Possible surgical complications
1. Shock
2. Hypoglycemia
3. Hemorrhage
4. Peptic ulcers
5. Adrenal crisis
6. Pneumothorax
7. Acute renal failure
8. Infection

♦ VIII. Hypophysectomy

A. Description—surgical removal of part or all of the pituitary gland

B. Preoperative nursing interventions
1. Complete patient and family preoperative teaching
    a. Determine the patient's understanding of the procedure
    b. Describe the OR, PACU, and preoperative and postoperative routines
    c. Demonstrate postoperative TCDB, splinting, and leg and ROM exercises
    d. Explain the postoperative need for drainage tubes, surgical dressings, oxygen therapy, I.V. therapy, and pain control
2. Complete a preoperative checklist
3. Administer preoperative medications, as prescribed
4. Allay the patient's and family's anxiety about surgery
5. Document the patient's history and physical assessment data base
6. Administer steroids, as prescribed
7. Administer antibiotics, as prescribed

C. Postoperative nursing interventions
1. Assess cardiac, respiratory, and neurologic status and fluid balance
2. Assess pain and administer postoperative analgesics, as prescribed
3. Assess for return of peristalsis: provide solid foods and liquids, as tolerated
4. Administer I.V. fluids
5. Allay the patient's anxiety
6. Inspect the surgical dressing or nasal drip pad and change, as directed
7. Reinforce TCDB
8. Keep the patient in semi-Fowler's position
9. Provide incentive spirometry

10. Maintain activity, as tolerated
11. Monitor VS, UO, I/O, CVP, laboratory studies, neurovital signs, daily weight, specific gravity, urine glucose and ketones, and pulse oximetry
12. Monitor and maintain the position and patency of the indwelling urinary catheter
13. Institute seizure precaution
14. Encourage the patient to express feelings about changes in body image and a fear of dying
15. Administer antibiotics, as prescribed

CLINICAL ALERT

16. Administer hormone replacements, as prescribed
17. Observe the patient for signs of increased intracranial pressure (ICP)
18. Check for rhinorrhea
19. Provide mouth and eye care
20. Avoid brushing the patient's teeth
21. Administer stool softeners, as prescribed
22. Individualize home care instructions
    a. Recognize the signs and symptoms of infection, seizure activity, and hormone deficiencies
    b. Avoid coughing, blowing nose, lifting, straining while defecating, and sneezing
    c. Comply with lifelong hormone replacement

D. Possible surgical complications
1. Diabetes insipidus
2. Increased ICP
3. Hemorrhage
4. Adrenal crisis
5. Thyroid storm
6. Meningitis
7. Diplopia

◆ IX. Thyroid and parathyroid surgeries

A. Description
1. Thyroidectomy: surgical removal of part or all of the thyroid gland
2. Parathyroidectomy: surgical removal of one or more parathyroid glands

B. Preoperative nursing interventions
1. Complete patient and family preoperative teaching
    a. Determine the patient's understanding of the procedure
    b. Describe the OR, PACU, and preoperative and postoperative routines
    c. Demonstrate postoperative TCDB, splinting, and leg and ROM exercises

       d. Explain the postoperative need for drainage tubes, surgical dressings, oxygen therapy, I.V. therapy, and pain control

   2. Complete a preoperative checklist

   3. Administer preoperative medications, as prescribed

   4. Allay the patient's and family's anxiety about surgery

   5. Document the patient's history and physical assessment data base

   6. Administer iodine preparations and antithyroid medications, as prescribed

  C. Postoperative nursing interventions

   1. Assess respiratory status

   2. Assess pain and administer postoperative analgesics, as prescribed

   3. Assess for return of peristalsis: provide solid foods and liquids, as tolerated

   4. Administer I.V. fluids

CLINICAL ALERT

   5. Allay the patient's anxiety

   6. Inspect the surgical dressing for bleeding, especially at the back of the neck, and change dressing, as directed

   7. Reinforce TCDB and splinting of incision

   8. Keep the patient in semi-Fowler's position, with neutral alignment and support to neck

   9. Provide incentive spirometry

  10. Maintain activity, as tolerated

  11. Provide humidified cold steam nebulizer

  12. Monitor VS, UO, I/O, CVP, laboratory studies, urine glucose and ketones, and pulse oximetry

CLINICAL ALERT

  13. Monitor and maintain position and patency of wound drainage tubes

  14. Maintain seizure precautions

CLINICAL ALERT

  15. Encourage the patient to express feelings about a fear of choking or loss of the voice

  16. Assess for tetany

  17. Assess for hoarseness and aphasia

  18. Assess for thyroid storm

  19. Have calcium gluconate and tracheostomy tray available

  20. Discourage talking

  21. Provide specific parathyroidectomy care

     a. Provide a high-calcium diet with vitamin D

     b. Administer calcium and vitamin D supplements, as prescribed

  22. Individualize home care instructions

     a. Recognize the signs and symptoms of infection, seizure activity, and hypothyroidism

     b. Alternate periods of talking with voice rest

     c. Complete incision care daily, as directed

     d. Complete ROM exercises of the neck daily

D. Possible surgical complications
1. Hypocalcemia
2. Laryngeal nerve damage
3. Hypothyroidism
4. Respiratory distress
5. Hemorrhage
6. Arrhythmias

◆ X. Hyperthyroidism

A. Definition—increased synthesis of thyroid hormone from overactivity (Graves' disease) or change in thyroid gland (toxic nodular goiter)

B. Possible etiology
1. Autoimmune disease
2. Genetic
3. Psychological or physiologic stress
4. Thyroid adenomas
5. Pituitary tumors
6. Infection

C. Pathophysiology
1. Thyroid-stimulating antibodies (TSAb) have a slow, sustained, stimulating effect on thyroid metabolism
2. Accelerated metabolism causes increased synthesis of thyroid hormone

D. Possible assessment findings
1. Anxiety
2. Flushed, smooth skin
3. Heat intolerance
4. Mood swings
5. Diaphoresis
6. Tachycardia
7. Palpitations
8. Dyspnea
9. Weakness
10. Increased hunger
11. Increased systolic blood pressure
12. Tachypnea
13. Fine hand tremors
14. Exophthalmos
15. Weight loss
16. Diarrhea
17. Hyperhidrosis
18. Bruit or thrill over thyroid

E. Possible diagnostic test findings
   1. Thyroid scan: nodules
   2. Blood chemistry: increased T_3, T_4, PBI, ^{131}Iodine; decreased TSH, cholesterol
   3. ECG: atrial fibrillation

F. Medical management
   1. Diet: high-protein, high-carbohydrate, high-calorie; restrict stimulants, such as coffee and caffeine
   2. I.V. therapy: heparin lock
   3. Activity: bed rest
   4. Monitoring: VS, I/O
   5. Laboratory studies: T_3, T_4
   6. Sedative: oxazepam (Serax)
   7. Radiation therapy
   8. Thioamides: methimazole (Tapazole), propylthiouracil (Propyl-Thyracil)
   9. Iodine preparations: potassium iodide (SSKI), radioactive iodine
   10. Adrenergic blocking agents: propranolol (Inderal), reserpine (Serpasil), guanethidine monosulfate (Ismelin)
   11. Vitamins: thiamine (vitamin B1), ascorbic acid (vitamin C)
   12. Digitalis glycoside: digoxin (Lanoxin)
   13. Glucocorticoids: cortisone acetate (Cortone), hydrocortisone sodium succinate (Solu-Cortef)
   14. I.V. glucose

CLINICAL ALERT

G. Nursing interventions
   1. Maintain the patient's diet
   2. Avoid stimulants, such as drugs and foods that contain caffeine
   3. Administer I.V. fluids
   4. Assess fluid balance
   5. Monitor and record VS, UO, I/O, and laboratory studies
   6. Administer medications, as prescribed
   7. Weigh the patient daily
   8. Provide rest periods
   9. Provide a quiet, cool environment
   10. Provide eye care
   11. Allay the patient's anxiety
   12. Encourage the patient to express feelings about changes in body image
   13. Provide postradiation nursing care
      a. Provide prophylactic skin and mouth perineal care
      b. Monitor dietary intake
      c. Provide rest periods

TEACHING TIPS
Patients with endocrine disorders

Be sure to include the following topics in your teaching plan when caring for patients with endocrine disorders.
- Follow-up appointments
- Optimal body weight maintenance
- Medication therapy including the action, adverse effects, and scheduling of medications
- Dietary recommendations and restrictions
- Fluid intake recommendations and restrictions
- Rest and activity patterns, including any limitations or restrictions
- Community agencies and resources for supportive services
- Ways to reduce stress
- Medical identification bracelet
- Safe, quiet environment

14. Individualize home care instructions (For teaching tips, see *Patients with endocrine disorders.*)
   a. Stop smoking
   b. Recognize the signs and symptoms of thyroid storm
   c. Adhere to activity limitations
   d. Avoid exposure to people with infections
   e. Monitor self for infection

CLINICAL ALERT

H. Possible medical complications
   1. Thyroid storm (thyroid crisis): tachycardia, delirium, agitation, coma, death, hyperpyrexia, dehydration, arrhythmias, diarrhea
   2. Cardiac arrhythmias
   3. Diabetes mellitus

I. Possible surgical intervention: subtotal thyroidectomy when euthyroid state is established (see page 211)

♦ XI. Hypothyroidism

A. Definition—underactive state of thyroid gland, resulting in absence or decreased secretion of thyroid hormone

B. Possible etiology
   1. Autoimmune disease: Hashimoto's thyroiditis
   2. Thyroidectomy
   3. Overuse of antithyroid drugs
   4. Malfunction of pituitary gland
   5. Use of radioactive iodine

C. Pathophysiology
  1. Thyroid gland fails to secrete a satisfactory quantity of thyroid hormone
  2. Hyposecretion of thyroid hormone results in overall decrease in metabolism

D. Possible assessment findings
  1. Fatigue
  2. Weight gain
  3. Dry, flaky skin
  4. Edema
  5. Cold intolerance
  6. Coarse hair
  7. Alopecia
  8. Thick tongue, swollen lips
  9. Mental sluggishness
  10. Menstrual disorders
  11. Constipation
  12. Hypersensitivity to narcotics, barbiturates, and anesthetics
  13. Anorexia
  14. Decreased diaphoresis
  15. Hypothermia

E. Possible diagnostic test findings
  1. Blood chemistry: decreased T_3, T_4, PBI, sodium; increased TSH, cholesterol
  2. RAIU: decreased
  3. ECG: sinus bradycardia

F. Medical management
  1. Diet: high-fiber, high-protein, low-calorie with increased fluid intake
  2. Activity: as tolerated
  3. Monitoring: VS, UO, and I/O
  4. Laboratory studies: T_3, T_4, and sodium
  5. Stool softener: docusate sodium (Colace)
  6. Thyroid hormone replacements: levothyroxine (Synthroid), liothyronine sodium (Cytomel), thyroglobulin (Proloid)

G. Nursing interventions
  1. Maintain the patient's diet
  2. Force fluids
  3. Assess fluid balance
  4. Monitor and record VS, UO, I/O, and laboratory studies
  5. Administer medications, as prescribed
  6. Encourage the patient to express feelings of depression
  7. Encourage physical activity and mental stimulation

8. Provide a warm environment

9. Avoid sedation: administer one-half to one-third the normal dose of sedatives or narcotics

10. Check for constipation and edema

11. Prevent skin breakdown

12. Provide frequent rest periods

13. Individualize home care instructions
    a. Exercise regularly
    b. Recognize the signs and symptoms of myxedema coma
    c. Monitor self for constipation
    d. Use additional protection in cold weather
    e. Limit activity in cold weather
    f. Avoid using sedatives
    g. Complete skin care daily

H. Possible medical complications
   1. Coronary artery disease
   2. Congestive heart failure (CHF)
   3. Acute organic psychosis
   4. Angina
   5. Myocardial infarction (MI)
   6. Myxedema coma: hypoventilation, hypothermia, respiratory acidosis, syncope, bradycardia, hypotension, seizures, and cerebral hypoxia

I. Possible surgical interventions: none

◆ XII. Thyroid cancer

A. Definition—malignant, primary tumor of the thyroid, which does not affect thyroid hormone secretion

B. Possible etiology
   1. Chronic overstimulation of the pituitary gland
   2. Chronic overstimulation of the thymus gland
   3. Neck radiation

C. Pathophysiology
   1. Unregulated cell growth and uncontrolled cell division result in the development of a neoplasm
   2. Papillary carcinoma: well-differentiated columnar cells form a solitary nodule in the thyroid gland that spreads to the cervical lymph nodes
   3. Follicular carcinoma: encapsulated, well-differentiated cells that invade blood vessels and lymphatics
   4. Anaplastic carcinoma: either squamous, spindle, or small round cells

5. Medullary carcinoma: solid, differentiated tumor arising from calcitonin-producing C cells

D. Possible assessment findings
   1. Enlarged thyroid gland
   2. Painless, firm, irregular, and enlarged thyroid nodule or mass
   3. Palpable cervical lymph nodes
   4. Dysphagia
   5. Hoarseness
   6. Dyspnea

E. Possible diagnostic test findings
   1. RAIU: "cold" nodule
   2. Thyroid biopsy: cytology positive for cancer cells
   3. Thyroid function tests: normal
   4. Blood chemistry: increased calcitonin, serotonin, and prostaglandins

F. Medical management
   1. Diet: high-protein, high-carbohydrate, high-calorie with supplemental feedings
   2. I.V. therapy: heparin lock
   3. Activity: as tolerated
   4. Monitoring: VS, I/O
   5. Laboratory studies: calcitonin, serotonin
   6. Radiation therapy
   7. Chemotherapy: chlorambucil (Leukeran), doxorubicin hydrochloride (Adriamycin), vincristine sulfate (Oncovin)
   8. Thyroid hormone replacements: levothyroxine (Synthroid), liothyronine sodium (Cytomel), thyroglobulin (Proloid)
   9. Pulse oximetry
   10. Antiemetics: prochlorperazine (Compazine), ondansetron (Zofran)

G. Nursing interventions

CLINICAL ALERT

   1. Maintain the patient's diet
   2. Assess respiratory status
   3. Assess ability to swallow
   4. Monitor and record VS, I/O, and laboratory studies
   5. Administer medications, as prescribed
   6. Encourage the patient to express feelings about fear of dying
   7. Provide postchemotherapeutic and postradiation nursing care
      a. Provide prophylactic skin, mouth, and perineal care
      b. Monitor dietary intake
      c. Administer antiemetics and antidiarrheals, as prescribed
      d. Monitor for bleeding, infection, and electrolyte imbalance
      e. Provide rest periods

8. Individualize home care instructions
   a. Provide information about the American Cancer Society
   b. Recognize the signs and symptoms of respiratory distress and difficulty swallowing

H. Possible medical complications
1. Laryngotracheal obstruction
2. Respiratory distress
3. Esophageal obstruction

I. Possible surgical interventions
1. Thyroidectomy (see page 211)
2. Modified neck dissection

◆ XIII. Simple goiter

A. Definition—enlarged thyroid gland

B. Possible etiology
1. Decreased iodine intake
2. Intake of goitrogenic foods: soybeans, peanuts, peaches, strawberries
3. Use of goitrogenic drugs: iodine, lithium, propylthiouracil
4. Genetic defects

C. Pathophysiology
1. Low levels of thyroid hormone stimulate increased secretion of TSH by the pituitary gland
2. TSH stimulation causes the thyroid to increase in size to compensate for the low levels of thyroid hormone

D. Possible assessment findings
1. Dysphagia
2. Enlarged thyroid gland
3. Dyspnea

E. Possible diagnostic test findings
1. Blood chemistry: normal or decreased T_4
2. RAIU: normal or increased
3. TSH: increased

F. Medical management
1. Diet: avoid goitrogenic foods, use iodized salt
2. Activity: as tolerated
3. Monitoring: VS, I/O
4. Laboratory studies: T_4
5. Thyroid hormone replacements: levothyroxine (Synthroid), liothyronine sodium (Cytomel), thyroglobulin (Proloid)
6. Avoid goitrogenic drugs such as sulfonamides, salicylates, and lithium

**CLINICAL
ALERT**

G. Nursing interventions
1. Maintain the patient's diet
2. Assess respiratory status
3. Monitor and record VS, I/O, and laboratory studies
4. Administer medications, as prescribed
5. Encourage the patient to express feelings about changes in body image
6. Assess the patient's ability to swallow
7. Individualize home care instructions regarding the signs and symptoms of respiratory distress and difficulty swallowing

H. Possible medical complications
1. Respiratory distress
2. Laryngotracheal obstruction

I. Possible surgical intervention: subtotal thyroidectomy (see page 211)

◆ **XIV. Hyperparathyroidism**

A. Definition—overactivity of one or more parathyroid glands, resulting in increased PTH secretion

B. Possible etiology
1. Chronic renal failure
2. Bone disease
3. Benign adenomas
4. Hypertrophy of parathyroid gland
5. Malignant tumors of parathyroid gland
6. Vitamin D deficiency
7. Malabsorption

C. Pathophysiology
1. Excessive secretion of PTH leads to bone demineralization and hypocalcemia
2. Hypercalcemia increases the risk of renal calculi

D. Possible assessment findings
1. Renal colic
2. Renal calculi
3. Arrhythmias
4. Constipation
5. Bowel obstruction
6. Anorexia
7. Weight loss
8. Nausea and vomiting
9. Depression
10. Mental dullness
11. Fatigue

12. Osteoporosis
13. Muscle weakness
14. Mood swings
15. Deep bone pain
16. Hematuria
17. Paresthesia
18. Thick nails
19. Pathologic fractures

E. Possible diagnostic test findings
1. ECG: shortened QT interval
2. Urine chemistry: decreased phosphorus; increased calcium
3. Blood chemistry: increased calcium, BUN, creatinine, chloride, alkaline phosphatase; decreased phosphorus
4. X-ray: osteoporosis

F. Medical management
1. Diet: low-calcium, high-fiber, high-phosphorus in small frequent feedings; increase fluid intake to 3,000 ml/day
2. I.V. therapy: heparin lock
3. Activity: as tolerated
4. Monitoring: VS, UO, and I/O
5. Laboratory studies: calcium, phosphorus, BUN, creatinine, potassium, and sodium
6. Radiation therapy
7. Treatments: strain urine, bed cradle
8. Analgesic: oxycodone hydrochloride (Tylox)
9. Diuretics: furosemide (Lasix), ethacrynic acid (Edecrin)
10. Antacid: aluminum hydroxide gel (AlternaGEL)
11. Estrogen: estrogen (Premarin)
12. Antineoplastic: plicamycin (Mithracin)
13. Phosphate salts: K-Phos, Neutra-Phos
14. Dialysis using calcium-free dialysate
15. I.V. saline

G. Nursing interventions
1. Maintain the patient's diet
2. Force fluids with acidifying solutions: cranberry juice
3. Administer I.V. fluids
4. Assess urinary status
5. Monitor and record VS, UO, I/O, and laboratory studies
6. Administer medications, as prescribed
7. Encourage the patient to express feelings about chronic illness
8. Encourage the patient to walk
9. Prevent falls

10. Strain urine

11. Assess bone and flank pain

12. Move the patient carefully to prevent pathologic fractures

13. Limit strenuous activity

14. Assess the patient for constipation

15. Provide postradiation nursing care
   a. Provide skin and mouth care
   b. Monitor dietary intake
   c. Provide rest periods

16. Individualize home care instructions
   a. Recognize the signs and symptoms of renal calculi
   b. Strain urine
   c. Prevent falls
   d. Prevent constipation

H. Possible medical complications
   1. Peptic ulcer
   2. Psychosis
   3. Arrhythmias
   4. Renal failure
   5. Pathologic fractures

I. Possible surgical intervention: parathyroidectomy (see page 211)

◆ XV. Hypoparathyroidism

A. Definition—decrease in PTH secretion

B. Possible etiology
   1. Thyroidectomy
   2. Autoimmune disease
   3. Parathyroidectomy
   4. Radiation
   5. Use of radioactive iodine
   6. Parathyroid tumor

C. Pathophysiology
   1. Decreased PTH decreases stimulation to osteoclasts, resulting in decreased release of calcium and phosphorus from bone
   2. Decreased circulating PTH reduces GI absorption of calcium and increases absorption of phosphorus
   3. Decreased blood calcium causes a rise in serum phosphates and decreased phosphate excretion by the kidney

D. Possible assessment findings
   1. Lethargy
   2. Calcification of ocular lens

3. Muscle and abdominal spasms

4. Trousseau's sign: positive

5. Chvostek's sign: positive

6. Tingling in fingers

7. Arrhythmias

8. Seizures

9. Visual disturbances: diplopia, photophobia, blurring

10. Dyspnea

11. Laryngeal stridor

12. Personality changes

13. Brittle nails

14. Alopecia

15. Deep tendon reflexes: increased

E. Possible diagnostic test findings

1. Blood chemistry: decreased PTH, calcium; increased phosphorus

2. Urine chemistry: decreased calcium

3. X-ray: calcification of basal ganglia; increased bone density

4. ECG: prolonged QT interval

5. Sulkowitch's test: decreased

F. Medical management

1. Diet: high-calcium, low-phosphorus, low-sodium with spinach restriction

2. Activity: as tolerated

3. I.V. therapy: heparin lock

4. Monitoring: VS, UO, and I/O

5. Laboratory studies: PTH, calcium, and phosphorus

6. Precautions: seizure

7. Antacid: aluminum hydroxide gel (AlternaGEL)

8. Sedative: phenobarbital (Luminal)

9. Anticonvulsants: phenytoin (Dilantin), $MgSO_4$ (Epsom salt)

10. Vitamins: ergocalciferol (vitamin D), dihydrotachysterol (Hytakerol)

11. Oral calcium salts: calcium gluconate (Kalcinate), calcium carbonate (Os-Cal)

12. Diuretic: chlorthalidone (Hygroton)

13. Hormone replacement: parathyroid extract (PTH)

14. I.V. calcium salts: calcium chloride or calcium gluconate

G. Nursing interventions

1. Maintain the patient's diet

2. Assess neurologic status

3. Maintain seizure precautions

4. Monitor and record VS, I/O, and laboratory studies

5. Administer medications, as prescribed

6. Allay the patient's anxiety
7. Keep tracheostomy tray and I.V. calcium gluconate available
8. Maintain a calm environment
9. Individualize home care instruction
    a. Recognize the signs and symptoms of seizure activity
    b. Follow dietary recommendations

H. Possible medical complications
  1. CHF
  2. Mental retardation
  3. Blindness

I. Possible surgical interventions: none

◆ XVI. Cushing's syndrome (hypercortisolism)

A. Definition
  1. Hyperactivity of the adrenal cortex that results in excessive secretion of glucocorticoids, particularly cortisol
  2. Possible increase in mineralocorticoids and sex hormones

B. Possible etiology
  1. Hyperplasia of the adrenal glands
  2. Hypothalamic stimulation of the pituitary gland
  3. Adenoma or carcinoma of the pituitary gland
  4. Exogenous secretion of ACTH by malignant neoplasms in the lungs or gallbladder
  5. Excessive or prolonged administration of glucocorticoids or ACTH
  6. Adenoma or carcinoma of the adrenal cortex

C. Pathophysiology
  1. Hypothalamic stimulation of the pituitary gland causes excessive secretion of ACTH
  2. Excessive secretion of ACTH causes increased plasma cortisol
  3. Secretion of hypothalamic corticotropin-releasing hormone (CRH) is not diminished by elevated blood cortisol levels

D. Possible assessment findings
  1. Weight gain
  2. HIRSUTISM
  3. Amenorrhea
  4. Weakness and fatigue
  5. Pain in joints
  6. Ecchymosis
  7. Edema
  8. Hypertension
  9. Mood swings
  10. Fragile skin

11. Purple striae on abdomen
12. Poor wound healing
13. Truncal obesity
14. Buffalo hump
15. Moon face
16. Gynecomastia
17. Enlarged clitoris
18. Decreased libido
19. Muscle wasting
20. Recurrent infections
21. Acne

E. Possible diagnostic test findings
   1. Dexamethasone suppression test: no decrease in 17-OHCS
   2. X-ray: pituitary or adrenal tumor; osteoporosis
   3. Angiography: pituitary or adrenal tumors
   4. CT scan: pituitary or adrenal tumors
   5. Urine chemistry: increased 17-OHCS and 17-KS; decreased specific gravity; glycosuria
   6. Blood chemistry: increased cortisol, aldosterone, sodium, ACTH, glucose; decreased potassium
   7. Ultrasonography: pituitary or adrenal tumors
   8. Hematology: increased WBCs, RBCs; decreased eosinophils
   9. GTT: hyperglycemia

F. Medical management
   1. Diet: low-sodium, low-carbohydrate, low-calorie, high-potassium, and high-protein
   2. Activity: as tolerated
   3. Monitoring: VS, I/O, UO, urine glucose and ketones, and specific gravity
   4. Laboratory studies: sodium, potassium, cortisol, BUN, glucose, WBCs, and RBCs
   5. Radiation therapy
   6. Diuretics: furosemide (Lasix), ethacrynic acid (Edecrin)
   7. Potassium supplements: potassium chloride (K-Lor), potassium gluconate (Kaon)
   8. Adrenal suppressants: metyrapone (Metopirone), aminoglutethimide (Cytadren)
   9. Hypoglycemics: short-acting (regular, Semilente); intermediate-acting (NPH, Lente); long-acting (PZI, Ultralente); tolbutamide (Orinase), chlorpropamide (Diabinese), acetohexamide (Dymelor), tolazamide (Tolinase), glyburide (DiaBeta, Micronase), glipizide (Glucotrol)

G. Nursing interventions
1. Maintain the patient's diet
2. Assess fluid balance
3. Monitor and record VS, UO, I/O, specific gravity, finger sticks, urine glucose and ketones, and laboratory studies
4. Assess edema
5. Check for infections of skin, respiratory, and urinary tracts
6. Protect the patient from falls and bruising
7. Protect from infection
8. Provide meticulous skin care
9. Limit water intake
10. Weigh the patient daily
11. Administer medications, as prescribed
12. Encourage the patient to express feelings about changes in body image and sexual function
13. Provide rest periods
14. Minimize environmental stress
15. Provide postradiation nursing care
    a. Provide prophylactic skin care
    b. Monitor dietary intake
    c. Provide rest periods
16. Individualize home care instructions
    a. Recognize the signs and symptoms of infection and fluid retention
    b. Avoid exposure to people with infections
    c. Monitor self for infection

H. Possible medical complications
1. Adrenal insufficiency
2. Infection
3. Peptic ulcers
4. Hypertension
5. Fractures
6. CHF
7. Psychosis
8. Arrhythmias
9. Diabetes mellitus
10. Arteriosclerosis
11. Nephrosclerosis

I. Possible surgical interventions
1. Adrenalectomy (see page 208)
2. Hypophysectomy (see page 210)

◆ XVII. Addison's disease

A. Definition—chronic hypoactivity of the adrenal cortex, resulting in insufficient secretion of glucocorticoids (cortisol) and mineralocorticoids (aldosterone)

B. Possible etiology
  1. Idiopathic atrophy of adrenal glands
  2. Surgical removal of adrenal glands
  3. Autoimmune disease
  4. Tuberculosis
  5. Metastatic lesions from lung cancer
  6. Pituitary hypofunction
  7. Histoplasmosis
  8. Trauma

C. Pathophysiology
  1. Autoimmune theory: body produces adrenocortical antibodies, resulting in adrenal hypofunction
  2. Decreased aldosterone causes disturbances in sodium, water, and potassium metabolism
  3. Decreased cortisol causes abnormal metabolism of fat, protein, and carbohydrate

D. Possible assessment findings
  1. Hypoglycemia
  2. Weakness and lethargy
  3. Bronzed skin pigmentation of nipples, scars, and buccal mucosa
  4. Dehydration
  5. Anorexia
  6. Thirst
  7. Decreased pubic and axillary hair
  8. Orthostatic hypotension
  9. Diarrhea
  10. Nausea
  11. Weight loss
  12. Depression

E. Possible diagnostic test findings
  1. Blood chemistry: decreased HCT, Hgb, cortisol, glucose, sodium, chloride, aldosterone; increased BUN, potassium
  2. Urine chemistry: decreased 17-KS and 17-OHCS
  3. BMR: decreased
  4. Fasting blood sugar (FBS): hypoglycemia
  5. ECG: prolonged PR and QT intervals

F. Medical management
1. Diet: high-carbohydrate, high-protein, high-sodium, low-potassium in small, frequent feedings before steroid therapy; high-potassium and low-sodium when on steroid therapy
2. I.V. therapy: hydration, electrolyte replacement; heparin lock
3. Activity: bed rest
4. Monitoring: VS, UO, I/O, and specific gravity
5. Laboratory studies: sodium, potassium, osmolality, cortisol, chloride, glucose, BUN, creatinine, Hgb, and HCT
6. I.V. saline
7. Vasopressor: phenylephrine hydrochloride (NeoSynephrine)
8. Antacids: magnesium and aluminum hydroxide (Maalox), aluminum hydroxide gel (Gelusil)
9. Mineralocorticoid (aldosterone): fludrocortisone acetate (Florinef)
10. Glucocorticoids: cortisone acetate (Cortone), hydrocortisone (Solu-Cortef)

G. Nursing interventions
1. Maintain the patient's diet
2. Administer I.V. fluids
3. Assess fluid balance
4. Monitor and record VS, UO, I/O, specific gravity, and laboratory studies
5. Weigh the patient daily
6. Administer medications, as prescribed
7. Allay the patient's anxiety
8. Protect the patient from falls
9. Encourage fluid intake
10. Assist with activities of daily living (ADLs)
11. Maintain a quiet environment
12. Individualize home care instructions
   a. Avoid strenuous exercise, particularly in hot weather
   b. Recognize the signs and symptoms of adrenal crisis
   c. Increase fluid intake in hot weather
   d. Carry injectable dexamethasone (Decadron)
   e. Avoid using over-the-counter drugs

CLINICAL ALERT

H. Possible medical complications
1. Addisonian crisis (adrenal crisis): marked hypotension, cyanosis, abdominal cramps, diarrhea, costovertebral tenderness, fever, confusion, coma
2. Arrhythmias
3. Hypovolemic shock
4. Renal failure

I. Possible surgical interventions: none

◆ XVIII. Pheochromocytoma

A. Definition—catecholamine-secreting neoplasm associated with hyperfunctioning adrenal medulla

B. Possible etiology
1. Genetics
2. Pregnancy
3. Trauma

C. Pathophysiology
1. Tumor in the adrenal medulla secretes large amounts of catecholamines (epinephrine and norepinephrine)
2. Increased catecholamines cause hypertension, increased BMR, and hyperglycemia

D. Possible assessment findings
1. Labile malignant hypertension
2. Throbbing headaches
3. Diaphoresis
4. Palpitations
5. Tachycardia
6. Excessive anxiety
7. Hyperactivity
8. Dilated pupils
9. Cold extremities
10. Weakness
11. Weight loss
12. Dyspnea
13. Vertigo
14. Angina
15. Nausea
16. Vomiting
17. Anorexia
18. Visual disturbances
19. Polyuria
20. Diarrhea
21. Tinnitus
22. Tremors

E. Possible diagnostic test findings
1. CT scan: adrenal tumor
2. Angiography: adrenal tumor
3. Magnetic resonance imaging (MRI): adrenal tumor
4. VMA: increased
5. ECG: tachycardia

6. Blood chemistries: increased BUN, creatinine, glucose, and catecholamines
7. Urine chemistries: increased glucose and catecholamines

F. Medical management
1. Diet: high-calorie, high-vitamin and mineral with restricted use of stimulants, such as caffeine beverages
2. Activity: as tolerated
3. Monitoring: VS, UO, I/O, and urine glucose and ketones
4. Position: semi-Fowler's
5. Laboratory studies: BUN, creatinine, and glucose
6. Sedative: oxazepam (Serax)
7. Alpha adrenergic blockers: phentolamine (Regitine), phenoxybenzamine hydrochloride (Dibenzyline)
8. Beta adrenergic blocker: propranolol (Inderal)
9. Vasodilator: nitroprusside sodium (Nipride)
10. Catecholamine inhibitor: metyrosine (Demser)

G. Nursing interventions
1. Maintain the patient's diet
2. Assess cardiovascular status
3. Keep the patient in semi-Fowler's position
4. Monitor and record VS, UO, I/O, orthostatic blood pressure, specific gravity, urine glucose and ketones, neurovital signs, and laboratory studies
5. Weigh the patient daily
6. Administer medications, as prescribed
7. Encourage the patient to express feelings about fear of dying
8. Protect the patient from falls
9. Minimize environmental stress

10. Provide rest periods
11. Keep phentolamine (Regitine) available
12. Provide postradiation nursing care
    a. Provide skin and mouth care
    b. Monitor dietary intake
    c. Provide rest periods
13. Individualize home care instructions
    a. Stop smoking
    b. Recognize the signs and symptoms of renal failure
    c. Monitor blood pressure, urine glucose, and ketones daily

H. Possible medical complications
1. Cardiac arrest
2. Cerebral hemorrhage
3. Blindness
4. Renal failure

    5. MI

    6. CHF

I. Possible surgical interventions

    1. Adrenal medulla resection after administration of phentolamine (Regitine)

    2. Adrenalectomy (see page 208)

♦ XIX. Hyperaldosteronism (primary aldosteronism, Conn's syndrome)

A. Definition—hypersecretion of aldosterone (mineralocorticoids) from adrenal cortex

B. Possible etiology

    1. Adenoma of adrenal cortex

    2. Adrenal hyperplasia

    3. Adrenal carcinoma

C. Pathophysiology: Aldosterone's primary effect on the renal tubules causes the kidneys to retain sodium and water and excrete potassium and hydrogen

D. Possible assessment findings

    1. Muscle weakness

    2. Polyuria

    3. POLYDIPSIA

    4. Metabolic alkalosis

    5. Hypertension

    6. Postural hypotension

    7. Headache

    8. Paresthesia

    9. Pyelonephritis

    10. Nocturia

    11. Chvostek's sign: positive

    12. Trousseau's sign: positive

E. Possible diagnostic test findings

    1. Blood chemistry: decreased potassium; increased sodium, carbon dioxide (CO_2)

    2. Arterial blood gases (ABGs): metabolic alkalosis

    3. Urine chemistry: increased aldosterone, protein, pH; decreased specific gravity

F. Medical management

    1. Diet: high-potassium, low-sodium

    2. Activity: as tolerated

    3. Monitoring: VS, U/O, and I/O

    4. Laboratory studies: potassium, sodium, calcium, and ABGs

5. Potassium salts: potassium chloride (KCl), potassium gluconate (Kaon)
6. Diuretics: spironolactone (Aldactone), acetazolamide (Diamox)
7. Calcium salts: calcium gluconate (Kalcinate), calcium carbonate (Os-Cal)

G. Nursing interventions
1. Maintain the patient's diet, as tolerated
2. Assess fluid balance
3. Monitor and record VS, UO, I/O, orthostatic blood pressure, specific gravity, and laboratory studies
4. Monitor laboratory results: ABGs, sodium, potassium, and calcium
5. Administer medications, as prescribed
6. Allay the patient's anxiety
7. Weigh the patient daily
8. Provide a quiet environment
9. Individualize home care instructions
    a. Recognize the signs and symptoms of fluid overload and muscle irritability
    b. Comply with medical follow-up

H. Possible medical complications
1. Neuropathy
2. Arrhythmias

I. Possible surgical intervention: adrenalectomy (see page 208)

◆ XX. Diabetes mellitus

A. Definition
1. Chronic disorder of carbohydrate metabolism with subsequent alteration of protein and fat metabolism
2. Results from a disturbance in the production, action, and rate of utilization of insulin
3. Five types of diabetes mellitus
    a. Type I (insulin-dependent diabetes mellitus [IDDM], or ketosis-prone): usually develops in childhood
    b. Type II (non-insulin-dependent diabetes mellitus [NIDDM], or ketosis-resistant): usually develops after age 30
    c. Gestational diabetes mellitus (GDM): occurs with pregnancy
    d. Secondary diabetes: induced by trauma, surgery, pancreatic disease or medications; can be treated as type I or type II
    e. Maturity-onset diabetes (MODY): type II that develops in teens and young adults under age 30

B. Possible etiology
   1. Failure of body to produce insulin
   2. Blockage of insulin supply
   3. Autoimmune disease
   4. Receptor defect in normally insulin-responsive cells
   5. Genetics
   6. Exposure to chemicals
   7. Hyperpituitarism
   8. Cushing's syndrome
   9. Hyperthyroidism
   10. Infection
   11. Surgery
   12. Stress
   13. Medications
   14. Pregnancy
   15. Trauma

C. Pathophysiology
   1. Type I (IDDM) results from an inability to produce endogenous insulin by the beta cells in the islets of Langerhans in the pancreas
   2. Type II (NIDDM) is a deficit in insulin release or an insulin-receptor defect in peripheral tissues
   3. Insulin deprivation of insulin-dependent cells leads to a marked decrease in the cellular rate of glucose uptake
   4. Glucogenesis increases because of decreased stimulation of glucose metabolism with resulting hyperglycemia and glycosuria
   5. Decreased insulin triggers release of free fatty acids that cannot be metabolized and are released as ketone bodies in blood urine
   6. Decreased insulin depresses protein synthesis, causing a release of amino acids that are converted by the liver into glucose and ketones
   7. The formation of urea results in overall nitrogen loss

D. Possible assessment findings
   1. Weight loss
   2. Anorexia
   3. POLYPHAGIA
   4. Acetone breath
   5. Weakness
   6. Fatigue
   7. Dehydration
   8. Pain
   9. Paresthesia
   10. POLYURIA
   11. Polydipsia
   12. Kussmaul's respirations

13. Multiple infections and boils
14. Flushed, warm, smooth, shiny skin
15. Atrophic muscles
16. Poor wound healing
17. Mottled extremities
18. Peripheral and visceral neuropathies
19. Retinopathy
20. Sexual dysfunction
21. Blurred vision

E. Possible diagnostic test findings
   1. Blood chemistry: increased glucose, potassium, chloride, ketones, cholesterol, and triglycerides; decreased CO_2; pH less than 7.4
   2. Urine chemistry: increased glucose, ketones
   3. FBS: increased
   4. GTT: hyperglycemia
   5. Postprandial blood sugar: hyperglycemia
   6. Glycosylated hemoglobin assay (HbA1c): increased

F. Medical management
   1. Diet: individually prescribed diet based on ideal weight, metabolic activity, and personal activity levels
      a. Use the American Diabetes Association's exchange list for meal planning to design a diet that will distribute an individual's caloric needs, carbohydrate, fat, and protein intake over 24 hours
      b. Avoid refined and simple sugars and saturated fats
      c. Limit cholesterol
      d. Include high fiber and high complex carbohydrates
   2. Activity: as tolerated
   3. Monitoring: VS, UO, and I/O
   4. Laboratory studies: glucose, potassium, HbA1c, and pH
   5. Hypoglycemics: short-acting (regular, Semilente); intermediate-acting (NPH, Lente); long-acting (PZI, Ultralente); tolbutamide (Orinase), chlorpropamide (Diabinese), acetohexamide (Dymelor), tolazamide (Tolinase), glyburide (DiaBeta, Micronase), glipizide (Glucotrol)
   6. Vitamin and mineral supplements

G. Nursing interventions
   1. Maintain the patient's diet
   2. Force fluids
   3. Assess acid-base and fluid balance
   4. Monitor and record VS, UO, I/O, finger sticks for blood glucose, and laboratory studies
   5. Administer medications, as prescribed

6. Encourage the patient to express feelings about diet, medication regimen, and body image changes
7. Encourage activity, as tolerated
8. Weigh the patient weekly
9. Provide meticulous skin and foot care
10. Monitor the patient for infection
11. Maintain a warm and quiet environment

12. Monitor wound healing
13. Observe for Somogyi phenomena and Shögren's syndrome
14. Provide information about the American Diabetes Association
15. Foster independence
16. Determine the patient's compliance to diet, exercise, and medication regimens
17. Individualize home care instructions
    a. Exercise regularly
    b. Stop smoking
    c. Recognize the signs and symptoms of hyperglycemia and hypoglycemia
    d. Monitor self for infection, skin breakdown, changes in peripheral circulation, poor wound healing, and numbness in extremities
    e. Know and use proper dietary substitutions if unable to take prescribed diet because of illness
    f. Adjust diet and insulin for changes in work, exercise, trauma, infection, fever, and stress
    g. Demonstrate administration of hypoglycemics
    h. Demonstrate home blood glucose monitoring technique (HBGM)
    i. Complete daily skin and foot care
    j. Carry an emergency supply of glucose
    k. Seek counseling for sexual dysfunction and feelings about body image changes
    l. Avoid use of over-the-counter medication
    m. Avoid alcohol
    n. Demonstrate use of the subcutaneous insulin infusion therapy (Insulin pump)
    o. Adhere to the treatment regimen to prevent complications

H. Possible medical complications
   1. Ketoacidosis (diabetic coma): abdominal pain; acetone breath; altered consciousness; hot, flushed skin; Kussmaul's respirations; nausea; vomiting; hypotension; oliguria; tachycardia
   2. Insulin reaction (hypoglycemia): hunger, weakness, hand tremors, pallor, tachycardia, diaphoresis, irritability, confusion, diplopia, slurred speech, headaches

3. Infections
4. Peripheral neuropathies
5. Glaucoma
6. Impotence
7. Coronary artery disease
8. Gangrene
9. Cerebrovascular accident (CVA)
10. Chronic renal failure
11. Hyperosmolar hyperglycemic nonketotic syndrome (HHNS): severe dehydration, severe hypotension, fever, stupor, and seizures
12. Hypovolemia
13. Diabetic retinopathy
14. Peripheral vascular disease

I. Possible surgical interventions: none

♦ XXI. Diabetes insipidus

A. Definition—deficiency of ADH (vasopressin) that is secreted by the posterior lobe of the pituitary gland (neurohypophysis)

B. Possible etiology
1. Trauma to posterior lobe of pituitary gland
2. Tumor of posterior lobe of pituitary gland
3. Brain surgery
4. Head injury
5. Idiopathic
6. Meningitis

C. Pathophysiology
1. Decreased ADH reduces the ability of distal and collecting renal tubules to concentrate urine
2. Copious, dilute urine and intense thirst result

D. Possible assessment findings
1. Polyuria (greater than 5 L/day)
2. Polydipsia (4 to 40 L/day)
3. Fatigue
4. Dehydration
5. Weight loss
6. Muscle weakness and pain
7. Headache
8. Tachycardia

E. Possible diagnostic test findings
1. Urine chemistry: specific gravity less than 1.004, osmolality 50 to 200 mOsm/kg
2. Blood chemistry: decreased ADH by radioimmunoassay

      3. Water deprivation test: inability to concentrate urine

F. Medical management
    1. Diet: regular with restriction of foods that exert a diuretic effect
    2. I.V. therapy: hydration, electrolyte replacement; heparin lock
    3. Activity: bed rest
    4. Monitoring: VS, UO, CVP, and I/O
    5. Laboratory studies: potassium, sodium, BUN, creatinine, specific gravity, and osmolality
    6. Treatments: indwelling urinary catheter
    7. ADH stimulant: carbamazepine (Tegretol)
    8. ADH replacement: lypressin (Diapid nasal spray)

G. Nursing interventions
    1. Maintain the patient's diet
    2. Force fluids
    3. Administer I.V. fluids
    4. Assess fluid balance
    5. Maintain patency of indwelling urinary catheter
    6. Monitor and record VS, UO, CVP, I/O, specific gravity, and laboratory studies
    7. Administer medications, as prescribed
    8. Allay the patient's anxiety
    9. Weigh the patient daily
   10. Individualize home care instructions
       a. Recognize the signs and symptoms of dehydration
       b. Increase fluid intake in hot weather
       c. Carry medications on person at all times

H. Possible medical complications
    1. Dehydration
    2. Arrhythmias
    3. Hypovolemic shock

I. Possible surgical intervention: hypophysectomy, when etiology is tumor (see page 210)

◆ XXII. Hyperpituitarism (acromegaly)

A. Definition—hypersecretion of growth hormone by the anterior pituitary gland (adenohypophysis)

B. Possible etiology
    1. Prolactin-secreting benign adenomas
    2. Growth-hormone secreting tumors
    3. Cushing's syndrome caused by pituitary dysfunction
    4. LH-, FSH-, or TSH-secreting adenomas
    5. Adrenalectomy

6. Pregnancy

C. Pathophysiology

1. Excessive secretion of growth hormone occurs after epiphyseal closing

2. Excessive secretion of growth hormone causes overdevelopment of cartilage, bone, soft tissue; thickens skin; and enlarges sweat glands, sebaceous glands, and gonads

3. Growth-hormone-induced hypermetabolism causes hormone alterations

D. Possible assessment findings

1. Coarse facial features
2. Enlarged tongue
3. Protruding jaw
4. Spiderlike fingers
5. Wide hands and feet
6. Weakness
7. Impotence
8. Infertility
9. Thick skin and nails
10. Diplopia
11. Cranial nerve palsies
12. Joint deformities
13. Pain in joints
14. Deepening of voice
15. Diaphoresis
16. Headache

E. Possible diagnostic test findings

1. Insulin tolerance test: hyperglycemia
2. CT scan: enlarged pituitary
3. Visual fields: hemianopia, diplopia
4. X-rays: thickened long bones and skull
5. Blood chemistry: increased phosphorus, prolactin, glucose, somatotropin; decreased FSH
6. Urine chemistry: increased calcium, glucose

F. Medical management

1. Activity: as tolerated
2. Monitoring: VS, UO, and I/O
3. Laboratory studies: glucose, potassium, and calcium
4. Radiation therapy via transphenoidal implant
5. Dopaminergics: levodopa (Larodopa), bromocriptine mesylate (Parlodel)

6. Hormones: somatotropin (Humatrope), ethinyl estradiol (Estinyl), testosterone (Delatestryl), levothyroxine sodium (Synthroid), liothyronine (Cytomel), diethylstilbestrol
7. Glucocorticoids: cortisone acetate (Cortone), hydrocortisone (Cortef), hydrocortisone sodium succinate (Solu-Cortef)
8. Ergot alkaloid: methysergide maleate (Sansert)
9. Mineralocorticoid: fludrocortisone acetate (Florinef)
10. Cryosurgery
11. Thermocoagulation
12. Ultrasound therapy

G. Nursing interventions
   1. Assess fluid balance
   2. Monitor and record VS, UO, I/O, urine glucose and ketones, finger sticks, and laboratory studies
   3. Administer medications, as prescribed
   4. Encourage the patient to express feelings about changes in body image and sexual dysfunction
   5. Maintain activity, as tolerated
   6. Provide skin care
   7. Position and support painful joints
   8. Protect the patient from falls
   9. Monitor for infection
   10. Provide postradiation nursing care
       a. Provide prophylactic skin and mouth care
       b. Monitor dietary intake
       c. Provide rest periods
   11. Individualize home care instructions
       a. Carry emergency adrenal hormone replacement drugs
       b. Wear medical alert bracelet

H. Possible medical complications
   1. Blindness
   2. Visual disturbances
   3. Diabetes mellitus
   4. Cushing's syndrome
   5. Hyperthyroidism
   6. Hypertension
   7. CHF
   8. Angina
   9. Cardiomyopathy
   10. Hyperparathyroidism
   11. Renal calculi
   12. Cardiac arrest

I. Possible surgical intervention: hypophysectomy (see page 210)

◆ **XXIII. Hypopituitarism (Simmonds' disease)**

A. Definition—hypofunction of anterior pituitary gland (adenohypophysis), resulting in insufficient or absent quantities of anterior pituitary gland hormones or target organ hormones

B. Possible etiology
1. Adenomas or carcinomas of pituitary gland
2. Postpartum hemorrhage
3. Head trauma
4. Necrosis of pituitary gland (Sheehan's syndrome)
5. Radiation of head
6. Hypophysectomy
7. Insufficient hypothalamic releasing factors

C. Pathophysiology
1. Decreased pituitary function results in decreased amounts of GH, TSH, and ACTH
2. With progressive loss of pituitary function, levels of FSH and LH also decrease

D. Possible assessment findings
1. Lethargy
2. Decreased strength
3. Decreased tolerance for cold temperatures
4. Hypothermia
5. Hypotension
6. Emaciation
7. Decreased axillary and pubic hair
8. Atrophy of gonads and thyroid
9. Impotence
10. Weight loss
11. Pallor
12. Decreased libido
13. Amenorrhea
14. Dry skin
15. Decreased perspiration
16. Recurrent infections
17. Headaches

E. Possible diagnostic test findings
1. Blood chemistry: decreased cortisol, growth hormone, ACTH, TSH, LH, FSH, glucose, and gonadotropins
2. RAIU: decreased
3. FBS: decreased glucose
4. GTT: decreased glucose
5. Hematology: decreased Hgb and HCT

      6. CT scan: adenohypophyseal tumor

      7. Visual fields: hemianopia and loss of color vision

      8. Angiography: adenohypophyseal tumor

      9. Urine chemistry: decreased gonadotropins, 17-OHCS, and 17-KS

    10. Skull X-ray: adenohypophyseal tumor

F. Medical management

    1. Diet: high-protein

    2. Activity: as tolerated

    3. Monitoring: VS, UO, I/O, and laboratory studies

    4. Radiation therapy

    5. Dopaminergics: levodopa (Larodopa), bromocriptine mesylate (Parlodel)

    6. Hormones: somatotropin (Humatrope), ethinyl estradiol (Estinyl), testosterone (Delatestryl), levothyroxine sodium (Synthroid), liothyronine (Cytomel)

    7. Glucocorticoids: cortisone acetate (Cortone), hydrocortisone (Cortef), hydrocortisone sodium succinate (Solu-Cortef)

G. Nursing interventions

    1. Maintain the patient's diet

    2. Assess fluid balance

    3. Monitor and record VS, UO, I/O, urine glucose and ketones, and laboratory studies

    4. Administer medications, as prescribed

    5. Encourage the patient to express feelings about changes in body image and sexual dysfunction

    6. Maintain activity, as tolerated

    7. Prevent falls

    8. Monitor for infection

    9. Maintain a warm environment

   10. Provide skin care

   11. Allay the patient's anxiety

   12. Reinforce the need to eat

   13. Provide postradiation nursing care

      a. Provide prophylactic skin care

      b. Monitor dietary intake

      c. Provide rest periods

   14. Individualize home care instructions

      a. Recognize the signs and symptoms of dehydration

      b. Avoid exposure to people with infections

      c. Monitor self for infection

H. Possible medical complications
   1. Death
   2. Hypothyroidism
   3. Adrenal insufficiency
I. Possible surgical interventions
   1. Hypophysectomy (see page 210)
   2. Resection of pituitary gland

POINTS TO REMEMBER

♦ Factors altering the function of the pituitary gland—the master gland—affect all hormonal activity.

♦ Changes in secondary sex characteristics and sexual function that accompany diseases of the endocrine system may embarrass some patients.

♦ Disturbances in mineralocorticoid and glucocorticoid secretion alter fluid and electrolyte balance.

♦ Diabetes insipidus is associated with a deficiency of ADH.

STUDY QUESTIONS

To evaluate your understanding of this chapter, answer the following questions in the space provided; then compare your responses with the correct answers in Appendix B, page 384.

1. What should the patient learn about hormone replacement after an adrenalectomy? _____

_____

_____

2. What type of diet and dietary supplements would be prescribed for the patient after a parathyroidectomy? _____

_____

_____

3. What are the possible assessment findings for hypothyroidism? _____

_____

_____

4. Which diagnostic tests would indicate that a patient has Cushing's syndrome? _____

_____

_____

5. Which acid-base imbalance is associated with hyperaldosteronism? _____

_____

_____

6. What are two key assessment findings for diabetes insipidus? _____

_____

_____

CRITICAL THINKING AND APPLICATION EXERCISES

1. Observe a glucose tolerance test. Prepare an oral presentation for your fellow students, describing the test and patient care before, during, and after the test.

2. Develop a chart comparing the major types of insulin.

3. Obtain a dietary history from a patient with diabetes. Using the patient's prescribed meal plan, assist him in choosing meals from the ADA exchange list.

4. Follow a patient with an endocrine disorder from admission through discharge. Develop a patient-specific plan of care, including any needs for follow-up and home care.

7

Renal and Urologic System

LEARNING OBJECTIVES

After studying this chapter, you should be able to:

- Describe the psychosocial impact of renal and urologic disorders.

- Differentiate between modifiable and nonmodifiable risk factors in the development of a renal or urologic disorder.

- List three probable and three possible nursing diagnoses for any patient with a renal or urologic disorder.

- Identify nursing interventions for a patient with a renal or urologic disorder.

- Identify three teaching topics to address for a patient with a renal or urologic disorder.

CHAPTER OVERVIEW

Caring for the patient with a renal or urologic disorder requires a sound understanding of renal and urologic anatomy and physiology and fluid balance. A thorough assessment is essential to planning and implementing appropriate patient care. The assessment includes a complete history, physical examination, diagnostic testing, identification of modifiable and nonmodifiable risk factors, and information related to the psychosocial impact of the disorder on the patient. Nursing diagnoses focus primarily on altered urinary elimination and body image disturbance. Nursing interventions are designed to assess patient hydration, maintain urinary output, and assist the patient to adjust to changes in body image and possible sexual dysfunction. Patient teaching — a crucial nursing activity — involves information about medical follow-up, medication regimens, signs and symptoms of possible complications, and reduction of modifiable risk factors through adherence to dietary and fluid recommendation and restrictions.

◆ I. Anatomy and physiology

A. Kidneys
  1. Two bean-shaped organs
  2. Four components: cortex, medulla, renal pelvis, and nephron
    a. Cortex
      (1) Makes up the outer layer of the kidney
      (2) Contains the glomeruli, proximal tubules of the nephron, and distal tubules of the nephron
    b. Medulla
      (1) Makes up the inner layer of the kidney
      (2) Contains the loops of Henle and the collecting tubules
    c. Renal pelvis: collects urine from the calices
    d. Nephron
      (1) Makes up the functional unit of the kidney
      (2) Contains the Bowman's capsule and the glomerulus
      (3) Contains the renal tubule, which consists of proximal convoluted tubule, loop of Henle, distal convoluted tubule, and collecting segments

B. Ureter
  1. This tubule extends from the renal pelvis to the bladder floor
  2. Ureter transports urine from the kidney to the bladder
  3. Ureterovesical sphincter prevents reflux of urine from the bladder into the ureter

C. Bladder
  1. Muscular, distendable sac that stores urine
  2. Total capacity of approximately 1 L

D. Urethra
  1. This tubule extends from the bladder to the urinary meatus
  2. Urethra transports urine from the bladder to the urinary meatus

E. Urine formation
  1. Blood from the renal artery is filtrated across the glomerular capillary membrane in the Bowman's capsule
  2. Filtration requires adequate intravascular volume and adequate cardiac output

3. Composition of formed filtrate is similar to blood plasma without proteins
4. Formed filtrate moves through the tubules of the nephron, which re-absorb and secrete electrolytes, water, glucose, amino acids, ammonia, and bicarbonate
5. Antidiuretic hormone (ADH) and aldosterone control the reabsorption of water and electrolytes

F. Blood pressure control
1. Regulation of fluid volume by the kidney affects blood pressure
2. Renin-angiotensin system is activated by decreased blood pressure
3. Renal disease can alter the renin-angiotensin system

G. Prostate gland
1. This fibrous capsule is connected to and surrounds the male urethra
2. Prostate gland contains ducts that secrete the alkaline portion of seminal fluid and that open into the prostatic portion of the urethra

◆ II. Assessment findings

A. History
1. Changes in pattern of urination: frequency, nocturia, hesitancy, urgency, dribbling, incontinence, and retention
2. Changes in appearance of urine: dilute, concentrated, HEMATURIA, and PYURIA
3. Dysuria
4. Pain
5. Chills and fever

B. Physical examination
1. Urine output changes: POLYURIA, OLIGURIA, and ANURIA
2. Specific gravity abnormalities
3. Hematuria
4. Urine pH abnormalities
5. Periorbital and peripheral edema
6. Bladder distention
7. Skin color changes
8. Intake and output (I/O) discrepancies
9. Muscle tremors
10. Pattern and character of respirations
11. Enlargement of prostate gland
12. Temperature changes
13. Weight changes

♦ III. Diagnostic tests and procedures

A. Urinalysis
  1. Definition and purpose
     a. Laboratory test of urine
     b. Microscopic examination for color, appearance, pH, specific gravity, protein, glucose, ketones, red blood cells (RBCs), white blood cells (WBCs), and casts
  2. Nursing interventions
     a. Wash perineal area
     b. Obtain first morning urine specimen

B. Urine culture and sensitivity
  1. Definition and purpose
     a. Laboratory test of urine
     b. Microscopic examination for bacteria
  2. Nursing interventions
     a. Clean perineal area and urinary meatus with bacteriostatic solution
     b. Collect midstream sample in sterile container

C. 24-hour urine collection
  1. Definition and purpose
     a. Laboratory test of urine
     b. Quantitative analysis of samples collected over 24 hours to determine kidney function
  2. Nursing interventions
     a. Instruct the patient to void and note time (collection starts with the next voiding)
     b. Place urine container on ice
     c. Measure each voided urine
     d. Instruct the patient to void at the end of the 24-hour period
     e. Note medications that might alter tests results

D. Blood chemistry
  1. Definition and purpose
     a. Laboratory test of blood sample
     b. Analysis for potassium, sodium, calcium, phosphorus, glucose, bicarbonate, blood urea nitrogen (BUN), creatinine, protein, albumin, and osmolality
  2. Nursing interventions
     a. Withhold food and fluids before the procedure, as directed
     b. Check the site for bleeding after the procedure

E. Kidneys, ureters, bladder (KUB) X-ray
  1. Definition and purpose
     a. Noninvasive examination of the renal system
     b. Radiographic picture of the kidneys, ureters, and bladder

2. Nursing interventions
   a. Schedule the X-ray before other examinations requiring contrast medium
   b. Ensure that the patient removes metallic belts

F. Excretory urography
  1. Definition and purpose
   a. Procedure using an injection of a radiopaque dye
   b. Fluoroscopic examination of kidneys, ureters, and bladder

  2. Nursing interventions before the procedure
   a. Note the patient's allergies to iodine, seafood, and radiopaque dyes
   b. Withhold food and fluids after midnight
   c. Administer laxatives, as prescribed
   d. Inform the patient about possible throat irritation and flushing of the face
  3. Nursing interventions after the procedure
   a. Instruct the patient to drink at least 1 qt (1 L) of fluids
   b. Check the venipuncture site for bleeding

G. Cystoscopy
  1. Definition and purpose
   a. Procedure using a cystoscope
   b. Direct visualization of the bladder
  2. Nursing interventions before the procedure
   a. Withhold food and fluids
   b. Allay the patient's anxiety
   c. Obtain written, informed consent
   d. Administer enemas and medications, as prescribed
  3. Nursing interventions after the procedure
   a. Administer analgesics and sitz baths, as prescribed
   b. Monitor I/O and vital signs (VS)
   c. Check the patient's urine for blood clots
   d. Force fluids

H. Renal angiography
  1. Definition and purpose
   a. Procedure using an injection of a radiopaque dye through a catheter
   b. Radiographic examination of the renal arterial supply
  2. Nursing interventions before the procedure
   a. Allay the patient's anxiety
   b. Inform the patient about a possible burning feeling after dye is injected
   c. Obtain written, informed consent
   d. Withhold food and fluids after midnight

CLINICAL ALERT

CLINICAL ALERT

e. Instruct the patient to void immediately before procedure

f. Administer enemas, as prescribed

g. Note the patient's allergies to iodine, seafood, and radiopaque dyes

3. Nursing interventions after the procedure

   a. Assess VS and peripheral pulses

   b. Inspect the catheter insertion site for bleeding

   c. Force fluids

I. Renal scan

  1. Definition and purpose

    a. Procedure using an I.V. injection of a radioisotope

    b. Visual imaging of blood flow distribution to the kidneys

  2. Nursing interventions before the procedure

    a. Assist with administering radioisotope as necessary

    b. Check the patient's history for allergies

  3. Nursing interventions after the procedure

    a. Assess the patient for signs of delayed allergic reaction, such as itching and hives

    b. Wear gloves when caring for incontinent patients and double-bag linens

J. Renal biopsy

  1. Definition and purpose

    a. Percutaneous procedure to remove a small amount of renal tissue

    b. Histologic evaluation

  2. Nursing interventions before the procedure

    a. Assess baseline clotting studies and VS

    b. Withhold food and fluids after midnight

    c. Obtain written, informed consent

  3. Nursing interventions after the procedure

    a. Monitor and record VS, hemoglobin (Hgb) and hematocrit (HCT)

    b. Check biopsy site for bleeding

K. Cystourethrogram

  1. Definition and purpose

    a. Procedure calling for the insertion of a catheter and the introduction of radiopaque dye

    b. Visualization of the bladder and ureters

  2. Nursing interventions

    a. Allay the patient's anxiety

    b. Note the patient's allergies to iodine, seafood, and radiopaque dyes before the procedure

    c. Advise the patient about voiding requirements during the procedure

    d. Monitor voiding after the procedure

   L. Cystometrogram (CMG)
     1. Definition and purpose
       a. Procedure to test the urinary bladder using a catheter
       b. Graphic recording of the pressures exerted at varying phases of filling of the bladder
     2. Nursing interventions before the procedure
       a. Allay the patient's anxiety
       b. Advise the patient about voiding requirements during the procedure
       c. Monitor voiding after the procedure

   M. Hematologic studies
     1. Definition and purpose
       a. Laboratory test of blood sample
       b. Analysis of blood sample for WBCs, RBCs, erythrocyte sedimentation rate (ESR), platelets, prothrombin time (PT), partial thromboplastin time (PTT), Hgb, and HCT
     2. Nursing interventions
       a. Explain the purpose of the procedure
       b. Check the venipuncture site for bleeding

♦ **IV. Psychosocial impact of renal and urologic disorders**

   A. Developmental impact
     1. Body image changes
     2. Feeling of lack of control over body functions
     3. Fear of rejection
     4. Embarrassment from changes in body function and structure
     5. Decreased self-esteem

   B. Economic impact
     1. Cost of renal dialysis and organ transplant
     2. Cost of hospitalizations and follow-up care
     3. Cost of medications
     4. Cost of special diet
     5. Disruption of employment

   C. Occupational and recreational impact
     1. Restrictions in physical activity
     2. Changes in leisure activity

   D. Social impact
     1. Changes in eating patterns
     2. Social isolation
     3. Changes in elimination patterns and modes
     4. Changes in sexual function

◆ V. Possible risk factors

A. Modifiable risk factors
1. Diet: high-sodium, high-calcium
2. Exposure to chemical and environmental pollutants
3. Smoking
4. Contact sports
5. Culturally based reluctance to discuss hygiene and health habits

B. Nonmodifiable risk factors
1. History of renal dysfunction
2. History of hypertension
3. Aging
4. Family history of renal disease

◆ VI. Nursing diagnostic categories

A. Probable nursing diagnostic categories
1. Risk for fluid volume deficit
2. Fluid volume excess
3. Altered urinary elimination
4. Pain
5. Sexual dysfunction
6. Body image disturbance
7. Self-esteem disturbance

B. Possible nursing diagnostic categories
1. Risk for impaired skin integrity
2. Noncompliance
3. Risk for activity intolerance
4. Anticipatory grieving
5. Impaired gas exchange

◆ VII. Kidney transplantation

A. Description—implantation of a kidney to a person who requires dialysis during the last stage of renal disease

B. Preoperative nursing interventions
1. Complete patient and family preoperative teaching
   a. Determine the patient's understanding of the procedure
   b. Describe the operating room (OR), postanesthesia unit (PACU), and preoperative and postoperative routines
   c. Demonstrate postoperative turning, coughing, and deep breathing (TCDB), splinting, leg exercises, and range-of-motion (ROM) exercises
   d. Explain the postoperative need for drainage tubes, surgical dressings, oxygen therapy, I.V. therapy, and pain control

2. Complete a preoperative checklist
3. Administer preoperative medications, as prescribed
4. Allay the patient's and family's anxiety about surgery
5. Document the patient's history and physical assessment data base
6. Verify histocompatibility tests
7. Administer immunosuppressive drugs, as prescribed, for 2 days before the transplantation
8. Maintain protective isolation
9. Administer transfusion therapy, as prescribed
10. Administer I.V. therapy, as prescribed
11. Monitor urinary output (UO)
12. Verify that hemodialysis was completed 24 hours before transplant

C. Postoperative nursing interventions
1. Assess cardiac and respiratory status and fluid balance
2. Assess pain and administer postoperative analgesics, as prescribed
3. Assess for return of peristalsis; give solid foods and liquids, as tolerated
4. Administer I.V. fluids and transfusion therapy, as prescribed
5. Allay the patient's anxiety
6. Inspect the surgical dressing and change, as directed
7. Reinforce TCDB and splinting of incision
8. Keep the patient in semi-Fowler's position
9. Provide incentive spirometry, intermittent positive pressure breathing (IPPB)
10. Maintain activity: as tolerated, increase walking
11. Monitor and record VS, UO, I/O, central venous pressure (CVP), laboratory studies, urine for blood, electrocardiogram (ECG), specific gravity, daily weight, pulse oximetry, and creatinine levels
12. Monitor and maintain position and patency of drainage tubes: indwelling urinary catheter, nasogastric (NG), wound drainage
13. Isolation precautions: protective
14. Encourage the patient to express feelings about chronicity of illness, fear of dying, guilt
15. Administer antifungals, as prescribed
16. Administer immunosuppressive agents with synthetic prostaglandins, as prescribed

CLINICAL ALERT

17. Administer corticosteroids, as prescribed
18. Assess for organ rejection
19. Monitor for infection
20. Provide mouth and skin care

21. Administer antibiotics, as prescribed
22. Administer antilymphocytic globulin (ALG) and antithymocytic globulin (ATG or RATG), as prescribed
23. Prepare for hemodialysis
24. Avoid prolonged periods of sitting
25. Promote live donor and recipient relationship
26. Monitor for depression
27. Monitor for edema of the scrotum, labia, or thigh ipsilateral to the graft
28. Assess the allograft site for pain and edema
29. Individualize home care instructions
    a. Recognize the signs and symptoms of rejection
    b. Avoid contact sports
    c. Complete incision care daily
    d. Adhere to a low-sodium and low-protein diet
    e. Monitor stool for occult blood

D. Possible surgical complications
   1. Renal graft rejection
   2. GI hemorrhage
   3. Acute renal failure
   4. Bladder and ureter fistulas
   5. Candidiasis of mouth
   6. Hypertension
   7. Cerebrovascular accident (CVA)
   8. Gastric ulcer
   9. Liver failure
   10. Depression
   11. Psychosis
   12. Congestive heart failure
   13. Hypovolemia

◆ VIII. Kidney surgery

A. Description
   1. Nephrectomy: surgical removal of the entire kidney
   2. Lithotomy: surgical removal of renal calculi

B. Preoperative nursing interventions
   1. Complete patient and family preoperative teaching
      a. Determine the patient's understanding of the procedure
      b. Describe the OR, PACU, and preoperative and postoperative routines

      c. Demonstrate postoperative TCDB, splinting, and leg and ROM exercises

      d. Explain the postoperative need for drainage tubes, surgical dressings, oxygen therapy, I.V. therapy, and pain control

  2. Complete a preoperative checklist

  3. Administer preoperative medications, as prescribed

  4. Allay the patient's and family's anxiety about surgery

  5. Document the patient's history and physical assessment data base

  6. Administer antibiotics, as prescribed

C. Postoperative nursing interventions

  1. Assess cardiac, respiratory, and neurologic status and fluid balance

  2. Assess pain and administer analgesics, as prescribed

  3. Assess for return of peristalsis; give solid foods, as tolerated, with increased fluids

  4. Administer I.V. fluids, transfusion therapy, and IVH, as prescribed

  5. Allay the patient's anxiety

  6. Inspect the surgical dressing and change, as directed

  7. Reinforce TCDB and splinting of incision

  8. Keep the patient in semi-Fowler's position

  9. Provide incentive spirometry

  10. Maintain activity: as tolerated, active and passive ROM exercises, increase walking

  11. Monitor and record VS, UO, I/O, CVP, laboratory studies, urine for blood, daily weight, specific gravity, and pulse oximetry

  12. Monitor and maintain position and patency of drainage tubes: NG, indwelling urinary catheter, wound drainage, nephrostomy, suprapubic, ureteral

  13. Encourage the patient to express feelings about changes in body image and a fear of dying

  14. Administer antibiotics, as prescribed

  15. Administer stool softeners, as prescribed

  16. Do not irrigate or manipulate the nephrostomy tube

  17. Apply antiembolism stockings

  18. Individualize home care instructions

      a. Recognize the signs and symptoms of renal failure

      b. Complete incision care daily

      c. Avoid using over-the-counter medications

      d. Increase fluid intake, especially cranberry juice

      e. Avoid lifting, straining, horseback riding, and contact sports

      f. Void frequently

D. Possible surgical complications

  1. Hemorrhage

  2. Atelectasis

3. Pneumothorax
4. Pneumonia
5. Paralytic ileus

◆ IX. Prostate surgery

A. Description
1. Transurethral resection of prostate (TURP): insertion of a resectoscope into the urethra to excise prostatic tissue
2. Suprapubic prostatectomy: low abdominal incision into the bladder to the anterior aspect of the prostate to remove large tumors of the prostate
3. Retropubic prostatectomy: low midline incision below the bladder into prostatic capsule to remove a mass in the pelvic area
4. Perineal prostatectomy: incision through the perineum to remove the prostate and surrounding tissue

B. Preoperative nursing interventions
1. Complete patient and family preoperative teaching
   a. Determine the patient's understanding of the procedure
   b. Describe the OR, PACU, and preoperative and postoperative routines
   c. Demonstrate postoperative TCDB, splinting, and leg and ROM exercises
   d. Explain the postoperative need for drainage tubes, surgical dressings, oxygen therapy, I.V. therapy, and pain control
2. Complete a preoperative checklist
3. Administer preoperative medications, as prescribed
4. Allay the patient's and family's anxiety about surgery
5. Document the patient's history and physical assessment data base
6. Administer antibiotics, as prescribed

C. Postoperative nursing interventions
1. Assess cardiac and respiratory status and fluid balance
2. Assess pain and administer postoperative analgesics, as prescribed
3. Assess for return of peristalsis; provide a high-protein, high-fiber, acid-ash diet, as tolerated, with increased fluids
4. Administer I.V. fluids
5. Allay the patient's anxiety
6. Inspect the surgical dressing and change, as directed
7. Reinforce TCDB and splinting of incision
8. Keep the patient in semi-Fowler's position
9. Provide incentive spirometry
10. Maintain activity: as tolerated, progressive ambulation
11. Monitor and record VS, UO, I/O, laboratory studies, urine for blood, stool counts, and pulse oximetry

12. Monitor and maintain position and patency of drainage tubes: NG, indwelling urinary catheter, wound drainage, suprapubic
13. Encourage the patient to express feelings about changes in body image and fear of sexual dysfunction
14. Administer stool softeners, as prescribed
15. Maintain closed continuous bladder irrigation
16. Administer antibiotics, as prescribed
17. Provide treatment: sitz baths
18. Administer anticholinergics, as prescribed

19. Administer antispasmodics, as prescribed
20. Avoid enemas and taking temperature rectally
21. Administer urinary antiseptics, as prescribed
22. Monitor urinary patterns after removal of catheters
23. Individualize home care instructions
    a. Recognize the signs and symptoms of bleeding and urinary tract obstruction
    b. Complete incision care daily
    c. Avoid using over-the-counter medications
    d. Avoid Valsalva's maneuver, lifting, exercising vigorously, or prolonged sitting in the car
    e. Increase fluid intake
    f. Complete perineal strengthening exercises daily
    g. Avoid alcohol and caffeine

D. Possible surgical complications
  1. Hemorrhage
  2. Shock
  3. Infection
  4. Epididymitis
  5. Impotence

♦ X. Urinary diversion

A. Description
  1. Ureterosigmoidostomy: ureters are excised from the bladder and implanted into the sigmoid colon; urine flows through the colon and is excreted through the rectum
  2. Nephrostomy: percutaneous insertion of catheter into kidney
  3. Ileal conduit: ureters are implanted into a segment of the ileum that has been resected from the intestinal tract with the formation of an abdominal stoma
  4. Cutaneous ureterostomy: ureters are excised from the bladder and brought through the abdominal wall to create a stoma

B. Preoperative nursing interventions
  1. Complete patient and family preoperative teaching
      a. Determine the patient's understanding of the procedure
      b. Describe the OR, PACU, and preoperative and postoperative routines
      c. Demonstrate postoperative TCDB, splinting, and leg and ROM exercises
      d. Explain the postoperative need for drainage tubes, surgical dressings, oxygen therapy, I.V. therapy, and pain control
  2. Complete a preoperative checklist
  3. Administer preoperative medications, as prescribed
  4. Allay the patient's and family's anxiety about surgery
  5. Document the patient's history and physical assessment data base
  6. Administer bowel preparation, as prescribed

C. Postoperative nursing interventions
  1. Assess renal status and fluid balance
  2. Assess pain and administer postoperative analgesics, as prescribed
  3. Assess for return of peristalsis; provide acid-ash diet, as tolerated, with increased fluids; avoid giving milk and dairy products
  4. Administer I.V. fluids
  5. Allay the patient's anxiety
  6. Inspect the surgical dressing and change, as directed
  7. Reinforce TCDB and splinting of incision
  8. Keep the patient in semi-Fowler's position
  9. Provide incentive spirometry
  10. Maintain activity: as tolerated, increased walking
  11. Monitor and record VS, UO, I/O, laboratory studies, daily weight, specific gravity, and pulse oximetry
  12. Monitor and maintain position and patency of drainage tubes: NG, indwelling urinary catheter, wound drainage
  13. Encourage the patient to express feelings about changes in body image, embarrassment, and sexual dysfunction
  14. Administer antibiotics, as prescribed
  15. Administer antispasmodics, as prescribed
  16. Apply and change ostomy bags
  17. Provide skin care, particularly around the stoma
  18. Apply antiembolism stockings
  19. Individualize home care instructions
      a. Recognize the signs and symptoms of stomal stenosis
      b. Complete stoma and skin care daily
      c. Use ostomy bags and leg bags
      d. Increase fluid intake
      e. Avoid enemas and laxatives
      f. Empty urinary diversion appliances frequently

D. Possible surgical complications
  1. Chronic renal failure
  2. Infection
  3. Urinary and rectal fistulas
  4. Hemorrhage
  5. Peritonitis
  6. Ureteral obstruction
  7. Stomal stenosis
  8. Bowel obstruction
  9. Renal calculi

◆ **XI. Cystitis**

A. Definition—inflammation of the urinary bladder related to a superficial infection that does not extend to the bladder mucosa

B. Possible etiology
  1. Stagnation of urine in the bladder
  2. Obstruction of the urethra
  3. Sexual intercourse
  4. Incorrect aseptic technique during catheterization
  5. Incorrect perineal care
  6. Kidney infection
  7. Radiation
  8. Diabetes mellitus
  9. Pregnancy

C. Pathophysiology
  1. Bacterial infection from a secondary source spreads to the bladder, causing an inflammatory response
  2. Cell destruction from trauma to the bladder wall, particularly the trigone area, initiates an acute inflammatory reaction

D. Possible assessment findings
  1. Frequency of urination
  2. Urgency of urination
  3. Burning or pain on urination
  4. Lower abdominal discomfort
  5. Dark, odoriferous urine
  6. Flank tenderness or suprapubic pain
  7. Nocturia
  8. Low-grade fever
  9. Urge to bear down on urination
  10. Dysuria
  11. Dribbling

TEACHING TIPS
Patients with renal or urologic disorders

Be sure to include the following topics in your teaching plan for patients with renal or urologic disorders:
- Follow-up appointments
- Smoking cessation
- Optimal body weight maintenance
- Medication therapy including the action, side effects, and scheduling of medications
- Infection control measures, including avoiding exposure to people with infections and monitoring self for infection
- Dietary recommendations and restrictions
- Fluid intake recommendations and restrictions
- Signs and symptoms of renal failure
- Rest and activity patterns, including limitations or restrictions
- Signs and symptoms of urinary tract infection
- Community agencies and resources for supportive services

E. Possible diagnostic test findings
   1. Urine culture and sensitivity: positive identification of organisms *(Escherichia coli, Proteus vulgaris, Streptococcus faecalis)*
   2. Urine chemistry: hematuria, pyuria; increased protein, leukocytes, specific gravity
   3. Cystoscopy: obstruction or deformity

F. Medical management
   1. Diet: acid-ash diet with increased intake of fluids and vitamin C
   2. Activity: as tolerated
   3. Monitoring: VS, UO, and I/O
   4. Laboratory studies: specific gravity, urine culture and sensitivity
   5. Treatment: sitz baths
   6. Antibiotics: trimethoprim and sulfamethoxazole (Bactrim), cephalexin (Keflex)
   7. Analgesic: oxycodone hydrochloride (Tylox)
   8. Urinary antiseptic: phenazopyridine (Pyridium)
   9. Antipyretic: acetaminophen (Tylenol)

G. Nursing interventions
   1. Maintain the patient's diet
   2. Force fluids (cranberry or orange juice) to 3 qt (3 L)/day
   3. Assess renal status
   4. Monitor and record VS, UO, I/O, and laboratory studies
   5. Administer medications, as prescribed
   6. Allay the patient's anxiety

7. Maintain treatments: sitz baths, perineal care
8. Encourage voiding every 2 to 3 hours
9. Individualize home care instructions (For teaching tips, see *Patients with renal or urologic disorders*, page 259)
   a. Avoid coffee, tea, alcohol, and cola
   b. Increase fluid intake to 3 qt/day using orange juice and cranberry juice
   c. Void every 2 to 3 hours and after intercourse
   d. Perform perineal care correctly
   e. Avoid bubble baths, vaginal deodorants, and tub baths

H. Possible medical complications
   1. Chronic cystitis
   2. Urethritis
   3. Pyelonephritis

I. Possible surgical interventions: none

◆ XII. Glomerulonephritis

A. Definition—inflammation of the capillary loops in the glomeruli of the kidney

B. Possible etiology
   1. Injected serum proteins
   2. Systemic lupus erythematosus
   3. Group A beta-hemolytic streptococcal infection

C. Pathophysiology
   1. Antigen-antibody complexes are filtered and trapped within the glomeruli, causing inflammation
   2. Inflammation occludes the glomeruli, causing decreased glomerular filtration and retention of protein wastes and electrolytes

D. Possible assessment findings
   1. Bradycardia
   2. Pharyngitis and tonsillitis
   3. Peripheral and periorbital edema
   4. Lethargy and malaise
   5. Anorexia
   6. Elevated temperature
   7. Hypertension
   8. Tea-colored urine
   9. Flank pain
   10. Dyspnea
   11. Visual disturbances
   12. Dizziness
   13. Oliguria

14. Seizures
15. Weight loss
16. Dehydration

E. Possible diagnostic test findings
   1. Urine chemistry: increased RBCs, WBCs, protein, casts, specific gravity
   2. Blood chemistry: increased BUN, creatinine; decreased protein, creatine clearance, C-reactive protein, albumin
   3. Hematology: decreased Hgb, HCT; increased ESR
   4. Renal biopsy: inflammation of the glomerular capillaries

F. Medical management
   1. Diet: high-carbohydrate, high-vitamin, with restricted intake of sodium, protein, potassium, and fluids
   2. I.V. therapy: heparin lock
   3. Activity: bed rest
   4. Monitoring: VS, UO, I/O, and ECG
   5. Laboratory studies: BUN, creatinine, specific gravity, sodium, potassium, glucose, Hgb, and HCT
   6. Antibiotics: penicillin V potassium (Pen-Vee K), ampicillin (Omnipen)
   7. Antihypertensives: diazoxide (Hyperstat), hydralazine hydrochloride (Apresoline)
   8. Digitalis glycoside: digoxin (Lanoxin)
   9. Immunosuppressants: cyclophosphamide (Cytoxan), azathioprine (Imuran)
   10. Antacids: magnesium and aluminum hydroxide (Maalox), aluminum hydroxide gel (AlternaGEL)
   11. Corticosteroid: prednisone (Deltasone)
   12. Diuretics: chlorthalidone (Hygroton), furosemide (Lasix)
   13. Peritoneal dialysis and hemodialysis
   14. Anticoagulants: warfarin sodium (Coumadin), heparin sodium (Lipo-Hepin)
   15. Precaution: seizure
   16. Plasmapheresis

G. Nursing interventions
   1. Maintain the patient's diet
   2. Restrict fluids
   3. Reinforce TCDB
   4. Assess renal, respiratory, cardiovascular, and neurologic status and fluid balance
   5. Monitor and record VS, UO, I/O, ECG, laboratory studies, urine glucose and ketones, hematuria, weight, and specific gravity
   6. Administer medications, as prescribed

7. Encourage the patient to express feelings about changes in body image

8. Maintain seizure precautions

9. Protect the patient from falls

10. Monitor for bleeding and infection

11. Provide skin and mouth care

12. Individualize home care instructions

a. Limit physical activity

b. Restrict protein and sodium intake

c. Monitor blood pressure and urine protein

H. Possible medical complications

1. Metabolic acidosis

2. Chronic renal failure

3. Hypertensive encephalopathy

4. Congestive heart failure (CHF)

5. Nephrotic syndrome

6. Pulmonary edema

I. Possible surgical interventions: none

◆ XIII. Pyelonephritis

A. Definition—inflammation of renal pelvis

B. Possible etiology

1. Enteric bacteria

2. Ureterovesical reflux

3. Urinary tract obstruction

4. Pregnancy

5. Trauma

6. Urinary tract infection

7. Incorrect aseptic technique

8. Diabetes mellitus

9. Staphylococcal or streptococcal infections

C. Pathophysiology

1. Bacterial infection from a secondary source spreads to the renal pelvis, causing an inflammatory response

2. Cell destruction from trauma to the renal pelvis initiates an inflammatory reaction

D. Possible assessment findings

1. Elevated temperature

2. Chills

3. Nausea and vomiting

4. Flank pain

5. Chronic fatigue

    6. Bladder irritability

    7. Hypertension

    8. Dysuria

    9. Burning on urination

    10. Frequency of urination

    11. Urgency of urination

    12. Headache

    13. Anorexia

    14. Weight loss

    15. Odoriferous, concentrated urine

E. Possible diagnostic test findings

    1. Excretory urography: atrophy, blockage, or deformity of kidney

    2. Urine culture and sensitivity: bacteria

    3. Urine chemistry: pyuria, hematuria; leukocytes, WBCs, and casts; specific gravity greater than 1.025; albuminuria

    4. Hematology: increased WBCs

    5. 24-hour urine collection: decreased creatinine clearance

F. Medical management

    1. Diet: soft, high-calorie, low-protein

    2. I.V. therapy: heparin lock, electrolyte and fluid replacement

    3. Activity: as tolerated

    4. Monitoring: VS, UO, I/O, urine pH, and specific gravity

    5. Laboratory studies: WBCs, urine protein, and urine culture and sensitivity

    6. Treatments: warm, moist compresses to flank

    7. Fluid intake: 3 qt (3 L)/day

    8. Analgesic: meperidine hydrochloride (Demerol)

    9. Antibiotics: cefazolin (Ancef), cefoxitin (Mefoxin), trimethoprim and sulfamethoxazole (Bactrim)

    10. Urinary antiseptic: phenazopyridine (Pyridium)

    11. Antiemetic: prochlorperazine (Compazine)

    12. Alkalinizers: potassium acetate, sodium bicarbonate

    13. Sedative: oxazepam (Serax)

    14. Peritoneal dialysis and hemodialysis

G. Nursing interventions

    1. Maintain the patient's diet

    2. Force fluids to 3 qt/day

    3. Assess renal status and fluid balance

    4. Monitor and record VS, UO, I/O, laboratory studies, daily weight, specific gravity, and urine for blood, protein, and pH

    5. Administer medications, as prescribed

    6. Allay the patient's anxiety

    7. Continue giving hot, moist compresses; warm baths

8. Prevent chilling
9. Provide rest periods
10. Provide skin, mouth, and perineal care
11. Encourage frequent voiding
12. Individualize home care instructions
    a. Void frequently
    b. Return to doctor immediately if symptoms reoccur
    c. Take prescribed medications for entire duration of prescription

H. Possible medical complications
   1. Chronic renal failure
   2. Hypertension
   3. Septicemia

I. Possible surgical interventions: none

♦ XIV. Urolithiasis

A. Definition—stones in kidney, ureters, or bladder

B. Possible etiology
   1. Diet high in calcium, vitamin D, milk, protein, oxalate, alkali
   2. Gout
   3. Hyperparathyroidism
   4. Urinary tract infection
   5. Urinary stasis
   6. Dehydration
   7. Idiopathic
   8. Immobility
   9. Genetics
   10. Hypercalcemia
   11. Urinary tract obstruction
   12. Leukemia
   13. Polycythemia vera
   14. Chemotherapy

C. Pathophysiology
   1. Crystalline substances that normally are dissolved and excreted in the urine form precipitates
   2. Stones are composed of calcium phosphate, oxalate, or uric acid

D. Possible assessment findings
   1. Flank pain
   2. Costovertebral tenderness
   3. Cool, moist skin
   4. RENAL COLIC
   5. Frequency of urination
   6. Urgency of urination

       7. Diaphoresis

       8. Chills and fever

       9. Pallor

     10. Nausea and vomiting

     11. Syncope

   •12. Dysuria

E. Possible diagnostic test findings

       1. KUB: stones

       2. Excretory Urography: stones

       3. Urine chemistry: pyuria, proteinuria, hematuria, presence of WBCs, increased specific gravity

       4. Cystoscopy: visualization of stones

       5. 24-hour urine collection: increased uric acid, oxalate, calcium, phosphorus, creatinine

       6. Blood chemistry: increased calcium, phosphorus, creatinine, BUN, uric acid, protein, alkaline phosphatase

F. Medical management

       1. Diet

          a. For calcium stones—acid-ash with limited intake of calcium and milk products

          b. For oxalate stones—alkaline-ash with limited intake of foods high in oxalate (cola, tea)

          c. For uric acid stones—alkaline-ash with limited intake of foods high in purine

       2. I.V. therapy: heparin lock, fluid replacement

       3. Activity: as tolerated

       4. Monitoring: VS, UO, I/O, and urine pH

       5. Laboratory studies: creatinine, BUN, phosphorus, calcium, and protein

       6. Treatments: strain urine, moist heat to flank, hot baths

       7. Force fluids to 3 qt (3 L)/day

       8. Antigout agent: sulfinpyrazone (Anturane)

       9. Analgesic: meperidine hydrochloride (Demerol)

     10. Antibiotics: cefazolin (Ancef), cefoxitin (Mefoxin)

     11. Antiemetic: prochlorperazine (Compazine)

     12. Acidifiers: ammonium chloride, methenamine mandelate (Mandelamine)

     13. Alkalinizers: potassium acetate, sodium bicarbonate

     14. Chemolysis

     15. Electrohydraulic lithotripsy

     16. Ultrasonic lithotripsy

     17. Laser impulse

     18. Extracorporeal shock wave lithotripsy

19. Percutaneous nephrostolithotomy (PCNL)
20. Prevention of cystinuria: tiopronin (Thiola)

G. Nursing interventions
  1. Maintain the patient's diet
  2. Force fluids to 3,000 ml/day
  3. Assess renal status
  4. Monitor and record VS, UO, I/O, daily weight, specific gravity, laboratory studies, and urine pH
  5. Administer medications, as prescribed
  6. Allay the patient's anxiety
  7. Continue straining urine and giving warm baths and warm soaks to flank
  8. Assess pain
  9. Individualize home care instructions
      a. Increase fluid intake especially during hot weather, illness, and exercise
      b. Void when urge is felt
      c. Test urine pH
      d. Increase fluids at night and void frequently

CLINICAL ALERT

H. Possible medical complications
  1. Chronic urinary tract infection
  2. Renal obstruction
  3. Ureterovesical reflux
  4. Hydronephrosis
  5. Pyelonephritis

I. Possible surgical intervention: lithotomy (see page 253)

◆ XV. Acute renal failure

A. Definition—sudden inability of the kidneys to regulate fluid and electrolyte balance and remove toxic products from the body

B. Possible etiology
  1. CHF
  2. Cardiogenic shock
  3. Hemorrhage
  4. Burns
  5. Septicemia
  6. Hypotension
  7. Acute tubular necrosis
  8. Acute vasoconstriction
  9. Endocarditis
  10. Malignant hypertension
  11. Diabetes mellitus

12. Dehydration
13. Tumor
14. Blood transfusion reaction
15. Cardiopulmonary bypass
16. Nephrotoxins: antibiotics, X-ray dyes, pesticides, anesthetics
17. Renal calculi
18. Benign prostatic hypertrophy
19. Acute glomerulonephritis
20. Trauma
21. Congenital deformity
22. Anaphylaxis
23. Collagen diseases

C. Pathophysiology
1. Decreased perfusion of the kidney results in decreased blood flow and glomerular filtrate, ischemia, and oliguria
2. Damaged nephrons are unable to absorb and secrete water, electrolytes, glucose, amino acids, ammonia, and bicarbonate
3. Disorder may progress from anuric or oliguric phase through diuretic phase to convalescence phase to recovery of function
4. Disorder may develop into chronic renal failure

D. Possible assessment findings
1. Urine output less than 400 ml/day for 1 to 2 weeks followed by diuresis (3 to 5 L/day) for 2 to 3 weeks
2. Lethargy
3. Drowsiness
4. Stupor
5. Coma
6. Irritability
7. Headache
8. Costovertebral pain
9. Circumoral numbness
10. Tingling extremities
11. Anorexia
12. Restlessness
13. Weight gain
14. Nausea and vomiting
15. Pallor
16. Epistaxis
17. Ecchymosis
18. Diarrhea or constipation
19. Stomatitis
20. Thick, tenacious sputum

E. Possible diagnostic test findings

1. Blood chemistry: increased potassium, phosphorus, magnesium, BUN, creatinine, and uric acid; decreased calcium, carbon dioxide (CO_2), and sodium
2. Hematology: decreased Hgb, HCT, erythrocytes; increased PT and PTT
3. Urine chemistry: albuminuria, proteinuria, increased sodium; casts, RBCs, and WBCs; specific gravity greater than 1.025, then fixed at less than 1.010
4. Excretory urography: decreased renal perfusion and function
5. Phenolsulfonphthalein (PSP): decreased
6. Arterial blood gases (ABGs): metabolic acidosis

F. Medical management

1. Diet: low-protein, increased-carbohydrate, moderate-fat, and moderate-calorie with potassium, sodium, and phosphorus intake regulated according to serum levels
2. I.V. therapy: electrolyte replacement, heparin lock
3. Position: semi-Fowler's
4. Activity: bed rest, active and passive ROM and isometric exercises
5. Monitoring: VS, UO, I/O, ECG, and CVP
6. Laboratory studies: BUN, creatinine, phosphorus, calcium, potassium, sodium, Hgb, HCT, and specific gravity
7. Nutritional support: total parental nutrition (TPN)
8. Treatments: indwelling urinary catheter, incentive spirometry, cooling blanket

9. Fluids: restrict intake to amount needed to replace fluid loss
10. Transfusion therapy: packed RBCs
11. Antibiotics: cefazolin (Ancef), cefoxitin (Mefoxin)
12. Analgesic: oxycodone hydrochloride (Tylox)
13. Diuretics: furosemide (Lasix), mannitol (Osmitrol)
14. Antacid: aluminum hydroxide gel (AlternaGEL)
15. Antiemetic: prochlorperazine (Compazine)
16. Cation exchange resins: sodium polystyrene sulfonate (Kayexalate)
17. Chelating agent: dimercaprol (BAL in Oil)
18. Beta adrenergic: dopamine hydrochloride (Intropin)
19. Anticonvulsant: phenytoin (Dilantin)
20. Peritoneal dialysis and hemodialysis
21. Antipyretic: acetaminophen (Tylenol)
22. Precaution: seizure
23. Alkalinizing agent: sodium bicarbonate
24. Continuous arteriovenous hemofiltration (CAVH)

G. Nursing interventions
    1. Maintain the patient's diet
    2. Restrict fluids
    3. Administer I.V. fluids
    4. Assess fluid balance, respiratory, cardiovascular, and neurologic status
    5. Keep the patient in semi-Fowler's position
    6. Monitor and record VS, UO, I/O, CVP, daily weight, specific gravity, laboratory studies, stool for occult blood, and urine glucose and ketones
    7. Administer TPN
    8. Administer medications, as prescribed
    9. Encourage the patient to express feelings about changes in body image
    10. Monitor for arrhythmias
    11. Provide cooling blanket
    12. Monitor the patient for infection
    13. Maintain a quiet environment
    14. Maintain seizure precautions
    15. Monitor the patient for bleeding
    16. Protect the patient from falls
    17. Encourage TCDB

CLINICAL ALERT

    18. Allay the patient's anxiety
    19. Observe for uremic frost
    20. Provide skin and mouth care using plain water
    21. Monitor neurovital signs
    22. Individualize home care instructions
       a. Avoid using over-the-counter medications
       b. Maintain a quiet environment

H. Possible medical complications
    1. Chronic renal failure
    2. Decubiti
    3. Contractures
    4. Atelectasis
    5. GI hemorrhage
    6. Convulsions
    7. Arrhythmias
    8. Cardiac arrest
    9. Pericarditis
    10. Potassium intoxication
    11. Pulmonary edema
    12. Pulmonary infection
    13. CHF
    14. Hypertension
    15. Anemia
    16. Metabolic acidosis

17. Peripheral neuropathy
18. Hypocalcemia

I. Possible surgical interventions: none

◆ XVI. Chronic renal failure

A. Definition—progressive, irreversible destruction of kidneys, resulting in loss of renal function

B. Possible etiology
1. Recurrent urinary tract infection
2. Exacerbations of nephritis
3. Urinary tract obstructions
4. Diabetes mellitus
5. Hypertension
6. Congenital abnormalities
7. Systemic lupus erythematosus
8. Nephrotoxins
9. Dehydration

C. Pathophysiology
1. Scarred nephrons are unable to absorb and secrete water, glucose, amino acids, ammonia, bicarbonate, and electrolytes
2. First stage: renal reserve is diminished, but metabolic wastes do not accumulate although renal damage exists
3. Second stage: renal insufficiency occurs and metabolic wastes begin to accumulate; kidneys are less able to correct metabolic imbalances
4. Third stage: uremia occurs with decreased urine output; increased accumulation of metabolic wastes; and disturbed fluid, electrolyte, and acid-base balances

D. Possible assessment findings
1. Muscle twitching
2. Paresthesia
3. Bone pain
4. Pruritus
5. Decreased urine output
6. Stomatitis
7. Lethargy
8. Seizures
9. Brittle nails and hair
10. Kussmaul's respirations
11. Uremic frost
12. Ecchymosis

E. Possible diagnostic test findings
1. Urine chemistry: proteinuria; increased WBCs, sodium; decreased and fixed specific gravity
2. Blood chemistry: increased BUN, creatinine, phosphorus, lipids; decreased calcium, CO_2, albumin
3. ABGs: metabolic acidosis
4. Hematology: decreased Hgb, HCT, platelets
5. Glucose tolerance test: decreased

F. Medical management
1. Diet: low-protein, low-sodium, low-potassium, low-phosphorus, with high-calorie and high-carbohydrate
2. Dietary restrictions: limit fluids
3. I.V. therapy: heparin lock
4. Activity: as tolerated
5. Monitoring: VS, UO, and I/O
6. Laboratory studies: BUN, creatinine, potassium, sodium, Hgb, HCT, glucose, albumin, and platelets
7. Treatment: tepid baths
8. Transfusion therapy: platelets
9. Antibiotics: cefazolin (Ancef), cefoxitin (Mefoxin)
10. Analgesic: oxycodone hydrochloride (Tylox)
11. Diuretic: furosemide (Lasix)
12. Antacids: aluminum hydroxide gel (AlternaGEL), magnesium and aluminum hydroxide (Maalox)
13. Antiemetic: prochlorperazine (Compazine)
14. Cation exchange resin: sodium polystyrene sulfonate (Kayexalate)
15. Chelating agent: dimercaprol (BAL)
16. Beta adrenergic: dopamine hydrochloride (Intropin)
17. Anticonvulsant: phenytoin (Dilantin)
18. Peritoneal dialysis and hemodialysis
19. Antipyretic: acetaminophen (Tylenol)
20. Precautions: seizure
21. Alkalinizing agent: sodium bicarbonate
22. Digitalis glycoside: digoxin (Lanoxin)
23. Stool softener: docusate sodium (Colace)
24. Antiarrhythmic: procainamide (Pronestyl)
25. Antianemics: ferrous sulfate (Feosol), iron dextran (Imferon), epoetin alfa (recombinant human erythropoietin, Epogen)
26. Vitamins: pyridoxine hydrochloride (vitamin B_6), ascorbic acid (vitamin C)
27. Calcium supplement: calcium carbonate (Os-Cal)

G. Nursing interventions
   1. Maintain the patient's diet
   2. Restrict fluids
   3. Assess renal, respiratory, and cardiovascular status and fluid balance
   4. Monitor and record VS, UO, I/O, ECG, specific gravity, daily weight, laboratory studies, neurovital signs, neurovascular checks, urine for glucose and ketones, and urine, stool, and emesis for occult blood
   5. Administer medications, as prescribed
   6. Encourage the patient to express feelings about chronicity of illness
   7. Provide treatment: tepid baths
   8. Maintain a cool and quiet environment
   9. Provide skin and mouth care using plain water
   10. Maintain seizure precautions
   11. Monitor for ecchymosis

   12. Monitor for infection
   13. Avoid giving the patient intramuscular injections
   14. Protect the patient from falls
   15. Individualize home care instructions
       a. Maintain a quiet environment
       b. Complete skin and mouth care daily

H. Possible medical complications
   1. Arrhythmias
   2. GI bleeding
   3. CHF
   4. Pericardial effusion
   5. Hyperphosphatemia
   6. Pleural effusion
   7. Dehydration
   8. Hyperparathyroidism
   9. Renal osteodystrophy
   10. Uremia
   11. Hypocalcemia

I. Possible surgical intervention: kidney transplantation (see page 251)

♦ XVII. Bladder cancer

A. Definition—malignant tumor that ulcerates mucosal lining of the bladder

B. Possible etiology
   1. Exposure to industrial chemicals
   2. Cigarette smoking
   3. Chronic bladder irritation
   4. Radiation

     5. Excessive intake of coffee, phenacetin, sodium, saccharin, sodium cyclamate

     6. Drug induced: cyclophosphamide (Cytoxan)

C. Pathophysiology

     1. Unregulated cell growth and uncontrolled cell division in bladder's transitional epithelium around trigone result in the development of a neoplasm

     2. Tumor metastasizes to ureters, prostate gland, vagina, rectum, and periaortic lymph nodes

D. Possible assessment findings

     1. Painless hematuria

     2. Dysuria

     3. Frequency of urination

     4. Anuria

     5. Urgency of urination

     6. Chills

     7. Flank or pelvic pain

     8. Elevated temperature

     9. Peripheral edema

E. Possible diagnostic test findings

     1. Cystoscopy: mass

     2. Excretory Urography: mass or obstruction

     3. KUB: mass or obstruction

     4. Cytologic exam: cytology positive for malignant cells

     5. Urine chemistry: hematuria

     6. Hematology: decreased RBCs, Hgb, HCT

F. Medical management

     1. I.V. therapy: heparin lock

     2. Activity: as tolerated

     3. Monitoring: VS, UO, and I/O

     4. Laboratory studies: Hgb and HCT

     5. Radiation therapy

     6. Chemotherapy

     7. Treatment: indwelling urinary catheter

     8. Transfusion therapy: packed RBCs

     9. Sedative: oxazepam (Serax)

     10. Antispasmodic: phenazopyridine (Pyridium)

     11. Antineoplastics: 5-fluorouracil (Adrucil), methotrexate (Rheumatrex), bleomycin (Blenoxane), thiotepa (Thiotepa), doxorubicin hydrochloride (Adriamycin)

     12. Antiemetics: prochlorperazine (Compazine), ondansetron (Zofran)

G. Nursing interventions
1. Maintain the patient's diet
2. Force fluids
3. Administer I.V. fluids
4. Assess renal status
5. Monitor and record VS, UO, I/O, and laboratory studies
6. Administer medications, as prescribed
7. Encourage the patient to express feelings about a fear of dying
8. Provide postchemotherapeutic and postradiation nursing care
   a. Provide prophylactic skin, mouth, and perineal care
   b. Monitor dietary intake
   c. Administer antiemetics and antidiarrheals, as prescribed
   d. Monitor the patient for bleeding, infection, and electrolyte imbalance
   e. Provide rest periods
9. Individualize home care instructions
   a. Provide information about the American Cancer Society
   b. Seek help from community agencies and resources for supportive services

H. Possible medical complications
1. Ureteral obstruction
2. Vesicorectal and vesicovaginal fistulas

I. Possible surgical interventions
1. Ureterosigmoidostomy (see page 256)
2. Ileal conduit (see page 256)
3. Cutaneous ureterostomy (see page 256)
4. Cystectomy
5. Transurethral resection (TUR) of bladder tumor

◆ XVIII. Benign prostatic hypertrophy (BPH)

A. Definition—hyperplasia of the lateral and subcervical lobes of the prostate gland that results in enlargement of the structure

B. Possible etiology
1. Unknown
2. Hormonal

C. Pathophysiology
1. Enlarged prostate gland compresses urethra, resulting in urinary obstruction and retention
2. Obstruction causes hydroureter and hydronephrosis

D. Possible assessment findings
1. Nocturia
2. Urgency, frequency, and burning on urination

    3. Decreased force and amount of stream

    4. Hesitancy

    5. Dysuria

    6. Urine retention

    7. Urinary tract infection

    8. Dribbling

E. Possible diagnostic test findings

    1. Rectal examination: enlarged prostate gland by palpation

    2. Urine chemistry: bacteria, hematuria, alkaline pH, increased specific gravity

    3. Blood chemistry: increased BUN, creatinine

    4. PSP: decreased

    5. Excretory urography: urethral obstruction, hydronephrosis

    6. Cystoscopy: enlarged prostate gland, obstructed urine flow, urinary stasis

    7. CMG: abnormal pressure recordings

    8. Urinary flow rate determination: volume small, flow pattern prolonged, peak flow low

F. Medical management

    1. Diet: force fluids

    2. Position: semi-Fowler's

    3. Activity: as tolerated

    4. Monitoring: VS, UO, and I/O

    5. Laboratory studies: BUN and creatinine

    6. Treatments: indwelling urinary catheter, hot baths

    7. Antibiotics: trimethoprim and sulfamethoxazole (Bactrim), cephalexin (Keflex)

    8. Analgesic: oxycodone hydrochloride (Tylox)

    9. Urinary antiseptic: phenazopyridine (Pyridium)

    10. Antianxiety: oxazepam (Serax)

    11. Alpha-blocker: phenoxybenzamine (Dibenzyline)

    12. Alpha-adrenergic antagonists: prazosin (Minipress), terazosin (Hytrin)

G. Nursing interventions

    1. Force fluids

    2. Assess fluid balance

    3. Keep the patient in semi-Fowler's position

    4. Monitor and record: VS, UO, I/O, and laboratory studies

    5. Administer medications, as prescribed

    6. Encourage the patient to express feelings about changes in body image and fear of sexual dysfunction

CLINICAL ALERT

    7. Maintain position and patency of indwelling urinary catheter to straight drainage

8. Maintain activity, as tolerated
9. Provide hot baths
10. Provide privacy while urinating
11. Monitor for urinary tract infection
12. Individualize home care instructions
    a. Recognize the signs and symptoms of urine retention
    b. Adhere to medical follow-up

H. Possible medical complications
1. Chronic renal failure
2. Hydronephrosis
3. Hydroureter
4. Renal calculi
5. Cystitis

I. Possible surgical interventions
1. Suprapubic cystotomy with insertion of suprapubic catheter
2. TURP (see page 255)
3. Prostatectomy (see page 255)
4. Transurethral dilation of prostate gland (TUDP)

◆ XIX. Prostatic cancer

A. Definition—malignant tumor of the prostate gland

B. Possible etiology
1. No known etiology
2. Associated risk factors: family history, age, black race, vasectomy, increased dietary fat

C. Pathophysiology
1. Unregulated cell growth and uncontrolled cell division result in the development of a neoplasm
2. Obstruction of urine flow occurs when the tumor encroaches on the bladder neck
3. Metastasis often occurs to bone, lymph nodes, brain, and lungs

D. Possible assessment findings
1. Difficulty and frequency of urination
2. Urine retention
3. Decreased size and force of urinary stream
4. Hematuria

E. Possible diagnostic test findings
1. Digital rectal examination: palpable firm nodule in gland or diffuse induration in posterior lobe
2. Serum acid phosphatase level: increased
3. Radioimmunoassay for acid phosphatase: increased
4. Prostatic-specific antigen (PSA): increased

     5. Transurethral ultrasound studies: mass or obstruction

     6. Prostate biopsy: cytology positive for cancer cells

     7. Excretory urograms: mass or obstruction

F. Medical management

     1. Diet: high-protein

     2. Dietary restrictions: caffeine, spicy foods

     3. Activity: as tolerated

     4. Monitoring: VS, UO, I/O

     5. Laboratory studies: BUN, creatinine, PSA

     6. I.V. therapy: heparin lock

     7. Analgesics: oxycodone hydrochloride (Tylox), meperidine hydro-chloride (Demerol)

     8. Corticosteroid: prednisone (Deltasone)

     9. Nonsteroidal anti-inflammatory drugs (NSAIDs): indomethacin (Indocin), ibuprofen (Motrin), sulindac (Clinoril)

    10. Stool softener: docusate sodium (Colace)

    11. Radiation therapy

    12. Chemotherapy

    13. Estrogen therapy: diethylstilbestrol (Stilphostrol)

    14. Radiation implant

    15. Antineoplastics: doxorubicin hydrochloride (Adriamycin), cisplatin (Platinol)

    16. Immunosuppressant: cyclophosphamide (Cytoxan)

    17. Nitrogen mustard: estramustine phosphate sodium (Emcyt)

    18. Treatment: Suprapubic or transurethral catheter

    19. Antiemetics: prochlorperazine (Compazine), ondansetron (Zofran)

G. Nursing interventions

     1. Maintain the patient's diet

     2. Monitor fluid intake

     3. Assess renal and fluid status

     4. Monitor and record VS, UO, I/O, and laboratory studies

     5. Administer medications, as prescribed

     6. Allay the patient's anxiety

     7. Maintain patency of the urinary catheter

     8. Encourage the patient to express feelings about the changes in body image and fear of sexual dysfunction

     9. Encourage ambulation

    10. Assess pain

    11. Provide postchemotherapeutic and postradiation nursing care

       a. Provide prophylactic skin, mouth, and perineal care

       b. Monitor dietary intake

       c. Administer antiemetics and antidiarrheals, as prescribed

       d. Provide rest periods

12. Individualize home care instructions
    a. Provide information about the American Cancer Society
    b. Seek help from community agencies and resources for supportive services
    c. Monitor effect of impotency on sexual activities
    d. Avoid prolonged sitting, standing, and walking
    e. Avoid straining during exercise and lifting
    f. Urinate frequently
    g. Avoid coffee and cola beverages
    h. Decrease fluid intake during evening hours
    i. Perform perineal exercises
    j. Complete catheter care, as directed
    k. Monitor self for bloody urine, pain, burning, frequency, decreased urine output, and loss of bladder control
    l. Use walker or cane, if needed

H. Possible medical complications: Metastatic cancer (bone, lymph nodes, brain, and lung)

I. Possible surgical interventions
    1. Radical prostatectomy (see page 255)
    2. Bilateral orchiectomy
    3. Cryosurgery
    4. Transurethral resection (see page 255)

POINTS TO REMEMBER

♦ Renal disease can alter the renin-angiotensin system, which controls blood pressure.

♦ Specific gravity of urine, the patient's daily weight, and accurate fluid output measurements are important objective assessments for renal function.

♦ After a kidney transplant, the nurse should assess the allograft site for rejection.

♦ The nurse should observe the patient with acute renal failure for uremic frost.

♦ The nurse should encourage the patient with a renal or urologic disorder to express feelings about changes in body function and fear of sexual dysfunction.

STUDY QUESTIONS

To evaluate your understanding of this chapter, answer the following questions in the space provided; then compare your responses with the correct answers in Appendix B, pages 384 and 385.

1. What urine and blood chemistry test results would be reported for a patient with glomerulonephritis? _____

_____

_____

2. Which foods can cause urolithiasis?_____

_____

_____

3. What type of diet would the doctor prescribe for a patient with acute renal failure?_____

_____

_____

4. What are the key assessment findings for BPH? _____

_____

_____

CRITICAL THINKING AND APPLICATION EXERCISES

1. Observe a cystoscopy. Prepare an oral presentation for your fellow students, describing the procedure and patient care before, during, and after the procedure.

2. Develop a dietary teaching plan for a patient with urolithiasis.

3. Interview a patient with a renal or urologic disorder. Evaluate the information for possible risk factors and identify ways to modify them.

4. Follow a patient with a renal or urologic disorder from admission through discharge. Develop a patient-specific plan of care, including any needs for follow-up and home care.

8

Musculoskeletal System

LEARNING OBJECTIVES

After studying this chapter, you should be able to:

♦ Describe the psychosocial impact of musculoskeletal disorders.

♦ Differentiate between modifiable and nonmodifiable risk factors in the development of a musculoskeletal disorder.

♦ List three probable and three possible nursing diagnoses for a patient with any musculoskeletal disorder.

♦ Identify nursing interventions for a patient with a musculoskeletal disorder.

♦ Identify three teaching topics for a patient with a musculoskeletal disorder.

CHAPTER OVERVIEW

Caring for the patient with a musculoskeletal disorder requires a sound understanding of musculoskeletal anatomy and physiology and body mechanics. A thorough assessment is essential to planning and implementing appropriate patient care. The assessment includes a complete history, physical examination, diagnostic testing, identification of modifiable and nonmodifiable risk factors, and information related to the psychosocial impact of the disorder on the patient. Nursing diagnoses focus primarily on impaired physical mobility and altered peripheral tissue perfusion. Nursing interventions are designed to maintain the patient's ability to carry out the activities of daily living and prevent further injury. Patient teaching — a crucial nursing activity — involves information about medical follow-up, medication regimens, signs and symptoms of possible complications, and reduction of modifiable risk factors through the use of proper body mechanics, the prevention of falls, and the participation in body flexibility and strength regimens.

◆ **I. Anatomy and physiology review**

A. Skeleton
1. Consists of 206 bones (long, short, flat, or irregular)
2. Stores calcium, magnesium, and phosphorus; marrow produces red blood cells (RBCs)
3. Works with muscles to provide support, locomotion, and protection of internal organs

B. Skeletal muscles
1. Provide body movement and posture by tightening and shortening
2. Attach to bones by tendons
3. Begin contracting with the stimulus of a muscle fiber by a motor neuron
4. Derive energy for muscle contraction from hydrolysis of adenosine triphosphate (ATP) to adenosine diphosphate (ADP) and phosphate
5. Retain some contraction to maintain muscle tone
6. Relax with the breakdown of acetylcholine by cholinesterase

C. Ligaments
1. Are tough bands of collagen fibers that connect bones
2. Encircle a joint to add strength and stability

D. Tendons
1. Are nonelastic collagen cords
2. Connect muscles to bones

E. Joints
1. Are the articulation of two bone surfaces
2. Provide stabilization and permit locomotion; degree of joint movement is called range of motion (ROM)

F. Synovium
1. Is the membrane that lines a joint's inner surfaces
2. Secretes synovial fluid and antibodies
3. Reduces friction in joints (in conjunction with cartilage)

G. Cartilage
  1. Serves as a smooth surface for articulating bones
  2. Absorbs shock to joints
  3. Atrophies with limited ROM or in the absence of weight bearing

H. Bursa
  1. Is a fluid-filled sac
  2. Serves as padding to reduce friction
  3. Facilitates the motion of body structures that rub against each other

♦ **II. Assessment findings**

A. History
  1. Pain
  2. Numbness
  3. Joint stiffness
  4. Swelling
  5. Fatigue
  6. Fever
  7. Difficulty with movement

B. Physical examination
  1. Abnormal vital signs (VS)
  2. Inflammation
  3. Edema
  4. Skin breakdown
  5. Skeletal deformity
  6. Limited ROM
  7. Poor posture
  8. Muscle weakness and rigidity
  9. Abnormal skin color and temperature
  10. Paresthesia
  11. Nodules
  12. Erythema
  13. Tophi
  14. Abnormal peripheral pulses
  15. Muscle spasms

♦ **III. Diagnostic tests and procedures**

A. Electromyography (EMG)
  1. Definition and purpose
    a. Test of muscle activity
    b. Graphical recording of the muscle at rest and during contraction

2. Nursing interventions
   a. Explain that the patient will be asked to flex and relax muscles during the procedure
   b. Instruct the patient that the procedure may cause some minor discomfort but is not painful
   c. Administer analgesics, as prescribed, after the procedure

B. Arthroscopy
   1. Definition and purpose—direct visualization of a joint after injection of local anesthesia
   2. Nursing interventions before the procedure
      a. Administer prophylactic antibiotics, as prescribed
      b. Explain the procedure, skin preparation, and use of local anesthetics

CLINICAL ALERT

   3. Nursing interventions after the procedure
      a. Apply a pressure dressing to the injection site
      b. Monitor neurovascular status
      c. Apply ice to the affected joint
      d. Limit weight bearing or joint use until allowed by the doctor
      e. Administer analgesics, as prescribed

C. Arthrocentesis
   1. Definition and purpose—needle aspiration of synovial fluid from a joint under local anesthesia to examine a specimen or remove the fluid
   2. Nursing interventions before the procedure
      a. Administer prophylactic antibiotics, as prescribed
      b. Explain the procedure to the patient

CLINICAL ALERT

   3. Nursing interventions after the procedure
      a. Maintain a pressure dressing on the aspiration site
      b. Monitor neurovascular status
      c. Apply ice to the affected area
      d. Limit weight bearing or joint use until allowed by the doctor
      e. Administer analgesics, as prescribed

D. Bone scan
   1. Definition and purpose
      a. Procedure using I.V. injection of a radioisotope
      b. Visual imaging of bone metabolism
   2. Nursing interventions before the procedure
      a. Determine the patient's ability to lie still during the scan
      b. Advise the patient that radioisotope will be injected intravenously
      c. Explain that the patient will be required to drink several glasses of fluid during the waiting period to enhance excretion of isotope not absorbed by bone tissue

E. Myelogram
   1. Definition and purpose
      a. Procedure using an injection of radiopaque dye by lumbar puncture
      b. Fluoroscopic visualization of the subarachnoid space, spinal cord, and vertebral bodies

   2. Nursing interventions before the procedure
      a. Note the patient's allergies to iodine, seafood, and radiopaque dyes
      b. Inform the patient about possible throat irritation and flushing of the face from the injection
   3. Nursing interventions after the procedure
      a. Maintain bed rest, with the patient lying flat
      b. Inspect the insertion site for bleeding
      c. Monitor neurovital signs
      d. Force fluids

F. X-ray examination
   1. Definition and purpose—noninvasive radiographic examination of bones and joints
   2. Nursing interventions
      a. Use caution when moving a patient with a suspected fracture
      b. Explain the procedure to the patient
      c. Make sure that the patient is not pregnant to prevent possible fetal damage from radiation exposure

G. Blood chemistry
   1. Definition and purpose
      a. Laboratory test of a blood sample
      b. Analysis for potassium, sodium, calcium, phosphorus, glucose, bicarbonate, blood urea nitrogen (BUN), creatinine, protein, albumin, osmolality, creatine kinase, serum aspartate aminotransferase (AST), aldolase, rheumatoid factor, complement fixation, lupus erythematosus cell preparation (LE prep), antinuclear antibody (ANA), anti-DNA, and C-reactive protein
   2. Nursing interventions
      a. Withhold food and fluid before the procedure
      b. Monitor the venipuncture site for bleeding after the procedure

H. Hematologic studies
   1. Definition and purpose
      a. Laboratory test of a blood sample
      b. Analysis for white blood cells (WBCs), RBCs, platelets, prothrombin time (PT), partial thromboplastin time (PTT), erythrocyte sedimentation rate (ESR), hemoglobin (Hgb), and hematocrit (HCT)

   2. Nursing interventions
      a. Note current drug therapy to anticipate possible interference with test results
      b. Assess the venipuncture site for bleeding after the procedure

♦ IV. Psychosocial impact of musculoskeletal disorders

A. Developmental impact
1. Decreased self-esteem
2. Fear of rejection
3. Changes in body image
4. Embarrassment from changes in body structure and function
5. Dependence

B. Economic impact
1. Disruption or loss of employment
2. Cost of vocational retraining
3. Cost of hospitalizations
4. Cost of home health care
5. Cost of special equipment

C. Occupational and recreational impact
1. Restrictions in work activity
2. Changes in leisure activity
3. Restrictions in physical activity

D. Social impact
1. Social isolation
2. Changes in role performance

♦ V. Possible risk factors

A. Modifiable risk factors
1. Occupations that require heavy lifting or use of machinery
2. Occupational or recreational activities that include repetitive motion of joints
3. Vegetarian diets
4. Immobility
5. Medication history
6. Stress
7. Contact sports
8. Obesity

B. Nonmodifiable risk factors
1. Aging
2. Menopause
3. Family history of musculoskeletal illness

4. History of musculoskeletal injury
5. History of immune disorders

♦ VI. Nursing diagnostic categories

A. Probable nursing diagnostic categories
1. Impaired physical mobility
2. Altered peripheral tissue perfusion
3. Impaired skin integrity
4. Acute pain
5. Toileting self-care deficit
6. Feeding self-care deficit
7. Bathing/hygiene self-care deficit

B. Possible nursing diagnostic categories
1. Sexual dysfunction
2. Powerlessness
3. Constipation
4. Body image disturbance
5. Social isolation
6. Risk for disuse syndrome
7. Chronic pain

♦ VII. Joint surgery

A. Description
1. Arthrodesis—surgical removal of cartilage from joint surfaces to fuse a joint into a functional position
2. Synovectomy—removal of the synovial membrane from a joint, using an arthroscope, to reduce pain
3. Arthroplasty (total joint replacement)—surgical replacement of a joint with a metal, plastic, or porous prosthesis

B. Preoperative nursing interventions
1. Complete patient and family preoperative teaching
   a. Determine the patient's understanding of the procedure
   b. Describe the operating room (OR), postanesthesia care unit (PACU), and preoperative and postoperative routines
   c. Demonstrate postoperative turning, coughing, and deep breathing (TCDB), splinting, and leg and ROM exercises
   d. Explain the postoperative need for drainage tubes, surgical dressings, oxygen therapy, I.V. therapy, and pain control
2. Complete a preoperative checklist
3. Administer preoperative medications, as prescribed
4. Allay the patient's and family's anxiety about surgery
5. Document the patient's history and physical assessment database
6. Administer antibiotics, as prescribed

C. Postoperative nursing interventions
   1. Assess cardiac and respiratory status
   2. Assess pain and administer postoperative analgesic, as prescribed
   3. Administer I.V. fluids and transfusion therapy, as prescribed
   4. Allay the patient's anxiety
   5. Inspect the surgical dressing and change, as directed
   6. Reinforce TCDB
   7. Keep the patient in semi-Fowler's position
   8. Provide incentive spirometry
   9. Maintain activity: active and passive ROM for unaffected limbs and isometric exercises, as tolerated
  10. Monitor VS, urine output (UO), intake and output (I/O), laboratory studies, neurovascular checks, and pulse oximetry
  11. Monitor and maintain the position and patency of wound drainage tubes
  12. Encourage the patient to express feelings about limited mobility
  13. Assess movement limitations
  14. Elevate the affected extremity
  15. Administer antibiotics, as prescribed
  16. Assess for return of peristalsis
  17. Give solid foods and liquids, as tolerated
  18. Administer stool softeners, as prescribed
  19. Provide routine cast care (arthrodesis)
  20. Provide specific care for total knee replacement
    a. Maintain continuous passive motion (CPM)
    b. Apply a knee immobilizer before getting the patient out of bed
    c. Administer anticoagulants, as prescribed
  21. Provide specific care for total hip replacement

CLINICAL ALERt

CLINICAL ALERT

    a. Maintain hips in abduction
    b. Limit hip flexion to 90 degrees when sitting
    c. Turn to the affected or unaffected side, as ordered
    d. Avoid sitting in low or soft chairs
    e. Do not allow patient to cross legs; possible dislodgement of prosthesis or dislocation may occur
    f. Have patient use elevated toilet seat
    g. Administer anticoagulants, as prescribed
  22. Individualize home care instructions
    a. Avoid jogging, jumping, and lifting, as prescribed
    b. Complete incision care daily, as prescribed
    c. Continue cast care, as directed

D. Possible surgical complications
   1. Infection
   2. Hemorrhage

♦ VIII. External fixation

A. Description—fracture immobilization in which transfixing pins are inserted through the bone above and below the fracture and then attached to a rigid external metal frame

B. Preoperative nursing interventions

1. Complete patient and family preoperative teaching
   a. Determine the patient's understanding of the procedure
   b. Describe the OR, PACU, and preoperative and postoperative routines
   c. Demonstrate postoperative TCDB, splinting, and leg and ROM exercises
   d. Explain the postoperative need for drainage tubes, surgical dressings, oxygen therapy, I.V. therapy, and pain control
2. Complete a preoperative checklist
3. Administer preoperative medications, as prescribed
4. Allay the patient's and family's anxiety about surgery
5. Document the patient's history and physical assessment database
6. Monitor for fracture complications
7. Maintain the position of the affected extremity with sandbags and pillows
8. Maintain traction or splint

C. Postoperative nursing interventions

1. Assess pain and administer postoperative analgesics, as prescribed
2. Assess for return of peristalsis; give solid foods and liquids, as tolerated
3. Administer I.V. fluids
4. Allay the patient's anxiety
5. Reinforce TCDB
6. Keep the patient in semi-Fowler's position
7. Provide incentive spirometry
8. Maintain activity: active and passive ROM for unaffected limbs, isometric exercises, and quadriceps setting, as tolerated
9. Monitor VS, UO, I/O, laboratory studies, and neurovascular checks
10. Encourage the patient to express feelings about changes in body image

11. Check wound and pin sites for infection
12. Provide pin care
13. Maintain balanced suspension traction
14. Do not readjust traction clamps
15. Individualize home care instructions
    a. Attend physical therapy sessions
    b. Maintain fixator, as set
    c. Complete pin care daily, as directed

D. Possible surgical complications
  1. Infection of wound and pin sites
  2. Osteomyelitis
  3. Hemorrhage
  4. Chronic pain

♦ **IX. Amputation**

  A. Description
    1. Surgical removal of all or part of a limb
    2. Two types of amputation
      a. Closed (flap)
      b. Open (guillotine)

  B. Preoperative nursing interventions
    1. Complete patient and family preoperative teaching
      a. Determine the patient's understanding of the procedure
      b. Describe the OR, PACU, and preoperative and postoperative routines
      c. Demonstrate postoperative TCDB, splinting, and leg and ROM exercises
      d. Explain the postoperative need for drainage tubes, surgical dressings, oxygen therapy, I.V. therapy, and pain control
    2. Complete a preoperative checklist
    3. Administer preoperative medications, as prescribed
    4. Allay the patient's and family's anxiety about surgery
    5. Document the patient's history and physical assessment database
    6. Administer antibiotics, as prescribed
    7. Prepare the patient for the possibility of phantom limb sensation or phantom pain

  C. Postoperative nursing interventions
    1. Assess cardiac and respiratory status
    2. Assess pain and administer postoperative analgesics, as prescribed
    3. Administer I.V. fluids and transfusion therapy, as prescribed
    4. Allay the patient's anxiety
    5. Inspect the ace wrap surgical dressing and change, as directed
    6. Reinforce TCDB
    7. Keep the patient in semi-Fowler's position
    8. Assess for return of peristalsis; give solid foods and liquids, as tolerated
    9. Provide incentive spirometry
    10. Maintain activity: active and passive ROM for unaffected limbs and isometric exercises, as tolerated
    11. Monitor VS, UO, I/O, laboratory studies, neurovascular checks, and pulse oximetry

12. Monitor and maintain the position and patency of wound drainage tubes
13. Encourage the patient to express feelings about changes in body image and phantom limb sensation and pain
14. Administer antibiotics, as prescribed
15. Elevate the affected extremity for 24 hours only
16. Rewrap the stump before getting the patient out of bed
17. Prevent hip flexion
18. Inspect the stump for bleeding, infection, and edema
19. Maintain a rigid dressing for the stump prosthesis
20. Irrigate the wound and change the ace wrap stump dressing, as directed
21. Reinforce physical therapy attendance
22. Provide trapeze
23. Individualize home care instructions
   a. Recognize the signs and symptoms of skin breakdown
   b. Complete stump care daily
   c. Use a prosthesis
   d. Maintain a stump conditioning program
   e. Avoid using powder or lotion on the stump
   f. Demonstrate proper wrapping of the stump
   g. Protect the stump from injury

D. Possible surgical complications
   1. Hemorrhage
   2. Infection
   3. Contractures
   4. Skin breakdown

♦ X. Release of transverse carpal ligament

A. Description—surgical ligation of the transverse carpal ligament to relieve compression of the median nerve in the carpal canal of the wrist

B. Postoperative nursing interventions
   1. Complete patient and family preoperative teaching
      a. Determine the patient's understanding of the procedure
      b. Describe the OR, PACU, and preoperative and postoperative routines
      c. Demonstrate postoperative TCDB, splinting, and leg and ROM exercises
      d. Explain the postoperative need for drainage tubes, surgical dressings, oxygen therapy, I.V. therapy, and pain control
   2. Complete a preoperative checklist
   3. Administer preoperative medications, as prescribed
   4. Allay the patient's and family's anxiety about surgery

    5. Document the patient's history and physical assessment database

    6. Use a splint to increase the patient's comfort

C. Postoperative nursing interventions

    1. Assess pain and administer postoperative analgesics, as prescribed

    2. Assess for return of peristalsis; give solid foods and liquids, as tolerated

    3. Administer I.V. fluids

    4. Allay the patient's anxiety

    5. Inspect the surgical dressing and change, as directed

    6. Reinforce TCDB

    7. Keep the patient in semi-Fowler's position

    8. Provide incentive spirometry

    9. Maintain activity: active and passive ROM and isometric exercises to affected and unaffected extremities, as tolerated

    10. Monitor VS, UO, I/O, laboratory studies, and neurovascular checks

    11. Elevate the hand and apply ice

    12. Administer steroids, as prescribed

    13. Administer antibiotics, as prescribed

    14. Assist with activities of daily living (ADLs)

    15. Prevent injury to the affected hand

    16. Apply splint

    17. Reinforce immobilization of the affected hand

    18. Individualize home care instructions

        a. Continue active ROM exercises of the affected hand

        b. Avoid heavy lifting

        c. Use a splint

        d. Monitor the affected hand for return of sensation and motor function

        e. Complete incision care daily, as directed

D. Possible surgical complications

    1. Infection

    2. Paralysis

◆ XI. Open reduction internal fixation of the hip (ORIF)

A. Description—surgical reduction and stabilization of a fracture, using orthopedic devices or hardware (such as Austin-Moore prosthesis, Smith-Petersen nail, Jewett nail, intramedullary nails, and compression screws)

B. Preoperative nursing interventions

    1. Complete patient and family preoperative teaching

        a. Determine the patient's understanding of the procedure

        b. Describe the OR, PACU, and preoperative and postoperative routines

    c. Demonstrate postoperative TCDB, splinting, and leg and ROM exercises

    d. Explain the postoperative need for drainage tubes, surgical dressings, oxygen therapy, I.V. therapy, and pain control

  2. Complete a preoperative checklist

  3. Administer preoperative medications, as prescribed

  4. Allay the patient's and family's anxiety about surgery

  5. Document the patient's history and physical assessment database

  6. Monitor the patient for fracture complications

  7. Keep the affected extremity in position with sandbags and pillows

  8. Maintain traction or splint

C. Postoperative nursing interventions

  1. Assess cardiac and respiratory status

  2. Assess pain and administer postoperative analgesics, as prescribed

  3. Assess for return of peristalsis; give solid foods and liquids, as tolerated

  4. Administer I.V. fluids and transfusion therapy, as prescribed

  5. Allay the patient's anxiety

  6. Inspect the surgical dressing and change, as directed

  7. Reinforce TCDB

  8. Keep the patient in semi-Fowler's position: no higher than 30 degrees

  9. Provide incentive spirometry

  10. Maintain activity: bed rest, active and passive ROM for unaffected limbs, isometric exercises, and progressive ambulation

  11. Monitor VS, UO, I/O, laboratory studies, neurovascular checks, and pulse oximetry

  12. Monitor and maintain the position and patency of drainage tubes

  13. Use abductor pillow and trochanter rolls

  14. Turn the patient to the affected or unaffected side, as ordered

  15. Maintain a high-fiber, low-calcium diet with increased fluid intake

  16. Apply antiembolism or pneumatic stockings

  17. Administer anticoagulants, as prescribed

  18. Administer antibiotics, as prescribed

  19. Administer stool softeners, as prescribed

  20. Use a fracture bedpan

  21. Provide heel and elbow protectors

  22. Individualize home care instructions

    a. Avoid jogging, jumping, lifting, crossing the legs, and sitting in soft or low chairs

    b. Complete incision care daily, as directed

    c. Apply antiembolism stockings

    d. Use an elevated toilet seat

D. Possible surgical complications
1. Osteomyelitis
2. Hemorrhage
3. Thrombophlebitis
4. Pneumonia
5. Avascular necrosis
6. Pulmonary embolism

♦ XII. Surgical intervention: Laminectomy

A. Description—surgical excision of vertebral posterior arch

B. Preoperative nursing interventions
1. Complete patient and family preoperative teaching
   a. Determine the patient's understanding of the procedure
   b. Describe the OR, PACU, and preoperative and postoperative routines
   c. Demonstrate postoperative TCDB, splinting, and leg and ROM exercises
   d. Explain the postoperative need for drainage tubes, surgical dressings, oxygen therapy, I.V. therapy, and pain control
2. Complete a preoperative checklist
3. Administer preoperative medications, as prescribed
4. Allay the patient's and family's anxiety about surgery
5. Document the patient's history and physical assessment database
6. Teach the patient the logrolling technique
7. Administer antibiotics, as prescribed

C. Postoperative nursing interventions
1. Assess neurologic and neurovascular status
2. Assess pain and administer postoperative analgesics, as prescribed
3. Assess for return of peristalsis; give solid foods and liquids, as tolerated
4. Administer I.V. fluids
5. Allay the patient's anxiety
6. Inspect surgical dressings for drainage of cerebrospinal fluid (CSF) and blood
7. Reinforce TCDB
8. Keep the patient in a flat position
9. Provide incentive spirometry
10. Maintain activity: active and passive ROM and isometric exercises
11. Monitor VS, UO, I/O, laboratory studies, and neurovascular checks

CLINICAL ALERT

12. Turn the patient by logrolling
13. Prevent flexion of the neck after cervical laminectomy
14. Administer muscle relaxants, as prescribed
15. Administer corticosteroids, as prescribed

16. Administer stool softeners, as prescribed
17. Individualize home care instructions
    a. Avoid lifting, driving, stooping, tub bathing, and repetitive bending, as prescribed
    b. Wear a supportive brace
    c. Complete exercises for the lower back daily
    d. Sleep on the side, with hips and knees flexed
    e. Sleep on a firm mattress
    f. Monitor lower extremities for numbness and decreased circulation
    g. Monitor ability to void
    h. Complete incision care daily, as directed

D. Possible surgical complications
    1. Urine retention
    2. Motor and sensory deficits
    3. Infection
    4. Muscle spasm
    5. Paralytic ileus

♦ XIII. Spinal fusion

A. Description—stabilization of spinous processes with bone chips from iliac crest or Harrington rod metallic implant

B. Preoperative nursing interventions
    1. Complete patient and family preoperative teaching
       a. Determine the patient's understanding of the procedure
       b. Describe the OR, PACU, and preoperative and postoperative routines
       c. Demonstrate postoperative TCDB, splinting, and leg and ROM exercises
       d. Explain the postoperative need for drainage tubes, surgical dressings, oxygen therapy, I.V. therapy, and pain control
    2. Complete a preoperative checklist
    3. Administer preoperative medications, as prescribed
    4. Allay the patient's and family's anxiety about surgery
    5. Document the patient's history and physical assessment database
    6. Administer antibiotics, as prescribed
    7. Teach the patient the logrolling technique

C. Postoperative nursing interventions
    1. Assess cardiac, respiratory, and neurologic status
    2. Assess pain and administer postoperative analgesics, as prescribed
    3. Assess for return of peristalsis; give solid foods and liquids, as tolerated
    4. Administer I.V. fluids
    5. Allay the patient's anxiety

6. Inspect the surgical dressing and change, as directed
7. Reinforce TCDB
8. Maintain the patient in the supine position
9. Provide incentive spirometry
10. Maintain activity: active and passive ROM and isometric exercises
11. Monitor VS, UO, I/O, and laboratory studies
12. Check neurovascular status: color, temperature, pulses, movement, and sensation in extremities
13. Administer antipyretics, as prescribed
14. Administer antibiotics, as prescribed

15. Administer corticosteroids, as prescribed
16. Turn the patient every 2 hours using the logrolling technique
17. Administer muscle relaxants, as prescribed
18. Administer stool softeners, as prescribed
19. Individualize home care instructions
    a. Avoid lifting, driving, stooping, tub bathing, repetitive bending, and prolonged sitting, as prescribed
    b. Walk regularly
    c. Note spinal flexion limitations
    d. Complete exercises for lower back daily
    e. Sleep on the side with hips and knees flexed
    f. Sleep on a firm mattress
    g. Monitor lower extremities for numbness and decreased circulation
    h. Monitor ability to void
    i. Complete incision care daily, as directed

D. Possible surgical complications
   1. Urine retention
   2. Infection
   3. Muscle spasm
   4. Motor and sensory deficits
   5. Paralytic ileus

◆ XIV. Rheumatoid arthritis

A. Definition—systemic inflammatory disease that affects the synovial lining of the joints

B. Possible etiology
   1. Unknown
   2. Autoimmune disease
   3. Genetic transmission

C. Pathophysiology
   1. Inflammation of the synovial membranes is followed by formation of PANNUS and destruction of cartilage, bone, and ligaments
   2. Pannus is replaced by fibrotic tissue and calcification, which causes SUBLUXATION of the joint

D. Possible assessment findings
   1. Fatigue
   2. Anorexia
   3. Malaise
   4. Elevated body temperature
   5. Painful, swollen joints
   6. Limited ROM
   7. Subcutaneous nodules
   8. Symmetrical joint swelling (mirror image of affected joints)
   9. Morning stiffness
   10. Paresthesia of the hands and the feet
   11. Crepitus
   12. Pericarditis
   13. Splenomegaly
   14. Leukopenia
   15. Enlarged lymph nodes

E. Possible diagnostic test findings
   1. X-rays: joint space narrowing, bone erosions
   2. Hematology: increased ESR, WBC, platelets
   3. Gamma globulin: increased IgM, IgG
   4. Synovial fluid analysis: increased WBC, decreased viscosity, opaque
   5. Latex fixation test: positive rheumatoid factor

F. Medical management
   1. Activity: as tolerated
   2. Monitoring: VS, UO, and I/O
   3. Analgesic: aspirin
   4. Nonsteroidal anti-inflammatory drugs (NSAIDs): indomethacin (Indocin), ibuprofen (Motrin), sulindac (Clinoril), piroxicam (Feldene), flurbiprofen (Ansaid), diclofenac sodium (Voltaren), naproxen (Naprosyn), diflunisal (Dolobid)
   5. Glucocorticoids: prednisone (Deltasone), hydrocortisone (Cortef)
   6. Antacids: magnesium and aluminum hydroxide (Maalox), aluminum hydroxide gel (Gelusil)
   7. Gold therapy: gold sodium thiomalate (Myochrysine)
   8. Physical therapy
   9. Heat therapy
   10. Cold therapy
   11. Plasmapheresis

TEACHING TIPS
Patients with musculoskeletal disorders

Be sure to include the following topics in your teaching plan when caring for patients with musculoskeletal disorders.
- Follow-up appointments
- Optimal body weight maintenance
- Medication therapy including the action, adverse effects, and scheduling of medications
- Use of assistive and adaptive devices, such as crutches, a walker, or a cane
- Signs and symptoms of soft tissue and bone infection
- Rest and activity patterns, including activity limitations or restrictions
- Signs and symptoms of motor, sensory, and circulatory deficits
- Safe environment
- Change in ADLs to compensate for limited ROM
- Proper body mechanics and correct posture
- Dietary recommendations and restrictions
- Community agencies and resources for supportive services
- Exercises for extremities
- Signs and symptoms of skin breakdown and contractures

12. Laboratory studies: ESR, WBC
13. Antirheumatic: hydroxychloroquine (Plaquenil)
14. Antimetabolite: methotrexate (Rheumatrex)

G. Nursing interventions
1. Assess neuromuscular status
2. Keep joints extended
3. Monitor and record VS, UO, I/O, and laboratory studies
4. Administer medications, as prescribed
5. Encourage the patient to express feelings about changes in body image and self-esteem
6. Provide skin care
7. Minimize environmental stress
8. Check joints for swelling, pain, and redness
9. Provide passive ROM exercises
10. Provide warm compresses and paraffin dips (heat therapy), as prescribed
11. Individualize home care instructions (For teaching tips, see *Patients with musculoskeletal disorders*)
    a. Provide information about the Arthritis Foundation
    b. Identify ways to reduce stress
    c. Avoid cold, stress, and infection
    d. Avoid unproven remedies

  e. Promote a quiet environment
  f. Complete skin and foot care daily

H. Possible medical complications: carpal tunnel syndrome

I. Possible surgical interventions
  1. Joint replacement (see page 286)
  2. Synovectomy (see page 286)

♦ **XV. Osteoarthritis (degenerative joint disease)**

A. Definition—degeneration of articular cartilage, usually affecting the weight-bearing joints (spine, knees, hips)

B. Possible etiology
  1. Aging
  2. Obesity
  3. Joint trauma
  4. Congenital abnormalities

C. Pathophysiology
  1. Cartilage softens with age, narrowing the joint space
  2. Normal use thins and erodes cartilage
  3. Cartilage flakes enter the synovial lining, which fibroses, thus limiting joint movement

D. Possible assessment findings
  1. Pain relieved by resting joints
  2. Joint stiffness
  3. Heberden's nodules
  4. Limited ROM
  5. CREPITATION
  6. Increased pain in damp, cold weather
  7. Enlarged, edematous joints
  8. Smooth, taut, shiny skin

E. Possible diagnostic test findings
  1. X-rays: joint deformity, narrowing of joint space, bone spurs
  2. Arthroscopy: bone spurs, narrowing of joint space
  3. Hematology: increased ESR

F. Medical management
  1. Diet: low-calorie, if not at optimal weight
  2. Activity: as tolerated
  3. Monitoring: VS, UO, and I/O
  4. Heat therapy
  5. Cold therapy
  6. Isometric exercises
  7. Weight reduction

8. Canes, walkers
9. Analgesic: aspirin
10. NSAIDs: indomethacin (Indocin), ibuprofen (Motrin), sulindac (Clinoril), piroxicam (Feldene), flurbiprofen (Ansaid), diclofenac (Voltaren), naproxen (Naprosyn), diflunisal (Dolobid)

G. Nursing interventions
1. Maintain the patient's diet
2. Assess musculoskeletal status
3. Keep joints extended
4. Monitor and record VS, UO, and I/O
5. Administer medications, as prescribed
6. Urge the patient to express feelings about changes in body image
7. Provide skin care
8. Provide rest periods
9. Determine degree of joint mobility
10. Maintain calorie count
11. Assess pain
12. Provide moist compresses and paraffin baths (heat therapy), as prescribed
13. Teach proper body mechanics
14. Provide passive ROM exercises
15. Individualize home care instructions
    a. Provide information about the Arthritis Foundation
    b. Avoid jogging, jumping, and lifting
    c. Identify ways to reduce stress
    d. Complete skin and foot care daily

H. Possible medical complications: contractures

I. Possible surgical interventions
1. Synovectomy (see page 286)
2. Arthrodesis (see page 286)
3. Joint replacement (see page 286)

◆ XVI. Gouty arthritis

A. Definition—inflammatory joint disease caused by the deposit of uric acid crystals

B. Possible etiology
1. Genetics
2. Decreased uric acid excretion
3. Chronic renal failure
4. Myxedema
5. Polycythemia vera
6. Hyperparathyroidism

C. Pathophysiology
  1. End product of purine metabolism is uric acid
  2. Abnormal purine metabolism results in decreased secretion of urates and increased blood levels of uric acid
  3. Uric acid forms a precipitate in areas where blood flow is slowest
  4. Genetic defect in purine metabolism can cause overproduction of uric acid

D. Possible assessment findings
  1. Joint pain
  2. Redness and swelling in joints
  3. Tophi in great toe, ankle, and outer ear
  4. Malaise
  5. Tachycardia
  6. Elevated skin temperature

E. Possible diagnostic test findings
  1. Hematology: increased ESR
  2. Blood chemistry: increased uric acid
  3. Synovial fluid analysis: sodium urate crystals

F. Medical management
  1. Diet: low-purine, alkaline-ash
  2. Dietary recommendations: increase fluid intake to 3 qt (3 L)/day
  3. Dietary restrictions: no shellfish, liver, sardines, anchovies, and kidneys; limited alcohol
  4. Activity: as tolerated
  5. Monitoring: VS, UO, and I/O
  6. Laboratory studies: uric acid, ESR
  7. Exercise program, including passive and active ROM exercises and ambulation, as tolerated
  8. Uricosuric agents: probenecid (Benemid), sulfinpyrazone (Anturane)
  9. Xanthine-oxidase inhibitor: allopurinol (Zyloprim)
  10. Antigout: colchicine (Colsalide)
  11. Analgesic: aspirin
  12. NSAIDs: indomethacin (Indocin), ibuprofen (Motrin), sulindac (Clinoril), piroxicam (Feldene), flurbiprofen (Ansaid), diclofenac (Voltaren), naproxen (Naprosyn), diflunisal (Dolobid)

G. Nursing interventions
  1. Maintain the patient's diet
  2. Force fluids to 3 qt (3 L)/day
  3. Assess integumentary status
  4. Monitor and record VS, UO, I/O, and laboratory studies
  5. Administer medications, as prescribed
  6. Allay the patient's anxiety

7. Provide skin care
8. Check joints for pain, edema, and ROM
9. Provide a bed cradle
10. Reinforce exercise of joints; show the patient how to perform the exercises
11. Individualize home care instructions
    a. Provide information about the Arthritis Foundation
    b. Recognize signs and symptoms of gout
    c. Limit alcohol intake
    d. Avoid fasting
    e. Identify ways to reduce stress
    f. Complete skin and foot care daily

H. Possible medical complications
    1. Renal calculi
    2. Cartilage damage

I. Possible surgical interventions—none

◆ XVII. Osteomyelitis

A. Definition—bacterial infection of bone and soft tissue

B. Possible etiology
    1. *Staphylococcus aureus*
    2. Hemolytic streptococcus
    3. Open trauma
    4. Infection

C. Pathophysiology
    1. Organism reaches bone through an open wound or via the bloodstream
    2. Infection causes bone destruction
    3. Bone fragments necrose (sequestra)
    4. New bone cells form over the sequestrum during healing, resulting in nonunion

D. Possible assessment findings
    1. Malaise
    2. Elevated body temperature
    3. Bone pain
    4. Tachycardia
    5. Localized edema and redness
    6. Muscle spasms
    7. Increased pain with movement

E. Possible diagnostic test findings
    1. Blood cultures: positive identification of organism
    2. Hematology: increased WBCs, ESR

    3. Wound culture: positive identification of organism

    4. Bone biopsy: positive

    5. Bone scan: positive

F. Medical management

    1. Diet: high-calorie, high-vitamin C and D, high-protein, and high-calcium

    2. I.V. therapy: heparin lock

    3. Activity: bed rest

    4. Monitoring: VS, UO, I/O, and neurovascular checks

    5. Laboratory studies: WBC, ESR

    6. Nutritional support: total parenteral nutrition (TPN)

    7. Special care: wound and skin

    8. Antibiotic: ciprofloxacin (Cipro)

    9. Analgesic: oxycodone (Tylox)

    10. Continuous wound irrigation

    11. Heat therapy

    12. Cast or splint for the affected body part

    13. Antipyretic: aspirin

G. Nursing interventions

    1. Maintain the patient's diet

    2. Force fluids to 3 qt (3 L)/day

    3. Administer I.V. fluids

    4. Assess integumentary status

    5. Maintain the patency of wound irrigation

    6. Monitor and record VS, UO, I/O, and laboratory studies

    7. Administer TPN

    8. Administer medications, as prescribed

    9. Encourage the patient to express feelings about changes in body image

    10. Provide skin care

    11. Turn the patient every 2 hours

    12. Immobilize the affected body part

    13. Maintain proper body alignment

    14. Maintain bed rest

    15. Provide cast and splint care

    16. Assess pain

    17. Individualize home care instructions

       a. Recognize the signs and symptoms of fractures

       b. Avoid exposure to people with infections

       c. Monitor self for infection

       d. Practice health routines that prevent infection

       e. Avoid weight bearing on the affected part

H. Possible medical complications
   1. Bone necrosis
   2. Pathological fractures
   3. Sepsis

I. Possible surgical interventions
   1. Incision and drainage of bone abscess
   2. Sequestrectomy
   3. Bone graft
   4. Bone segment transfer

◆ XVIII. Osteoporosis

A. Definition
   1. Osteoporosis is a metabolic bone dysfunction that results in reduced bone mass and increased porosity
   2. Metabolic illnesses or medications that cause osteoporosis increase the risk of skeletal fracture

B. Possible etiology
   1. Lowered estrogen levels
   2. Immobility
   3. Liver disease
   4. Calcium deficiency
   5. Vitamin D deficiency
   6. Protein deficiency
   7. Bone marrow disorders
   8. Lack of exercise
   9. Increased phosphorus
   10. Cushing's syndrome
   11. Hyperthyroidism

C. Pathophysiology
   1. Rate of bone resorption exceeds the rate of bone formation
   2. Increased phosphate stimulates parathyroid activity, which increases bone resorption
   3. Estrogens decrease bone resorption

D. Possible assessment findings
   1. Dowager's hump (kyphosis)
   2. Back pain: thoracic and lumbar
   3. Loss of height
   4. Unsteady gait
   5. Joint pain
   6. Weakness

E. Possible diagnostic test findings
   1. X-ray: thin, porous bone; increased vertebral curvature
   2. Photon absorptiometry: decreased bone mineral content

F. Medical management
   1. Diet: high in calcium, protein, vitamins, minerals, and boron
   2. Dietary restrictions: limit caffeine and alcohol
   3. Activity: as tolerated
   4. Monitoring: VS, UO, and I/O
   5. Laboratory studies: calcium, phosphorus
   6. Estrogen: estradiol (Estrace)
   7. Calcium supplement: calcium carbonate (Os-Cal)
   8. Vitamin and mineral supplements
   9. Exercise program
   10. Thiazide diuretic: hydrochlorothiazide (Aldactazide, Dyazide)
   11. NSAIDs: indomethacin (Indocin), ibuprofen (Motrin), sulindac (Clinoril), piroxicam (Feldene), flurbiprofen (Ansaid), diclofenac sodium (Voltaren), naproxen (Naprosyn), diflunisal (Dolobid)

G. Nursing interventions
   1. Maintain the patient's diet
   2. Assess musculoskeletal status
   3. Monitor and record VS, UO, I/O, and laboratory studies
   4. Administer medications, as prescribed
   5. Encourage the patient to express feelings about changes in body image
   6. Individualize home care instructions
      a. Reinforce the importance of following an exercise program
      b. Teach proper body mechanics and posture
      c. Provide information about the Osteoporosis Foundation
   7. Assess pain

H. Possible medical complication: pathologic fractures

I. Possible surgical interventions: none

◆ XIX. Osteogenic sarcoma (osteosarcoma)

A. Definition—malignant bone tumor that invades the ends of long bones

B. Possible etiology
   1. Osteoblastic activity
   2. Osteolytic activity

C. Pathophysiology
   1. Unregulated cell growth and uncontrolled cell division result in the development of a neoplasm
   2. Tumor arises from osteoblasts and dissolves the bone and soft tissue
   3. Tumor may spread to the lung

D. Possible assessment findings
 1. Pain
 2. Limited movement
 3. Pathologic fractures
 4. Soft tissue mass over the tumor site
 5. Warm tissue over the tumor site
 6. Elevated body temperature

E. Possible diagnostic test findings
 1. Bone scan: mass
 2. Biopsy: cytology positive for cancer cells
 3. Computerized tomography (CT) scan: mass
 4. Blood chemistry: increased alkaline phosphatase
 5. Bone marrow aspiration: cancer cells

F. Medical management
 1. Diet: high-protein
 2. I.V. therapy: heparin lock
 3. Activity: as tolerated
 4. Monitoring: VS, UO, and I/O
 5. Laboratory studies: calcium, phosphorus
 6. Antiemetics: prochlorperazine (Compazine), ondansetron (Zofran)
 7. Nutritional support: TPN
 8. Radiation therapy
 9. Analgesics: oxycodone (Tylox), meperidine hydrochloride (Demerol)
 10. Antineoplastics: cyclophosphamide (Cytoxan), vincristine sulfate (Oncovin)
 11. Antidiarrheals: attapulgite (Kaopectate), loperamide (Imodium)

G. Nursing interventions
 1. Maintain the patient's diet
 2. Assess integumentary and musculoskeletal status
 3. Monitor and record VS, UO, I/O, and laboratory studies
 4. Administer TPN
 5. Administer medications, as prescribed
 6. Encourage the patient to express feelings about changes in body image and a fear of dying
 7. Provide postchemotherapeutic nursing care
    a. Provide prophylactic skin, mouth, and perineal care
    b. Monitor dietary intake
    c. Administer antiemetics and antidiarrheals, as prescribed
    d. Monitor for bleeding, infection, and electrolyte imbalance
    e. Provide rest periods
 8. Assess pain

9. Individualize home care instructions
   a. Provide information about the American Cancer Society
   b. Recognize signs and symptoms of a fracture
   c. Avoid exposure to people with infections
   d. Monitor self for infections
   e. Monitor pain control interventions
   f. Complete skin care daily

H. Possible medical complications
   1. Metastasis
   2. Pathológic fractures

I. Possible surgical intervention: amputation (see page 289)

◆ XX. Carpal tunnel syndrome

A. Definition—chronic compression neuropathy of the median nerve at the wrist

B. Possible etiology
   1. Strenuous and repetitive use of the hands
   2. Fractures and dislocations of the wrist
   3. Bruising of the wrist
   4. Menopause
   5. Genetics
   6. Pregnancy
   7. Tenosynovitis
   8. Rheumatoid arthritis
   9. Acromegaly
   10. Hyperparathyroidism
   11. Obesity
   12. Gout
   13. Amyloidosis

C. Pathophysiology
   1. Median nerve supplies sensory innervation to the palmar surface of the thumb and the first three fingers
   2. Median nerve also supplies motor innervation to the wrist and finger flexion
   3. Compression of the median nerve in the space between the inelastic transverse carpal ligament and the bones of the wrist (carpal tunnel) leads to pain and numbness in the thumb, index, middle, and half of the ring finger

D. Possible assessment findings
   1. Nocturnal pain and paresthesia in the thumb and first three fingers, relieved by shaking the hand
   2. Burning and tingling of the hand

3. Impaired sensation in the hand
4. Pain radiating to forearm, shoulder, neck, and chest
5. THENAR atrophy
6. Loss of fine motor movement of the hand

E. Possible diagnostic test findings
   1. Tinel's sign: positive
   2. Motor nerve velocity studies: segmental, distal, median, and motor conduction delay, and conduction block at wrist

F. Medical management
   1. Diet: low-sodium
   2. Dietary restrictions: limit fluids
   3. Position: avoid flexion of the wrist, elevate the hand
   4. Activity: avoid using the hand
   5 Monitoring: VS, UO, I/O, and neurovascular checks
   6. Hand splint
   7. Analgesic: acetaminophen (Tylenol)
   8. Diuretic: furosemide (Lasix)
   9. Glucocorticoid: cortisone (Cortone)
   10. NSAIDs: indomethacin (Indocin), ibuprofen (Motrin), sulindac (Clinoril), piroxicam (Feldene), flurbiprofen (Ansaid), diclofenac sodium (Voltaren), naproxen (Naprosyn), diflunisal (Dolobid)
   11. Vitamin: pyridoxine hydrochloride (Vitamin B_6)

G. Nursing interventions
   1. Maintain the patient's diet
   2. Assess neurovascular status
   3. Elevate the patient's hand
   4. Monitor and record VS
   5. Administer medications, as prescribed
   6. Encourage the patient to express feelings about inability to use the hand and to perform job requirements
   7. Provide skin care
   8. Provide ROM exercises to the splinted hand
   9. Protect the hand from cold, burns, abrasions, local trauma, and chemical irritations

CLINICAL ALERT

   10. Avoid manual activity that includes dorsiflexion and volar flexion of the wrist
   11. Individualize home care instructions
       a. Maintain ROM exercises for the hand
       b. Avoid activities that increase pain
       c. Alternate rest periods with activities involving the hand
       d. Protect the hand from trauma

e. Splint the hand
f. Consider vocational retraining, if appropriate
g. Complete skin care daily

H. Possible medical complications
1. Contracture
2. Loss of thumb abduction and opposition ("ape hand")
3. Trophic changes of tips of thumbs and index and middle fingers

I. Possible surgical intervention: carpal tunnel release (see page 290)

♦ **XXI. Herniated nucleus pulposa (HNP, "slipped disk")**

A. Definition
1. Rupture of intervertebral disk
2. Two types of ruptured disk
   a. Lumbrosacral (L4, L5)
   b. Cervical (C5, C6, C7)

B. Possible etiology
1. Accidents
2. Back or neck strain
3. Congenital bone deformity
4. Degeneration of disk
5. Weakness of ligaments
6. Heavy lifting
7. Trauma

C. Pathophysiology
1. Protrusion of the nucleus pulposus into the spinal canal compresses the spinal cord or nerve roots
2. Compression of the spinal cord or nerve roots causes pain, numbness, and loss of motor function

D. Possible assessment findings
1. Lumbrosacral
   a. Acute pain in the lower back radiating across the buttock and down the leg
   b. Weakness, numbness, and tingling of the foot and leg
   c. Pain on ambulation
2. Cervical
   a. Neck stiffness
   b. Weakness, numbness, and tingling of the hand
   c. Neck pain that radiates down the arm to the hand
   d. Weakness of affected upper extremities
   e. Atrophy of biceps and triceps
   f. Straightening of normal lumbar curve with scoliosis away from the affected side

E. Possible diagnostic test findings
   1. Lasègue's sign: positive
   2. CSF analysis: increased protein
   3. Myelogram: compression of spinal cord
   4. EMG: spinal nerve involvement
   5. X-ray: narrowing of disk space
   6. Deep tendon reflexes: depressed or absent upper extremity reflexes or Achilles reflex

F. Medical management
   1. Diet: calories according to metabolic needs; increase fiber; force fluids
   2. Position: semi-Fowler's
   3. Activity: bed rest; active and passive ROM and isometric exercises
   4. Monitoring: VS, UO, I/O, neurovascular checks, and laboratory studies
   5. Heating pad; moist, hot compresses
   6. Orthopedic devices: back brace, cervical collar
   7. Analgesic: oxycodone hydrochloride (Tylox)
   8. Antacids: magnesium and aluminum hydroxide (Maalox), aluminum hydroxide gel (Gelusil)
   9. Stool softener: docusate sodium (Colace)
   10. Pelvic traction
   11. Cervical traction
   12. Muscle relaxants: diazepam (Valium), cyclobenzaprine hydrochloride (Flexeril)
   13. Chemonucleolysis using chymopapain (Discase)
   14. NSAIDs: indomethacin (Indocin), ibuprofen (Motrin), sulindac (Clinoril), piroxicam (Feldene), flurbiprofen (Ansaid), diclofenac sodium (Voltaren), naproxen (Naprosyn), diflunisal (Dolobid)
   15. Corticosteroid: cortisone (Cortone)
   16. Transcutaneous electrical nerve stimulation (TENS)

G. Nursing interventions
   1. Maintain the patient's diet; increase fluid intake
   2. Assess neurovascular status
   3. Keep the patient in semi-Fowler's position with moderate hip and knee flexion
   4. Monitor and record VS, UO, I/O, and laboratory studies
   5. Administer medications, as prescribed
   6. Encourage the patient to express feelings about changes in body image and about fears of disability
   7. Provide skin and back care
   8. Turn the patient every 2 hours, using the logrolling technique
   9. Maintain bed rest and body alignment

10. Maintain traction, braces, and cervical collar
11. Promote independence in ADLs
12. Apply bedboards
13. Individualize home care instructions
   a. Exercise regularly, with special attention to exercises that strengthen and stretch the muscles
   b. Avoid lifting, sleeping prone, climbing stairs, and riding in a car, as prescribed
   c. Avoid flexion, extension, or rotation of the neck
   d. Use one pillow
   e. Use a back brace or cervical collar

H. Possible medical complications
   1. Upper respiratory infection
   2. Urinary tract infection
   3. Thrombophlebitis
   4. Chronic pain
   5. Muscle atrophy
   6. Progressive paralysis
   7. Urine retention

I. Possible surgical interventions
   1. Laminectomy (see page 293)
   2. Spinal fusion (see page 294)
   3. Microdiskectomy
   4. Percutaneous lateral diskectomy

◆ **XXII. Fractures**

A. Definition
   1. Break in the continuity of bone
   2. Types of fractures
      a. Complete
      b. Incomplete
      c. Comminuted
      d. Greenstick
      e. Simple
      f. Compound
      g. Transverse
      h. Spiral
      i. Oblique
      j. Depressed
      k. Compression
      l. Avulsion
      m. Pathologic

    3. Types of hip fractures
      a. Intracapsular
      b. Extracapsular
      c. Intertrochanteric

B. Possible etiology
    1. Trauma
    2. Osteoporosis
    3. Multiple myeloma
    4. Bone tumors
    5. Immobility
    6. Malnutrition
    7. Cushing's syndrome
    8. Osteomyelitis
    9. Steroid therapy
   10. Aging

C. Pathophysiology
    1. Fracture occurs when stress placed on the bone is more than the bone can withstand
    2. Localized tissue injury results in muscle spasm, edema, hemorrhage, compressed nerves, and ecchymosis

D. Possible assessment findings
    1. Pain aggravated by motion
    2. Tenderness over the fracture site
    3. Loss of function or motion
    4. Edema
    5. Crepitus
    6. Ecchymosis
    7. Deformity
    8. False motion
    9. Paresthesia
   10. Affected leg that appears shorter (fractured hip)

E. Possible diagnostic test findings
    1. X-ray: break in continuity of bone
    2. Hematology: decreased Hgb and HCT

F. Medical management
    1. Diet: high-protein, high-vitamin, and low-calcium; increase fluid intake
    2. Position: elevate a fractured leg; keep the patient flat with the leg abducted for a fractured hip
    3. Activity: as tolerated for extremity fractures; active and passive ROM exercises for unaffected limbs for fractured hip; isometric exercises

4. Monitoring: VS, UO, I/O, and neurovascular checks
5. Laboratory studies: Hgb, HCT, phosphorus, and calcium
6. Cast care, pin care, ice packs, incentive spirometry, abductor pillow (fractured hip)
7. Analgesic: oxycodone hydrochloride (Tylox)
8. Skin traction: Buck's, Bryant's, or Russell's
9. Skeletal traction: Thomas splint with Pearson attachment, Steinmann pin, Kirschner wire, or Crutchfield tongs (fractured neck)
10. Closed reduction with hip spica cast (fractured hip)
11. Cast or closed reduction (fracture)

G. Nursing interventions
1. Maintain the patient's diet; increase fluid intake
2. Assess neurovascular and respiratory status
3. Keep the patient in a flat position with the foot of the bed elevated 25 degrees (fractured hip)
4. Keep the legs abducted (fractured hip)
5. Elevate a fractured extremity
6. Monitor and record VS, UO, I/O, and laboratory studies
7. Administer medications, as prescribed
8. Allay the patient's anxiety
9. Provide skin, pin, and cast care
10. Turn the patient to the affected or unaffected side every 2 hours, as ordered (fractured hip)
11. Keep the hip extended (fractured hip)
12. Maintain activity, as tolerated (fractures)
13. Promote independence in ADLs
14. Provide active and passive ROM and isometric exercises for unaffected limbs

CLINICAL ALERT

15. Provide a trapeze
16. Maintain traction to ensure proper body alignment and promote healing
17. Keep side rails up
18. Provide appropriate sensory stimulation with frequent reorientation
19. Provide TCDB and incentive spirometry
20. Prevent constipation, as prescribed
21. Maintain proper body alignment
22. Inspect pin sites for infection
23. Provide diversional activities
24. Provide heel and elbow protectors and sheepskin
25. Apply antiembolism stockings
26. Use the logrolling technique to turn the patient

27. Individualize home care instructions
    a. Complete cast care (fracture)
    b. Attend physical therapy sessions
    c. Avoid weight bearing on affected limb
    d. Complete skin and foot care daily

H. Possible medical complications
    1. Deep vein thrombosis

CLINICAL ALERT

    2. Anemia
    3. Fat embolism
    4. Pulmonary embolism
    5. Renal lithiasis
    6. Pneumonia

CLINICAL ALERT

    7. Urinary tract infections
    8. Compartment syndrome (fracture)
    9. Hypovolemic shock
    10. Nonunion
    11. Osteomyelitis (fracture)
    12. Avascular necrosis of the femoral head (fractured hip)
    13. Pressure sores

I. Possible surgical interventions
    1. ORIF (see page 291)
    2. External fixation for fractures (see page 288)

◆ XXIII. Systemic lupus erythematosus (SLE)

A. Definition—chronic connective tissue disease involving multiple organ systems

B. Possible etiology
    1. Unknown
    2. Genetic
    3. Autoimmune disease
    4. Viral
    5. Drug-induced: procainamide (Pronestyl) and hydralazine (Apresoline)

C. Pathophysiology
    1. Defect in the body's immunologic mechanism produces serum autoantibodies directed against components of the patient's cell nuclei
    2. Deposits of antigen or antibody complexes affect connective cells throughout the body, including blood vessels, mucous membranes, joints, skin, kidneys, muscles, brain, and heart

D. Possible assessment findings
    1. Oral and nasopharyngeal ulcerations

    2. Alopecia

    3. Photosensitivity

    4. Early morning joint stiffness

    5. Low-grade fever

    6. Butterfly erythema on face

    7. Erythema on palms

    8. Muscle pain

    9. Abdominal pain

    10. Malaise and weakness

    11. Weight loss

    12. Lymphadenopathy

    13. Anorexia

E. Possible diagnostic test findings

    1. Hematology: decreased Hgb, HCT, WBC, platelets; increased ESR

    2. Rheumatoid factor: positive

    3. LE prep: positive

    4. Urine chemistry: proteinuria, hematuria

    5. Blood chemistry: decreased complement fixation

    6. ANA test: positive

F. Medical management

    1. Diet: high in iron, protein, and vitamins (especially vitamin C)

    2. I.V. therapy: heparin lock

    3. Activity: as tolerated

    4. Monitoring: VS, UO, and I/O

    5. Laboratory studies: Hgb, HCT, WBC, platelets, ESR, BUN, and creatinine

    6. Plasmapheresis

    7. Special care: seizure precautions

    8. Analgesic: acetaminophen (Tylenol)

    9. Antacids: magnesium and aluminum hydroxide (Maalox), aluminum hydroxide gel (Gelusil)

    10. Corticosteroid: prednisone (Deltasone)

    11. Antimalarial: hydroxychloroquine (Plaquenil)

    12. Antipyretic: aspirin

    13. NSAIDs: indomethacin (Indocin), ibuprofen (Motrin), sulindac (Clinoril), piroxicam (Feldene), flurbiprofen (Ansaid), diclofenac sodium (Voltaren), naproxen (Naprosyn), diflunisal (Dolobid)

    14. Antianemics: ferrous sulfate (Feosol), ferrous gluconate (Fergon)

    15. Immunosuppressants: azathioprine (Imuran), cyclophosphamide (Cytoxan)

    16. Vitamins and minerals

    17. Surgical placement of shunt for dialysis, if needed

G. Nursing interventions

1. Avoid foods high in L-canavanine
2. Assess musculoskeletal and renal status
3. Monitor and record VS, UO, I/O, laboratory studies, and daily weight
4. Administer medications, as prescribed
5. Encourage the patient to express feelings about changes in body image and the chronicity of the disease
6. Avoid exposing the patient to sunlight
7. Minimize environmental stress
8. Maintain seizure precautions
9. Provide rest periods
10. Prevent infection
11. Maintain a quiet environment
12. Do not use dusting powder on the patient
13. Promote independence in ADLs
14. Provide postchemotherapeutic nursing care
    a. Provide prophylactic skin, mouth, and perineal care
    b. Monitor dietary intake
    c. Administer antiemetics and antidiarrheals, as prescribed
    d. Monitor for bleeding, infection, and electrolyte imbalance
15. Individualize home care instructions
    a. Provide information about the Lupus Foundation
    b. Stop smoking
    c. Identify ways to reduce stress
    d. Recognize the signs and symptoms of renal failure
    e. Avoid exposure to people with infections
    f. Monitor self for infection
    g. Monitor self for fatigue and joint pain
    h. Complete mouth care daily
    i. Avoid over-the-counter medications
    j. Avoid exposure to sunlight
    k. Do not use hair spray or hair coloring
    l. Do not take oral contraceptives
    m. Use liquid cosmetics to cover rashes
    n. Maintain a quiet environment

H. Possible medical complications

1. Necrosis of glomerular capillaries
2. Inflammation of cerebral and ocular blood vessels
3. Necrosis of lymph nodes
4. Vasculitis of gastrointestinal tract and pleura
5. Degeneration of the skin's basal layer

      6. Congestive heart failure (CHF)
      7. Seizures
      8. Depression
      9. Infection
     10. Peripheral neuropathy

  I. Possible surgical interventions: none

POINTS TO REMEMBER

♦ Metabolic illnesses or medications that cause osteoporosis increase the risk of skeletal fracture.

♦ Alterations in mobility that result from a musculoskeletal disorder may affect a patient's developmental, economic, occupational, recreational, and social activities.

♦ Pain control is a primary focus for the nursing management of a patient with a musculoskeletal disorder.

STUDY QUESTIONS

To evaluate your understanding of this chapter, answer the following questions in the space provided; then compare your responses with the correct answers in Appendix B, page 385.

1. How should the patient be positioned after a total hip replacement? _____

   _____

   _____

2. What is a key home care instruction for a patient with an external fixation?

   _____

   _____

3. How does the pain of rheumatoid arthritis differ from that of osteoarthritis? _____

   _____

   _____

4. Which pharmacologic agents are used to treat gouty arthritis? _____

   _____

   _____

5. What is the pathophysiologic basis for osteomyelitis?_____

_____

_____

6. What are the assessment findings for HNP? _____

_____

_____

CRITICAL THINKING AND APPLICATION EXERCISES

1. Observe an ORIF. Prepare an oral presentation for your fellow students, describing the procedure and patient care before, during, and after the procedure.

2. Develop a chart comparing the major antiinflammatory agents used for musculoskeletal disorders.

3. Write a dietary teaching plan for a patient with gout.

4. Interview a patient with a musculoskeletal disorder. Evaluate the information for possible risk factors and identify ways to modify them.

5. Follow a patient with a musculoskeletal disorder from admission through discharge. Develop a patient-specific plan of care, including any needs for follow-up and home care.

CHAPTER

9

Integumentary System

LEARNING OBJECTIVES

After studying this chapter, you should be able to:

♦ Describe the psychosocial impact of integumentary disorders.

♦ Differentiate between modifiable and nonmodifiable risk factors in the development of an integumentary disorder.

♦ List three probable and three possible nursing diagnoses for a patient with any integumentary disorder.

♦ Identify nursing interventions for a patient with an integumentary disorder.

♦ Identify three teaching topics for a patient with an integumentary disorder.

CHAPTER OVERVIEW

Caring for the patient with an integumentary disorder requires a sound understanding of integumentary anatomy and physiology and the management of modifiable risk factors. A thorough assessment is essential to planning and implementing appropriate patient care. The assessment includes a complete history, physical examination, diagnostic testing, identification of modifiable and nonmodifiable risk factors, and information related to the psychosocial impact of the disorder on the patient. Nursing diagnoses focus primarily on impaired skin integrity and body image disturbance. Nursing interventions are designed to support healing of the skin, prevent further injury to the affected area and help patients adjust to the changes in body image. Patient teaching — a crucial nursing activity — involves information about medical follow-up, medication regimens, signs and symptoms of possible complications, and reduction of modifiable risk factors through the use of techniques that prevent skin damage and infection.

◆ I. Anatomy and physiology review

A. Skin: first line of defense against microorganisms; composed of three layers
   1. Epidermis
      a. Outer avascular layer composed of dense squamous cells that constantly shed
      b. Keratinocytes and melanocytes in this layer
   2. Dermis
      a. Origin of hair, nails, sebaceous glands, eccrine sweat glands, apocrine sweat glands
      b. Collagen layer that supports the epidermis and contains nerves and blood vessels
   3. Subcutaneous tissue (hypodermis)
      a. Third layer of skin is composed of loose connective tissue filled with fatty cells
      b. It provides heat, insulation, shock absorption, and a reserve of calories

B. Hair
   1. Protects and covers the body, except for the palms, lips, soles of the feet, nipples, and external genitalia
   2. Hormones stimulate differential growth

C. Nails
   1. Composed of dead cells filled with keratin
   2. Protect the tips of the fingers and toes

D. Glandular appendages
   1. Three types are sebaceous, eccrine, and apocrine
   2. Sebaceous glands (oil), which lubricate hair and epidermis, are stimulated by sex hormones
   3. Eccrine sweat glands regulate body temperature through water secretion
   4. Apocrine sweat glands are located in the axilla, nipple, anal, and pubic areas and secrete odorless fluid; decomposition of this fluid by bacteria causes odor

◆ II. Assessment findings

A. History
  1. Change in skin color, texture, and temperature
  2. Perspiration or dryness
  3. Itching
  4. Brittle, thick, or soft nails
  5. Fever
  6. Hair loss
  7. Rash

B. Physical examination
  1. Pattern of pigmentation and hair distribution
  2. Skin texture, turgor, color, and temperature
  3. Peripheral edema
  4. TROPHIC changes: skin, hair, and nails
  5. Skin lesions: type, shape, and character
  6. PRURITUS
  7. NEVI and scars
  8. Elevated body temperature
  9. Erythema
  10. Petechiae and ecchymosis

◆ III. Diagnostic tests and procedures

A. Blood chemistry
  1. Definition and purpose
     a. Laboratory test of a blood sample
     b. Analysis for potassium, sodium, calcium, phosphorus, ketones, glucose, osmolality, chloride, blood urea nitrogen (BUN), and creatinine
  2. Nursing interventions
     a. Withhold food and fluids before the procedure, as directed
     b. Check the site for bleeding after the procedure

B. Hematologic studies
  1. Definition and purpose
     a. Laboratory test of a blood sample
     b. Analysis for red blood cells (RBCs), white blood cells (WBCs), erythrocyte sedimentation rate (ESR), platelets, prothrombin time (PT), partial thromboplastin time (PTT), hemoglobin (Hgb), hematocrit (HCT)
  2. Nursing interventions: check the site for bleeding

C. Skin biopsy (punch biopsy)
  1. Definition and purpose
      a. Procedure using a circular punch instrument to remove a small amount of skin tissue
      b. Histologic evaluation
  2. Nursing interventions: check the site for bleeding and infection

D. Skin testing
  1. Definition and purpose
      a. Procedure using a patch, scratch, or intradermal technique
      b. Administration of an allergen to the skin's surface or into the dermis
  2. Nursing interventions
      a. Keep the area dry
      b. Record the site, date, and time of test
      c. Inspect the site for erythema, papules, VESICLES, edema, and induration
      d. Record the date and time for follow-up site reading

E. Skin scrapings
  1. Definition and purpose
      a. Procedure calling for cells scraped by a scalpel and covered with potassium hydroxide
      b. Microscopic examination of scales, nails, and hair
  2. Nursing interventions: check scraping site for bleeding and infection

F. Skin studies
  1. Definition and purpose
      a. Laboratory test
      b. Microscopic examination of skin, including gram stain, culture and sensitivity, cytology, and immunofluorescence (IF)
  2. Nursing interventions
      a. Follow laboratory procedure guidelines
      b. Note current antibiotic therapy

G. Wood's light
  1. Definition and purpose
      a. Procedure using ultraviolet (UV) light
      b. Direct examination of skin
  2. Nursing interventions
      a. Explain procedure
      b. Allay the patient's anxiety

◆ IV. Psychosocial impact of integumentary disorders

A. Developmental impact
   1. Changes in body image
   2. Fear of rejection
   3. Changes in role performance
   4. Decreased self-esteem

B. Economic impact
   1. Cost of cosmetics
   2. Disruption or loss of employment
   3. Cost of hospitalizations and follow-up care
   4. Cost of medications

C. Occupational and recreational impact
   1. Restrictions in physical activity
   2. Changes in leisure activity

D. Social impact
   1. Social isolation
   2. Sexual dysfunction

◆ V. Possible risk factors

A. Modifiable risk factors
   1. Infection
   2. Occupation
   3. Exposure to chemical and environmental pollutants
   4. Exposure to radiation
   5. Exposure to sun
   6. Personal hygiene habits
   7. Climate
   8. Use of cosmetics and soaps
   9. Stress
   10. Nutritional deficiencies
   11. Medications
   12. Crowded living conditions
   13. Skin moles

B. Nonmodifiable risk factors
   1. Aging
   2. History of endocrine, vascular, or immune disorders
   3. Family history of skin disease or allergies
   4. History of allergies
   5. Exposure to communicable disease
   6. Pregnancy
   7. Menopause

◆ VI. Nursing diagnostic categories

A. Probable nursing diagnostic categories
   1. Impaired skin integrity
   2. Body image disturbance
   3. Self-esteem disturbance
   4. Pain
   5. Sensory/perceptual alteration: tactile

B. Possible nursing diagnostic categories
   1. Ineffective breathing pattern
   2. Ineffective individual coping
   3. Risk for fluid volume deficit
   4. Risk for infection
   5. Anxiety
   6. Social isolation

◆ VII. Skin graft

A. Description
   1. Replacement of damaged skin with healthy skin to protect underlying structures or to reconstruct areas for cosmetic or functional purposes
   2. Split-thickness graft: graft of half of the epidermis, which is removed by a dermatome
   3. Full-thickness graft: graft of the entire epidermis
   4. Pinch graft: graft of a small piece of skin, obtained by elevating the skin with a needle and removing it with scissors

B. Preoperative nursing interventions
   1. Complete patient and family preoperative teaching
      a. Determine the patient's understanding of the procedure
      b. Describe the operating room (OR), postanesthesia care unit (PACU), and preoperative and postoperative routines
      c. Demonstrate postoperative turning, coughing, and deep breathing (TCDB), splinting, leg exercises, and range-of-motion (ROM) exercises
      d. Explain the postoperative need for drainage tubes, surgical dressings, oxygen therapy, I.V. therapy, and pain control
   2. Complete a preoperative checklist
   3. Administer preoperative medications, as prescribed
   4. Allay the patient's and family's anxiety about surgery
   5. Document the patient's history and physical assessment database
   6. Prepare the donor and graft sites

C. Postoperative nursing interventions
1. Assess pain and administer postoperative analgesics, as prescribed
2. Assess for return of peristalsis; provide solid foods and liquids, as tolerated
3. Administer I.V. fluids
4. Allay the patient's anxiety
5. Provide hydrotherapy, as directed
6. Reinforce TCDB
7. Provide incentive spirometry
8. Maintain activity: as tolerated, active and passive ROM and isometric exercises
9. Avoid weight bearing on the extremity with the graft site
10. Monitor and record vital signs (VS), urinary output (UO), intake and output (I/O), and neurovascular checks distal to the recipient site
11. Elevate and immobilize the graft site
12. Encourage the patient to express feelings about changes in body image

CLINICAL ALERT

13. Administer antibiotics, as prescribed
14. Assess the graft site for infection, hematoma, and fluid accumulation under the graft; keep the graft and donor sites free from pressure
15. Keep the donor site dry and open to air
16. Prevent scratching
17. Apply heat lamp to the donor site
18. Apply sterile saline or antibiotic solution to the graft site, as ordered
19. Change graft site dressing, as ordered
20. Individualize home care instructions
    a. Continue physical therapy

CLINICAL ALERT

    b. Apply lubricating lotion to the graft site
    c. Protect the graft site from direct sunlight
    d. Demonstrate cosmetic camouflage techniques

D. Possible surgical complications
1. Infection of the graft and donor sites
2. Graft rejection or failure
3. Hematoma under the graft
4. Fluid accumulation under the graft

♦ VIII. Contact dermatitis

A. Definition—inflammatory response of the skin after contact with a specific antigen

B. Possible etiology
1. Mechanical, biological, and chemical irritants
2. Cosmetics and hair dyes
3. Detergents, cleaning agents, and soaps
4. Insecticides

5. Poison ivy

6. Wool

C. Pathophysiology

1. Contact with an antigen triggers a localized inflammatory response

2. Inflammatory response produces skin changes

D. Possible assessment findings

1. Pruritus and burning

2. Erythema at point of contact

3. Localized edema

4. Vesicles and papules

5. LICHENIFICATION

6. Pigmentation changes

7. Eczema

8. Scaling

E. Possible diagnostic test findings

1. Skin test (patch): positive to specific antigen

2. Visual examination: area of dermatitis correlates with area of antigen contact

F. Medical management

1. Position: elevation of extremity

2. Activity: as tolerated

3. Monitoring: VS and neurovascular checks

4. Treatments: cool, wet dressings with aluminum acetate solution (Burow's solution), tepid baths, and bed cradle

5. Antibiotic: ampicillin (Omnipen)

6. Antipruritic: diphenhydramine hydrochloride (Benadryl)

7. Corticosteroid: hydrocortisone (Cort-Dome)

8. Antihistamine: diphenhydramine hydrochloride (Benadryl)

9. Antianxiety agents: diazepam (Valium), oxazepam (Serax)

G. Nursing interventions

1. Assess neurovascular status

2. Maintain elevation of affected extremity

3. Monitor and record VS and neurovascular checks

4. Administer medications, as prescribed

5. Encourage the patient to express feelings about changes in physical appearance

6. Provide tepid baths, bed cradle, and cool, wet dressings

7. Avoid soaps

8. Avoid using heating pads or blankets

CLINICAL ALERT 9. Avoid temperature extremes

10. Prevent scratching and rubbing of affected area: increases risk of further irritation, inflammation, and possible infection

TEACHING TIPS
Patients with integumentary disorders

Be sure to include the following topic areas in your teaching plan when caring for patients with integumentary disorders.
- Follow-up appointments
- Smoking cessation
- Optimal body weight maintenance
- Medication therapy, including the action, adverse effects, and scheduling of medications
- Prevention of skin damage and irritation, including:
  – extreme temperatures
  – skin dryness
  – cool environment
  – sunlight and wind
  – scratching and rubbing
  – trauma
  – detergents and soaps
- Dressing changes, as directed
- Infection control measures
- Avoidance of over-the-counter skin medications
- Daily skin care
- Signs and symptoms of skin infection
- Community agencies and resources for supportive services
- Fluid intake

    11. Maintain a cool environment

    12. Provide diversional activities

    13. Individualize home care instructions: avoid causative agent (For teaching tips, see *Patients with integumentary disorders*)

H. Possible medical complications: infection

I. Possible surgical interventions: none

◆ IX. Psoriasis

A. Definition—chronic, noninfectious skin inflammation that occurs in patches

B. Possible etiology
    1. Stress
    2. Epidermal trauma
    3. Streptococcal infection
    4. Changes in climate
    5. Genetics
    6. Anxiety

      7. Alcoholism

      8. Rheumatoid arthritis

      9. Drug induced: lithium, propranolol

     10. Hormones

     11. Obesity

C. Pathophysiology

    1. Loss of normal regulatory mechanisms of cell division leads to rapid multiplication of epidermal cells that interferes with formation of normal protective layer of skin

    2. Papules coalesce to form plaques

D. Possible assessment findings

    1. Pruritus

    2. Shedding, scaling plaques

    3. Yellow discoloration and thickening of nails

    4. Erythema

    5. Papules on sacrum, nails, palms

E. Possible diagnostic test finding: plaques, on visual examination

F. Medical management

    1. Monitoring: VS and neurovascular checks

    2. Treatments: bed cradle, daily soaks, and tepid, wet compresses

    3. Corticosteroids: triamcinolone acetonide (Kenalog) covered with occlusive dressing, betamethasone valerate (Valisone)

    4. Antipsoriatics: anthralin (Anthra-Derm), coal tar (Estar), followed by exposure to UV light, etretinate (Tegison)

    5. Antimetabolite: methotrexate (Amethopterin)

    6. Photochemotherapy (PUVA therapy): methoxsalen (Oxsoralen) followed by exposure to black light

    7. Keratolytics: benzoyl peroxide (Benzagel), salicylic acid (Keratex, Salacid)

    8. Antimicrobial: sulfasalazine (Azulfidine)

    9. Diet: high-protein, high-calorie, frequent feedings

G. Nursing interventions

    1. Assess neurovascular status

    2. Monitor and record VS and neurovascular checks

    3. Administer medications, as prescribed

    4. Encourage the patient to express feelings about changes in body image

    5. Administer UV light and PUVA therapy

    6. Apply occlusive dressings

    7 Prevent scratching

    8. Help the patient to remove scales during soaks

    9. Provide information about the National Psoriasis Foundation

10. Maintain the patient's diet
11. Individualize home care instructions
    a. Identify ways to reduce stress
    b. Wear light cotton clothing over affected areas

H. Possible medical complications
  1. Depression
  2. Infection
  3. Rheumatoid arthritis

I. Possible surgical interventions: none

◆ X. Herpes zoster (shingles)

A. Definition—acute viral infection of nerve structure caused by varicella zoster

B. Possible etiology
  1. Cytotoxic drug-induced immunosuppression
  2. Hodgkin's disease
  3. Exposure to varicella zoster
  4. Debilitating disease

C. Pathophysiology
  1. Activation of dormant varicella zoster virus causes an inflammatory reaction
  2. Affected areas include spinal and cranial sensory ganglia and posterior gray matter of the spinal cord

D. Possible assessment findings
  1. Neuralgia
  2. Malaise
  3. Pruritus
  4. Burning
  5. Unilaterally clustered skin vesicles along peripheral sensory nerves on trunk, thorax, or face
  6. Erythema
  7. Fever
  8. Anorexia
  9. Headache
  10. Paresthesia
  11. Edematous skin

E. Possible diagnostic test findings
  1. Antinuclear antibody (ANA): positive
  2. Skin cultures and stains: identification of organism
  3. Visual examination: vesicles along peripheral sensory nerves

F. Medical management
   1. Activity: as tolerated
   2. Monitoring: VS, seventh cranial nerve function, and neurovascular checks
   3. Treatments: air mattress, acetic acid compresses, tepid baths, and bed cradle
   4. Analgesics: acetaminophen (Tylenol), oxycodone hydrochloride (Tylox)
   5. Antianxiety agents: diazepam (Valium), hydroxyzine (Vistaril)
   6. Antipruritic: diphenhydramine hydrochloride (Benadryl)
   7. Corticosteroids: hydrocortisone (Cortef), triamcinolone acetonide (Kenalog)
   8. Nerve block using lidocaine (Xylocaine)
   9. Antiviral agents: acyclovir (Zovirax), vidarabine monohydrate (Vira-A), interferon (Roferon-A)
  10. Laboratory studies: culture and sensitivity

G. Nursing interventions
   1. Assess pain
   2. Monitor and record VS, laboratory results, and seventh cranial nerve function
   3. Administer medications, as directed
   4. Encourage the patient to express feelings about changes in physical appearance and recurrent nature of the illness
   5. Provide acetic acid compresses, tepid baths, bed cradle, and air mattress
   6. Prevent scratching and rubbing of affected areas
   7. Allay the patient's anxiety
   8. Individualize home care instructions
      a. Recognize the signs and symptoms of hearing loss
      b. Avoid wool and synthetic clothing
      c. Wear lightweight, loose cotton clothing
      d. Keep blisters intact

H. Possible medical complications
   1. Infection
   2. Posttherapeutic neuralgia
   3. Ophthalmic herpes zoster
   4. Facial paralysis
   5. Vertigo
   6. Tinnitus
   7. Hearing loss
   8. Visceral dissemination

I. Possible surgical interventions: none

♦ **XI. Burns**

   A. Definition—destruction of epidermis, dermis, and subcutaneous layers of skin

   B. Possible etiology
      1. Radiation: X-ray, sun, nuclear reactors
      2. Mechanical: friction
      3. Chemical: acids, alkalies, vesicants
      4. Electrical: lightning, electrical wires
      5. Thermal: flame, frostbite, scald

   C. Pathophysiology
      1. Cell destruction causes loss of intracellular fluid and electrolytes
      2. Amount of cell destruction is directly related to extent (area) and degree (depth) of burn
      3. First-degree (superficial partial thickness) involves epidermal layer
      4. Second-degree (dermal partial thickness) involves epidermal and dermal layers
      5. Third-degree (full thickness) involves epidermal, dermal, subcutaneous layers, and nerve endings

   D. Possible assessment findings
      1. First-degree
         a. Erythema
         b. Edema
         c. Pain
         d. Blanching
      2. Second-degree
         a. Pain
         b. Oozing, fluid-filled vesicles
         c. Erythema
         d. Shiny, wet subcutaneous layer after vesicles rupture
      3. Third-degree
         a. Eschar
         b. Edema
         c. Little or no pain

   E. Possible diagnostic test findings
      1. Blood chemistry: increased potassium; decreased sodium, albumin, complement fixation, immunoglobulins
      2. Arterial blood gases (ABGs): metabolic acidosis
      3. 24-hour urine collection: decreased creatinine clearance, negative nitrogen balance
      4. Hematology: increased Hgb, HCT; decreased fibrinogen, platelets, WBCs

   5. Urine chemistry: hematuria, myoglobinuria

   6. Visual examination: extent of burn determined by Rule of Nines, Lund and Browder chart

F. Medical management

   1. Withhold oral food and fluids until allowed by the doctor

   2. Diet: high in protein, fat, calories, carbohydrates; small, frequent feedings

   3. I.V. therapy: hydration and electrolyte replacement using Evan, Brooke, Parkland, or Massachusetts General Hospital protocols; heparin lock

   4. Oxygen therapy

   5. Intubation and mechanical ventilation

   6. Gastrointestinal decompression: nasogastric (NG) tube, Miller-Abbott tube

   7. Position: semi-Fowler's

   8. Activity: bed rest

   9. Monitoring: VS, UO, electrocardiogram (ECG), hemodynamic variables, I/O, neurovital signs, neurovascular checks, and stool for occult blood

  10. Laboratory studies: potassium, sodium, glucose, osmolality, creatinine, BUN, Hgb, HCT, platelets, WBCs, ABGs, culture and sensitivity

  11. Nutritional support: total parental nutrition (TPN), NG feedings

  12. Treatments: indwelling urinary catheter, postural drainage, chest physiotherapy (CPT), incentive spirometry, bed cradle, intermittent positive pressure breathing (IPPB), suction, Jobst clothing, and Hubbard tank bath

  13. Precaution: protective; standard

  14. Transfusion therapy: fresh frozen plasma (FFP), platelets, packed RBCs, plasma

  15. Antibiotic: gentamicin sulfate (Garamycin)

  16. Anti-infectives: mafenide (Sulfamylon), silver sulfadiazine (Silvadene), silver nitrate, povidone-iodine (Betadine)

  17. Antianxiety: diazepam (Valium)

  18. Antitetanus: tetanus toxoid

  19. Analgesic: morphine sulfate (Roxanol)

  20. Antacids: magnesium and aluminum hydroxide (Maalox), aluminum hydroxide gel (AlternaGEL)

  21. Histamine antagonists: cimetidine (Tagamet), ranitidine (Zantac)

  22. Vitamins: phytonadione (AquaMEPHYTON), cyanocobalamin (vitamin B_{12})

  23. Colloid: 5% albumin (Albuminar)

  24. Diuretic: mannitol (Osmitrol)

  25. Sedative: oxazepam (Serax)

26. Digitalis glycoside: digoxin (Lanoxin)
27. Escharotomy
28. Biological dressings
29. Early excisional therapy
30. Specialized bed: Air fluidized (Clinitron, Skytron, Fluid Air)
31. Pulse oximetry
32. Mucosal barrier fortifier: sucralfate (Carafate)

G. Nursing interventions
1. Maintain the patient's diet; withhold food and fluids, as ordered
2 Administer I.V. fluids
3. Administer oxygen
4. Provide suction, TCDB, IPPB, CPT, and postural drainage
5. Assess respiratory status and fluid balance
6. Assess pain
7. Maintain position, patency, and low suction of NG tube
8. Keep the patient in semi-Fowler's position
9. Monitor and record VS, UO, I/O, laboratory studies, hemodynamic variables, neurovital signs, stool for occult blood, specific gravity, calorie count, daily weight, neurovascular checks, and pulse oximetry
10. Provide tracheostomy care or endotube care
11. Administer TPN

CLINICAL ALERT

12. Administer medications, as prescribed
13. Encourage the patient to express feelings about disfigurement, immobility from scarring, and a fear of dying
14. Allay the patient's anxiety
15. Provide treatments: ROM exercises, tanking, bed cradle, splints, and Jobst clothing
16. Elevate affected extremities
17. Maintain a warm environment during acute period
18. Maintain protective and standard precautions
19. Provide skin and mouth care
20. Assess bowel sounds
21. Individualize home care instructions
    a. Follow dietary recommendations and restrictions
    b. Avoid wearing restrictive clothing
    c. Lubricate healing skin with cocoa butter
    d. Use splints and Jobst clothing
    e. Seek help from community agencies and resources

H. Possible medical complications
1. Paralytic ileus
2. Curling's ulcer
3. Acute renal failure

4. Pneumonia
5. Congestive heart failure
6. Septicemia
7. Pulmonary edema
8. Hypovolemic shock

I. Possible surgical intervention: skin grafting (see page 323)

♦ XII. Skin cancer

A. Definition
   1. Malignant primary tumor of the epidermal layer of the skin
   2. Three types of skin cancer
      a. Basal cell epithelioma
      b. Melanoma
      c. Squamous cell carcinoma

B. Possible etiology
   1. Heredity
   2. Chemical irritants
   3. Ultraviolet rays
   4. Radiation
   5. Friction or chronic irritation
   6. Immunosuppressive drugs
   7. Precancerous lesions: leukoplakia, nevi, senile keratoses
   8. Infrared heat or light

C. Pathophysiology
   1. Unregulated cell growth and uncontrolled cell division result in the development of a neoplasm
   2. Basal cell epithelioma: basal cell keratinization causes tumor growth in basal layer of the epidermis
   3. Melanoma: tumor arises from melanocytes of the epidermis
   4. Squamous cell carcinoma: tumor arises from keratinocytes

D. Possible assessment findings
   1. Basal cell epithelioma: waxy nodule with telangiectasis
   2. Melanoma: irregular, circular bordered lesion with hues of tan, black, or blue
   3. Squamous cell carcinoma: small, red, nodular lesion that begins as an erythematous macule or plaque with indistinct margins
   4. Pruritus
   5. Local soreness
   6. Change in color, size, or shape of preexisting lesion
   7. Oozing, bleeding, crusting lesion

E. Possible diagnostic test findings (skin biopsy): cytology positive for cancer cells

F. Medical management
1. I.V. therapy: heparin lock
2. Monitoring: VS
3. Radiation therapy
4. Cryosurgery with liquid nitrogen
5. Chemosurgery with zinc chloride
6. Curettage and electrodesiccation
7. Immunotherapy for melanoma: bacille Calmette-Guérin (BCG) vaccine
8. Alkylating agents: carmustine (BiCNU), dacarbazine (DTIC-Dome)
9. Antineoplastics: hydroxyurea (Hydrea), vincristine sulfate (Oncovin)
10. Antimetabolite: fluorouracil (Adrucil)
11. Antiemetics: prochlorperazine (Compazine), ondansetron (Zofran)

G. Nursing interventions
1. Monitor and record VS
2. Administer medications, as prescribed
3. Encourage the patient to express feelings about changes in body image and a fear of dying
4. Provide postchemotherapeutic and postradiation nursing care
   a. Provide prophylactic skin, mouth, and perineal care
   b. Monitor dietary intake
   c. Administer antiemetics and antidiarrheals, as prescribed
   d. Monitor for bleeding, infection, and electrolyte imbalance
   e. Provide rest periods
5. Assess lesions
6. Individualize home care instructions
   a. Avoid contact with chemical irritants
   b. Use sun-screening lotions and layered clothing when outdoors
   c. Monitor self for lesions and moles that do not heal or that change characteristics
   d. Have moles removed that are subject to chronic irritation
   e. Provide information about the Skin Cancer Foundation
   f. Seek help from community agencies and resources

H. Possible medical complications: metastasis (melanoma)

I. Possible surgical interventions
1. Surgical excision of tumor
2. Melanoma: bone marrow transplant (see page 346)

POINTS TO REMEMBER

♦ Infection is a common complication of integumentary disorders.

♦ The patient's embarrassment from skin changes can cause social isolation.

♦ Many risk factors associated with integumentary disorders are modifiable.

♦ Burns can cause intracellular fluid loss and electrolyte imbalances.

STUDY QUESTIONS

To evaluate your understanding of this chapter, answer the following questions in the space provided; then compare your responses with the correct answers in Appendix B, page 385.

1. Which key nursing assessment should be performed after a skin graft? _____

_____

_____

2. Which medications might the doctor prescribe for a patient with contact dermatitis? _____

_____

_____

3. What are the possible assessment findings for a second-degree burn? _____

_____

_____

4. What are the possible modifiable risk factors for skin cancer? _____

_____

_____

CRITICAL THINKING AND APPLICATION EXERCISES

1. Observe a skin graft. Prepare an oral presentation for your fellow students, describing the procedure and patient care before, during, and after the procedure.

2. Develop a chart summarizing the major care areas involved with a patient with second and third degree burns.

3. Interview a patient with skin cancer. Evaluate the information for possible risk factors and identify ways to modify them.

4. Follow a patient with an integumentary disorder from admission through discharge. Develop a patient-specific plan of care, including any needs for follow-up and home care.

Hematologic and Lymphatic Systems

CHAPTER OVERVIEW

Caring for the patient with a hematologic or lymphatic disorder requires a sound understanding of cardiovascular and lymphatic anatomy and physiology, hemodynamics, and fluid balance. A thorough assessment is essential to planning and implementing appropriate patient care. The assessment includes a complete history, physical examination, diagnostic testing, identification of modifiable and nonmodifiable risk factors, and information related to the psychosocial impact of the disorder on the patient. Nursing diagnoses focus primarily on activity intolerance, risk for infection, and anxiety. Nursing interventions are designed to monitor bleeding, prevent infection, and assist the patient to adjust to the effects of chronic illness. Patient teaching — a crucial nursing activity — involves information about medical follow-up, medication regimens, signs and symptoms of possible complications, and reduction of modifiable risk factors through adherence to infection control measures and changing behaviors that lead to increased bleeding.

◆ I. Anatomy and physiology review

A. Lymphatic vessels
1. Consist of capillary-like structures that are permeable to large molecules
2. Prevent edema by moving fluid and proteins from interstitial spaces to venous circulation
3. Reabsorb fats from the small intestine

B. Lymph nodes
1. Tissue that filters out bacteria and other foreign cells
2. Regional grouping of lymph nodes: cervicofacial, supraclavicular, axillary, epitrochlear, inguinal, and femoral

C. Lymph
1. Fluid found in interstitial spaces
2. Composition of lymph: water and end products of cell metabolism

D. Spleen
1. The largest lymphatic organ
2. Filters blood
3. Traps formed particles
4. Destroys bacteria
5. Serves as blood reservoir
6. Forms lymphocytes and monocytes

E. Erythrocytes: red blood cells (RBCs)
1. RBCs are formed in the bone marrow
2. RBCs contain hemoglobin (Hgb)
3. Oxygen binds with Hgb to form oxyhemoglobin

F. Thrombocytes (platelets)
1. Formed in the bone marrow
2. Function in the coagulation of blood

G. Leukocytes: white blood cells (WBCs)
1. WBCs are formed in the bone marrow and lymphatic tissue
2. WBCs include granulocytes and agranulocytes
3. Provide immunity and protection from infection by phagocytosis

H. Plasma
  1. Liquid portion of the blood
  2. Composition of plasma: water, protein (albumin and globulin), glucose, and electrolytes

I. ABO blood groups
  1. System of antigens located on the surface of RBCs that determines blood type
  2. Blood types: A antigen, B antigen, AB antigens, O (zero) antigens
  3. Universal donor: blood type O
  4. Universal recipient: blood type AB

J. Coagulation
  1. Blood clotting
  2. Series of reactions involving the conversion of prothrombin to thrombin to fibrinogen to fibrin to form a clot

K. Bone marrow
  1. Two types exist: red and yellow
  2. Hematopoiesis is carried out by red marrow
  3. Hematopoiesis produces erythrocytes, leukocytes, and thrombocytes
  4. Red bone marrow is a source of lymphocytes and macrophages
  5. Yellow bone marrow is red bone marrow that has changed to fat

L. Liver
  1. The largest organ in the body
  2. Produces bile (main function), which emulsifies fats and stimulates peristalsis
  3. Conveys bile to the duodenum at the sphincter of Oddi through the common bile duct
  4. Metabolizes carbohydrates, fats, and proteins
  5. Synthesizes coagulation factors VII, IX, X, and prothrombin
  6. Stores vitamins A, D, B_{12}, and iron
  7. Detoxifies chemicals
  8. Excretes bilirubin
  9. Receives dual blood supply from portal vein and hepatic artery
  10. Produces and stores glycogen
  11. Promotes erythropoiesis when bone marrow production is insufficient

♦ **II. Assessment findings**

A. History
  1. Enlarged glands
  2. Pain
  3. Fatigue and weakness
  4. Bleeding
  5. Pallor

6. Lassitude
7. Shortness of breath
8. Fainting
9. Vertigo
10. Jaundice
11. Night sweats
12. Fever
13. Weight loss
14. Tachycardia
15. Activity intolerance
16. Frequent infections
17. Melena
18. Headache

B. Physical examination
1. Lymph node enlargement
2. Anemia
3. ECCHYMOSIS
4. Skin: pallor, cyanosis, jaundice, PETECHIAE
5. Gingivitis
6. Ophthalmoscopic exam: bleeding fundi
7. Sclera: jaundice, capillary hemorrhage
8. Hepatomegaly
9. Sternal tenderness
10. Splenomegaly
11. Myocardial hypertrophy
12. EPISTAXIS
13. Dyspnea on exertion

♦ III. Diagnostic tests and procedures

A. Blood chemistry
1. Definition and purpose
   a. Laboratory test of a blood sample
   b. Analysis for potassium, calcium, blood urea nitrogen (BUN), creatinine, protein, albumin, and bilirubin
2. Nursing interventions
   a. Withhold food and fluids, as directed, before the procedure
   b. Check the site for bleeding after the procedure

B. Hematologic studies
1. Definition and purpose
   a. Laboratory test of a blood sample
   b. Analysis for WBCs, RBCs, erythrocyte sedimentation rate (ESR), Hgb, and hematocrit (HCT)

      2. Nursing interventions
         a. Note current drug therapy before the procedure
         b. Check the site for bleeding after the procedure

C. Lymphangiography
    1. Definition and purpose
       a. Procedure involving an injection of radiopaque dye through a catheter
       b. Radiographic picture of lymphatic system and dissection of lymph vessel

CLINICAL ALERT

    2. Nursing interventions before the procedure
       a. Note the patient's allergies to iodine, seafood, and radiopaque dyes
       b. Inform the patient of possible throat irritation and flushing of the face after injection of the dye
       c. Obtain written, informed consent
       d. Withhold food and fluids, as directed
    3. Nursing interventions after the procedure
       a. Assess vital signs (VS) and peripheral pulses
       b. Check catheter insertion site for bleeding
       c. Force fluids
       d. Advise the patient that skin, stool, and urine will have a blue discoloration

D. Bone marrow examination (aspiration or biopsy)
    1. Definition and purpose
       a. Procedure involving the percutaneous removal of bone marrow
       b. Examination of erythrocytes, leukocytes, thrombocytes, and precursor cells
    2. Nursing interventions before the procedure
       a. Obtain written, informed consent
       b. Determine the patient's ability to lie still during aspiration
    3. Nursing interventions after the procedure
       a. Maintain pressure dressing
       b. Check the aspiration site for bleeding and infection

E. Schilling test
    1. Definition and purpose
       a. Procedure involving administration of oral radioactive cyanocobalamin and intramuscular cyanocobalamin
       b. Microscopic examination of a 24-hour urine sample for cyanocobalamin (vitamin B_{12})
    2. Nursing interventions before the procedure
       a. Withhold food and fluids after midnight
       b. Obtain written, informed consent

3. Nursing interventions after the procedure
  a. Instruct the patient to save all voided urine for 24 hours
  b. Keep urine at room temperature

F. Gastric analysis
  1. Definition and purpose
    a. Procedure involving the aspiration of stomach contents through a nasogastric (NG) tube
    b. Fasting analysis of gastric secretions to measure acidity and diagnose pernicious anemia
  2. Nursing interventions before the procedure
    a. Withhold food and fluids
    b. Instruct the patient not to smoke for 8 to 12 hours before the test
    c. Withhold medications that can affect gastric secretions
  3. Nursing interventions after the procedure
    a. Obtain vital signs
    b. Assess for reactions to gastric acid stimulant, if used

G. Urine urobilinogen
  1. Definition and purpose
    a. Laboratory test of a 2-hour or a 24-hour urine sample
    b. Microscopic examination to diagnose hemolytic jaundice
  2. Nursing interventions
    a. Use bottle with a preservative and refrigerate specimen
    b. Note salicylate use
    c. Start urine collection in the afternoon when food is being digested for a 2-hour specimen
    d. Begin the 24-hour collection after the first voided specimen in the morning

H. Erythrocyte life span determination
  1. Definition and purpose
    a. Procedure involving reinjection of the patient's blood that has been tagged with chromium 51
    b. Measurement of the life span of circulating RBCs
  2. Nursing interventions
    a. Inform the patient that frequent blood samples will be drawn over a 2-week period
    b. Check the venipuncture site for bleeding
    c. Apply a pressure dressing after the procedure

I. Bence Jones protein assay
  1. Definition and purpose
    a. Procedure involving a 24-hour urine sample
    b. Microscopic examination for the Bence Jones protein to diagnose multiple myeloma

2. Nursing interventions
   a. Withhold all medications for 48 hours before the test
   b. Instruct the patient to void and note the time (collection of urine starts with the next voiding)
   c. Place urine container on ice
   d. Measure each voided urine
   e. Instruct the patient to void at the end of the 24-hour period
   f. Note any medications that might interfere with the test

J. Romberg test
   1. Definition and purpose
      a. Physical test
      b. Examination to assess loss of balance in pernicious anemia
   2. Nursing interventions
      a. Explain the procedure
      b. Monitor for imbalance
      c. Prevent the patient from falling

K. Erythrocyte fragility test
   1. Definition and purpose
      a. Laboratory test of a blood sample
      b. Analysis to measure the rate at which RBCs burst in varied hypotonic solutions
   2. Nursing interventions
      a. Explain the procedure
      b. Send the specimen to the laboratory

L. Rumpel-Leede capillary fragility tourniquet test
   1. Definition and purpose
      a. Crude physical test
      b. Examination of vascular resistance, platelet number, and function
   2. Nursing interventions: Explain that a blood pressure cuff will be placed on the arm for 5 minutes, followed by counting of petechiae

M. Bone scan
   1. Definition and purpose
      a. Procedure using an I.V. injection of radioisotope
      b. Visual imaging of bone metabolism
   2. Nursing interventions before the procedure: determine the patient's ability to lie still

N. Coagulation studies
   1. Definition and purpose
      a. Laboratory tests of a blood sample
      b. Analysis for platelet function, platelet count, prothrombin time (PT), partial thromboplastin time (PTT), coagulation time, and bleeding time

2. Nursing interventions
   a. Note current drug therapy before procedure
   b. Check the site for bleeding after the procedure

♦ IV. Psychosocial impact of hematologic and lymphatic disorders

A. Developmental impact
   1. Fear of dying
   2. Decreased self-esteem
   3. Fear of rejection

B. Economic impact
   1. Disruption or loss of employment
   2. Cost of hospitalization
   3. Cost of medications

C. Occupational and recreational impact
   1. Restrictions in work activity
   2. Changes in leisure activity

D. Social impact
   1. Changes in role performance
   2. Social isolation

♦ V. Possible risk factors

A. Modifiable risk factors
   1. Exposure to chemical and environmental pollutants
   2. Sexual activity patterns
   3. History of aspirin use
   4. Alcohol consumption
   5. Drug toxicity
   6. Diet
   7. Exposure to occupational radiation or radiation therapy

B. Nonmodifiable risk factors
   1. Ethnic background
   2. Aging
   3. Malabsorption syndromes
   4. History of liver disease
   5. History of malignancy

♦ VI. Nursing diagnostic categories

A. Probable nursing diagnostic categories
   1. Risk for activity intolerance
   2. Ineffective breathing pattern

3. Chronic pain
4. Impaired gas exchange

B. Possible nursing diagnostic categories
1. Risk for infection
2. Altered nutrition: less than body requirements
3. Altered oral mucous membrane
4. Body image disturbance
5. Self-esteem disturbance
6. Anxiety
7. Social isolation
8. Risk for impaired skin integrity

◆ VII. Splenectomy

A. Description—surgical removal of the spleen

B. Preoperative nursing interventions
1. Complete patient and family preoperative teaching
   a. Determine the patient's understanding of the procedure
   b. Describe the operating room (OR), postanesthesia care unit (PACU), and preoperative and postoperative routines
   c. Demonstrate postoperative turning, coughing, and deep breathing (TCDB), splinting, leg exercises, and range-of-motion (ROM) exercises
   d. Explain the postoperative need for drainage tubes, surgical dressings, oxygen therapy, I.V. therapy, and pain control
2. Complete a preoperative checklist
3. Administer preoperative medications, as prescribed
4. Allay the patient's and family's anxiety about surgery
5. Document the patient's history and physical assessment database
6. Monitor PT, PTT, HCT, Hgb, and platelet count
7. Administer vitamin K
8. Verify inoculation with polyvalent pneumococcal vaccine 2 weeks before procedure
9. Administer antibiotics, as prescribed

CLINICAL ALERT

C. Postoperative nursing interventions
1. Assess cardiac, respiratory, and neurologic status
2. Assess pain and administer postoperative analgesics, as prescribed
3. Assess for return of peristalsis; provide solid foods and liquids, as tolerated
4. Administer I.V. fluids, total parenteral nutrition (TPN), and transfusion therapy, as prescribed
5. Allay the patient's anxiety
6. Inspect the surgical dressing and change, as directed
7. Reinforce TCDB and splinting of incision

8. Keep the patient in semi-Fowler's position
9. Provide incentive spirometry
10. Increase activity as tolerated
11. Monitor and record VS, urinary output (UO), intake and output (I/O), laboratory studies, and pulse oximetry
12. Monitor and maintain position and patency of drainage tubes: wound drainage
13. Apply abdominal binder
14. Monitor for abdominal distention
15. Individualize home care instructions
    a. Complete incision care daily
    b. State the need for prophylactic use of antibiotics
    c. Avoid contact sports

D. Possible surgical complications
1. Pneumococcal pneumonia
2. Infection
3. Hemorrhage
4. Sepsis
5. Disseminated intravascular coagulation (DIC)
6. Atelectasis
7. Subphrenic abscess
8. Thrombophlebitis

◆ VIII. Bone marrow transplant

A. Description
1. Bone marrow is aspirated from multiple sites along the iliac crest of the donor
2. Donor bone marrow is infused intravenously into the recipient

B. Preoperative nursing interventions
1. Complete patient and family preoperative teaching
    a. Determine the patient's understanding of the procedure
    b. Describe the OR, PACU, and preoperative and postoperative routines
    c. Demonstrate postoperative TCDB, splinting, and leg and ROM exercises
    d. Explain the postoperative need for drainage tubes, surgical dressings, oxygen therapy, I.V. therapy, and pain control
2. Complete a preoperative checklist
3. Administer preoperative medications, as prescribed
4. Allay the patient's and family's anxiety about surgery
5. Document the patient's history and physical assessment database
6. Verify bone marrow compatibility
7. Administer chemotherapy for 3 days before the transplant

    8. Maintain the radiation treatment schedule

    9. Maintain protective isolation or the use of a laminar air flow room

   10. Monitor for infection

C. Postoperative nursing interventions

    1. Assess cardiac and respiratory status

    2. Administer I.V. fluids

    3. Allay the patient's anxiety

    4. Keep the patient in semi-Fowler's position

    5. Maintain activity, as tolerated

    6. Monitor and record VS; UO; I/O; central venous pressure (CVP); laboratory studies; urine, stool, and emesis for occult blood; daily weight; specific gravity; urine glucose, ketones, and protein; and pulse oximetry

    7. Precautions: protective

    8. Encourage the patient to express feelings about a fear of dying

    9. Administer antibiotics, as prescribed

   10. Provide postchemotherapeutic and postradiation nursing care

      a. Provide prophylactic skin, mouth, and perineal care

      b. Monitor dietary intake

      c. Administer antiemetics and antidiarrheals, as prescribed

      d. Monitor for bleeding, infection, and electrolyte imbalance

      e. Provide rest periods

   11. Inspect for bruising and petechiae

   12. Administer immunosuppressants, as prescribed

   13. Individualize home care instructions

      a. Recognize the signs and symptoms of infection and bleeding

      b. Identify changes in vision

D. Possible surgical complications

    1. Marrow graft rejection

    2. Graft versus host disease

    3. Cataracts

    4. Stomatitis

    5. Hemorrhage

◆ IX. Agranulocytosis (granulocytopenia)

A. Definition—profound decrease in the number of granulocytes

B. Possible etiology

    1. Idiopathic

    2. Exposure to chemicals

    3. Drug induced: chloramphenicol (Chloromycetin), chlorpromazine (Thorazine), phenytoin (Dilantin)

    4. Chemotherapy

    5. Radiation

      6. Radioisotopes

      7. Hemodialysis

      8. Viral infection

C. Pathophysiology

      1. Number of granulocytes is reduced because of increased utilization, lack of maturation, or shortened life span

      2. The reduced number of granulocytes diminishes resistance to disease

D. Possible assessment findings

      1. Fatigue

      2. Malaise

      3. Elevated temperature

      4. Chills

      5. Sore throat

      6. Multiple infections

      7. Weakness

      8. Dysphagia

      9. Enlarged cervical lymph nodes

      10. Tachycardia

      11. Ulcerations of oral mucosa and throat

E. Possible diagnostic test findings

      1. Hematology: decreased WBCs, granulocytes; increased ESR

      2. Bone marrow biopsy: absence of polymorphonuclear leukocytes

      3. Culture and sensitivity: positive identification of organisms

F. Medical management

      1. Diet: high-protein, high-vitamin, high-calorie, bland, and soft

      2. I.V. therapy: heparin lock

      3. Position: semi-Fowler's

      4. Activity: bed rest and active and passive ROM exercises

      5. Monitoring: VS, UO, and I/O

      6. Laboratory studies: WBCs, granulocytes, and urine and blood for culture and sensitivity

      7. Treatment: saline gargles

      8. Precautions: protective

      9. Transfusion therapy: packed WBCs and whole blood

      10. Antibiotics: ticarcillan (Ticar), tobramycin sulfate (Nebcin)

      11. Antipyretic: acetaminophen (Tylenol)

      12. Sedative: oxazepam (Serax)

      13. Stool softener: docusate sodium (Colace)

      14. Analgesic: ibuprofen (Motrin)

      15. Antifungal: fluconazole (Diflucan)

      16. Hematopoietic growth factor: epoetin alfa (Epogen)

G. Nursing interventions
   1. Maintain the patient's diet
   2. Force fluids
   3. Provide TCDB
   4. Assess respiratory status
   5. Keep the patient in semi-Fowler's position
   6. Monitor and record: VS, UO, I/O, laboratory studies, and stool count
   7. Administer medications, as prescribed
   8. Encourage the patient to express feelings about imposed isolation
   9. Maintain bed rest
   10. Provide tepid baths and saline gargles
   11. Maintain protective precautions
   12. Administer transfusion therapy, as prescribed
   13. Provide gentle mouth and skin care
   14. Monitor for infection

CLINICAL ALERT

   15. Avoid enemas and rectal temperatures
   16. Avoid raw fruits and vegetables
   17. Avoid exposure to flowers and plants in room
   18. Individualize home care instructions (For teaching tips, see *Patients with hematologic or lymphatic disorders*, page 350)
      a. Avoid using over-the-counter medications
      b. Prevent constipation

H. Possible medical complications
   1. Sepsis
   2. Rectal abscess
   3. Pneumonia
   4. Hemorrhagic necrosis of mucous membranes
   5. Parenchymal liver damage

I. Possible surgical intervention: splenectomy (see page 345)

◆ X. Leukemia

A. Definition
   1. Uncontrolled proliferation of WBC precursors that fail to mature
   2. Three types
      a. Acute myelogenous (AML)
      b. Chronic lymphocytic (CLL)
      c. Chronic myelocytic (CML)

B. Possible etiology
   1. Unknown
   2. Genetics
   3. Virus

TEACHING TIPS

Patients with hematologic or lymphatic disorders

Be sure to include the following topics in your teaching plan when caring for patients with hematologic or lymphatic disorders.

- Follow-up appointments
- Smoking cessation
- Optimal body weight maintenance
- Medication therapy, including the action, adverse effects, and scheduling of medications
- Infection control measures
- Signs and symptoms of infection and bleeding
- Daily skin, mouth, and foot care
- Dietary recommendations and restrictions
- Avoidance of over-the-counter medications
- Prevention of constipation
- Medical identification bracelet
- Safe environment
- Independence in ADLs
- Reactions to limitation on lifestyle and ADLs
- Rest and activity patterns, including any limitations or restrictions
- Community agencies and resources for supportive services

4. Exposure to chemicals
5. Radiation
6. Altered immune system
7. Chemotherapy
8. Polycythemia vera

C. Pathophysiology
   1. Normal hemopoietic cells are replaced by leukemic cells in bone marrow
   2. Immature forms of WBCs circulate in the blood, infiltrating the liver, spleen, and lymph nodes

D. Possible assessment findings
   1. Petechiae
   2. Ecchymosis
   3. Frequent infections
   4. Elevated temperature
   5. Enlarged lymph nodes, spleen, and liver
   6. Joint, abdominal, and bone pain
   7. Gingivitis
   8. Night sweats

9. Stomatitis
10. Prolonged menses
11. Hematemesis
12. Melena
13. Jaundice
14. Tachycardia
15. Hypotension
16. Epistaxis
17. Generalized pain

E. Possible diagnostic test findings
   1. Hematology: decreased HCT, Hgb, RBCs, platelets; increased ESR, immature WBCs, bleeding time
   2. Bone marrow biopsy: large number of immature leukocytes

F. Medical management
   1. Diet: high-protein, high-vitamin and mineral, high-calorie, low-roughage, bland and soft in small, frequent feedings
   2. I.V. therapy: hydration and heparin lock
   3. Oxygen therapy
   4. Position: semi-Fowler's
   5. Activity: bed rest and active and passive ROM and isometric exercises
   6. Monitoring: VS, UO, and I/O
   7. Laboratory studies: Hgb, HCT, WBCs, platelets, BUN, creatinine, and surveillance cultures
   8. Nutritional support: TPN
   9. Radiation therapy
  10. Chemotherapy
  11. Treatments: sitz baths, bed cradle, and tepid baths
  12. Precautions: protective or laminar air flow room
  13. Transfusion therapy: platelets, packed RBCs, and whole blood
  14. Antibiotics: doxorubicin (Adriamycin), plicamycin (Mithracin)
  15. Antipyretic: acetaminophen (Tylenol)
  16. Stool softener: docusate sodium (Colace)
  17. Analgesic: ibuprofen (Motrin)
  18. Antigout: allopurinol (Zyloprim)
  19. Tranquilizer: oxazepam (Serax)
  20. Systemic alkalinizer: sodium bicarbonate
  21. Antimetabolites: fluorouracil (Adrucil), methotrexate sodium (Mexate)
  22. Alkylating agents: busulfan (Myleran), chlorambucil (Leukeran)
  23. Antineoplastics: vinblastine (Velban), vincristine sulfate (Oncovin)
  24. Enzyme: L-asparaginase (Elspar)

25. Estrogen: diethylstilbestrol (DES)
26. Progestin: medroxyprogesterone (Provera)
27. IgG antibody: immune globulin I.V. (Gammagard)
28. Antiemetic: prochlorperazine (Compazine)
29. Leukopheresis
30. Antifungal: fluconazole (Mycostatin)
31. Hematopoietic growth factor: epoetin alfa (Neupogen)

G. Nursing interventions

1. Maintain the patient's diet
2. Force fluids
3. Administer I.V. fluids
4. Administer oxygen
5. Provide TCDB
6. Assess cardiovascular, neurologic, respiratory, and renal status and fluid balance
7. Keep the patient in semi-Fowler's position
8. Monitor and record VS, UO, I/O, laboratory studies, daily weight, and urine, stool, and emesis for occult blood
9. Administer TPN
10. Administer transfusion therapy, as prescribed
11. Administer medications, as prescribed
12. Encourage the patient to express feelings about changes in body image and a fear of dying
13. Maintain bed rest
14. Provide treatments: sitz baths, bed cradle, and tepid baths

CLINICAL ALERT

15. Allay the patient's anxiety
16. Monitor for bleeding and infection
17. Maintain protective precautions

CLINICAL ALERT

18. Provide gentle mouth and skin care
19. Avoid giving the patient intramuscular injections and enemas and taking temperature rectally
20. Avoid using straight razors on the patient
21. Provide postchemotherapeutic and postradiation nursing care
    a. Provide prophylactic skin, mouth, and perineal care
    b. Monitor dietary intake
    c. Administer antiemetics and antidiarrheals, as prescribed
    d. Monitor for bleeding, infection, and electrolyte imbalance
    e. Provide rest periods
22. Individualize home care instructions
    a. Provide information about the American Cancer Society
    b. Recognize the signs and symptoms of occult blood
    c. Prevent constipation
    d. Use an electric razor

    e. Avoid using over-the-counter medications

    f. Monitor stool for occult blood

    g. Increase fluid intake

H. Possible medical complications

    1. Gross systemic hemorrhage

    2. Acute renal failure

    3. Cerebrovascular accident (CVA)

    4. Thrombocytopenia

    5. Perirectal abscess

    6. Gastrointestinal bleeding

    7. Fungal and bacterial infection

    8. Meningitis

I. Possible surgical intervention: bone marrow transplant (see page 346)

♦ XI. Lymphomas

A. Definition

    1. Hodgkin's disease: proliferation of malignant Reed-Sternberg cells within lymph nodes

    2. Malignant lymphoma: malignant tumors of lymph nodes and lymphatic tissues that cannot be classified as Hodgkin's disease

    3. Classes of malignant lymphoma: B-lymphocyte malignancies, T-lymphocyte malignancies, and histiocyte malignancies

B. Possible etiology

    1. Unknown

    2. Viral

    3. Genetic (Hodgkin's disease)

    4. Environmental (Hodgkin's disease)

    5. Immunologic

C. Pathophysiology

    1. Reed-Sternberg cells proliferate in a single lymph node and travel contiguously through the lymphatic system to other lymphatic nodes and organs (Hodgkin's disease)

    2. Immune system cell tumors occur throughout lymph nodes and lymphatic organs in unpredictable patterns (malignant lymphoma)

D. Possible assessment findings

    1. Enlarged, nontender, firm, and movable lymph nodes in lower cervical regions (Hodgkin's disease)

    2. Recurrent, intermittent fever

    3. Night sweats

    4. Weight loss

    5. Malaise

    6. Lethargy

      7. Severe pruritus

      8. Dyspnea (Hodgkin's disease)

      9. Anorexia

     10. Bone pain (Hodgkin's disease)

     11. Cough

     12. Recurrent infection

     13. Hepatomegaly

     14. Splenomegaly

     15. Dysphagia (Hodgkin's disease)

     16. Edema and cyanosis of face and neck (Hodgkin's disease)

     17. Prominent, painless, generalized LYMPHADENOPATHY (malignant lymphoma)

E. Possible diagnostic test findings

      1. Bone marrow aspiration and biopsy: small, diffuse lymphocytic or large, follicular-type cells (malignant lymphoma)

      2. Hematology: decreased Hgb, HCT, platelets (malignant lymphoma and Hodgkin's disease); increased ESR (Hodgkin's disease and malignant lymphoma); increased leukocytes, gammaglobulin (Hodgkin's disease)

      3. Lymphangiogram: positive lymph node involvement (Hodgkin's disease)

      4. Lymph node biopsy: positive for Reed-Sternberg cells (Hodgkin's disease)

      5. Chest X-ray: lymphadenopathy (Hodgkin's disease)

      6. Blood chemistry: increased alkaline phosphatase, copper (Hodgkin's disease)

      7. Stage I: asymptomatic; malignant cells found in a single lymph node

      8. Stage II: symptomatic; malignant cells found in two or three adjacent lymph nodes on the same side of the diaphragm

      9. Stage III: symptomatic; malignant cells widely disseminated to lymph nodes on both sides of the diaphragm and to organs

     10. Stage IV: symptomatic; malignant cells found in one or more extra-lymphatic organs or tissues with or without lymphatic involvement

F. Medical management

      1. Diet: high-protein, high-calorie, high-vitamin and mineral, high-iron, high-calcium, bland, and soft

      2. I.V. therapy: heparin lock

      3. Oxygen therapy

      4. Position: semi-Fowler's

      5. Activity: bed rest and active and passive ROM exercises

      6. Monitoring: VS, UO, and I/O

      7. Laboratory studies: Hgb, HCT, WBCs, and platelets

8. Radiation therapy
9. Precautions: protective
10. Transfusion therapy: packed RBCs
11. MOPP chemotherapy protocol (Hodgkin's disease): mechlore-thamine (Mustargen), vincristine sulfate (Oncovin), procarbazine (Matulane), prednisone (Deltasone)
12. ABVD chemotherapy protocol (Hodgkin's disease): doxorubicin (Adriamycin), bleomycin (Blenoxane), vinblastine (Velban), dacar-bazine (DTIC-Dome)
13. Analgesic: meperidine hydrochloride (Demerol)
14. Sedative: oxazepam (Serax)
15. Stool softener: docusate sodium (Colace)
16. Antipruritic: diphenhydramine (Benadryl)
17. CVP chemotherapy protocol (malignant lymphoma): cyclophos-phamide (Cytoxan), vincristine sulfate (Oncovin), prednisone (Deltasone)
18. CHOP chemotherapy protocol (malignant lymphoma): cyclophos-phamide (Cytoxan), doxorubicin (Adriamycin), vincristine sulfate (Oncovin), prednisone (Deltasone)
19. Antiemetic: prochlorperazine (Compazine)

G. Nursing interventions
1. Maintain the patient's diet
2. Force fluids
3. Administer I.V. fluids
4. Administer oxygen
5. Provide TCDB
6. Assess respiratory, cardiovascular, and neurologic status and fluid balance
7. Keep the patient in semi-Fowler's position
8. Monitor and record VS, UO, I/O, laboratory studies, and specific gravity
9. Administer medications, as prescribed
10. Encourage the patient to express feelings about changes in body image and a fear of dying
11. Maintain bed rest
12. Give frequent baths with mild soap
13. Provide mouth and skin care
14. Administer transfusion therapy, as prescribed
15. Allay the patient's anxiety

16. Avoid giving aspirin to the patient
17. Avoid using straight razors on the patient
18. Provide postchemotherapeutic and postradiation nursing care
   a. Provide prophylactic skin, mouth, and perineal care
   b. Monitor dietary intake

      c. Administer antiemetics and antidiarrheals, as prescribed

      d. Monitor for bleeding, infection, and electrolyte imbalance

      e. Provide rest periods

19. Monitor for jaundice and infection
20. Maintain protective precautions
21. Individualize home care instructions

      a. Provide information about the American Cancer Society

      b. Recognize the signs and symptoms of motor and sensory deficits

      c. Increase fluid intake

      d. Use electric razors

      e. Avoid using over-the-counter medications

      f. Avoid taking aspirin

H. Possible medical complications

1. Metastasis (Hodgkin's disease)
2. Hypersplenism
3. Pleural effusion (Hodgkin's disease)
4. Herpes zoster (Hodgkin's disease)
5. Depression
6. Pancytopenia (Hodgkin's disease)
7. Pneumonitis (Hodgkin's disease)
8. Paraplegia
9. Pericarditis (Hodgkin's disease)
10. Nephritis (Hodgkin's disease)
11. Hypothyroidism (Hodgkin's disease)
12. Neuralgia (Hodgkin's disease)
13. Obstructive jaundice (Hodgkin's disease)
14. Infections: viral, bacterial, fungal (malignant lymphoma)
15. Intestinal obstruction (malignant lymphoma)
16. Leukemia (malignant lymphoma)
17. Superior vena cava obstruction (malignant lymphoma)

I. Possible surgical interventions: splenectomy (see page 345)

◆ XII. Acquired immunodeficiency syndrome (AIDS)

A. Definition

1. Defect in T-cell mediated immunity that allows the development of fatal opportunistic infections
2. Caused by human immunodeficiency virus (HIV)
3. An illness characterized by laboratory evidence of HIV infection co-existing with one or more indicator diseases, such as herpes simplex virus, cytomegalovirus, mycobacteria, candidal infection, *Pneumocystis carinii,* Kaposi's sarcoma, wasting syndrome, and dementia

B. Possible etiology
  1. Exposure to blood containing HIV: transfusions, contaminated needles, handling of blood, in utero
  2. Exposure to semen and vaginal secretions containing HIV: sexual intercourse, handling of semen and vaginal secretions

C. Pathophysiology
  1. HIV is transmitted by contact with infected blood or body fluids
     a. HIV-infected lymphocytes are carried in semen, vaginal secretions, and blood
     b. Infected lymphocytes in semen and vaginal secretions are transferred through minute breaks in the skin and mucosa
     c. Infected lymphocytes in blood are transferred via transfusion, fetal circulation, and minute breaks in the skin and mucosa
  2. HIV, a retrovirus, selectively infects human cells containing CD_4 antigen on their surface, the majority of which are T_4 lymphocytes
  3. HIV virus reproduces within the T_4 lymphocytes and destroys them
  4. The destruction of the T4 lymphocytes diminishes resistance to disease

D. Possible assessment findings
  1. Fatigue, weakness, anorexia, weight loss, recurrent diarrhea, fever, lymphadenopathy, pallor, night sweats, malnutrition
  2. Disorientation, confusion, dementia
  3. Opportunistic infections

E. Possible diagnostic test findings
  1. Hematology: decreased WBCs, RBCs, platelets
  2. Blood chemistry: increased transaminase, alkaline phosphatase, gamma globulin; decreased albumin
  3. Enzyme linked immunosorbent assay (ELISA): positive HIV antibody titer
  4. Western blot: positive
  5. $CD4^+$ level: less than 200

F. Medical management
  1. Diet: high-calorie, high-protein in small, frequent feedings
  2. I.V. therapy: hydration, electrolyte replacement, and heparin lock
  3. Oxygen therapy
  4. Position: semi-Fowler's
  5. Activity: as tolerated, active and passive ROM exercises
  6. Monitoring: VS, UO, I/O, and neurovital signs
  7. Laboratory studies: WBCs, RBCs, platelets, and albumin
  8. Nutritional support: TPN
  9. Treatments: chest physiotherapy (CPT), postural drainage, and incentive spirometry
  10. Precautions: standard

11. Transfusion therapy: fresh frozen plasma (FFP), platelets, and packed RBCs
12. Antibiotics: aerosolized pentamidine (NebuPent), trimethoprim and sulfamethoxazole (Bactrim)
13. Antivirals: dapsone, didanosine (Videx), ganciclovir (Cytovene), zidovudine (Retrovir, AZT), acyclovir (Zovirax), pentamidine (Pentam)
14. Plasmapheresis
15. Interferon
16. Interleukin II
17. Specialized bed: active or static, low air loss (Kin Air, Biodyne)
18. Antifungals: fluconazole (Diflucan), amphotericin B (Fungizone)
19. Pulse oximetry
20. Antiemetic: prochlorperazine (Compazine)

G. Nursing interventions
1. Maintain the patient's diet
2. Force fluids
3. Administer I.V. fluids
4. Administer oxygen
5. Provide incentive spirometry and TCDB
6. Assess respiratory and neurologic status and fluid balance
7. Keep the patient in semi-Fowler's position
8. Monitor and record VS, UO, I/O, laboratory studies, daily weight, specific gravity, and pulse oximetry
9. Administer TPN
10. Administer medications, as prescribed
11. Encourage the patient to express feelings about changes in body image, a fear of dying, and social isolation
12. Maintain activity, as tolerated
13. Allay the patient's anxiety
14. Provide rest periods

CLINICAL ALERT

15. Provide skin and mouth care
16. Maintain standard precautions
17. Monitor for opportunistic infections
18. Caution the patient to avoid anal sex
19. Caution an I.V. drug user to clean drug paraphernalia with bleach
20. Make referrals to community agencies for support
21. Individualize home care instructions
    a. Refrain from donating blood
    b. Avoid using alcohol and recreational drugs
    c. Use condoms during sexual intercourse

H. Possible medical complications
   1. *Pneumocystis carinii* pneumonia
   2. Cryptococcal meningitis
   3. Burkitt's lymphoma
   4. Encephalopathy
   5. Depression
   6. Herpes simplex virus
   7. Cytomegalovirus infection
   8. Epstein-Barr virus
   9. Oral and esophageal candidiasis
   10. Kaposi's sarcoma
   11. Toxoplasmosis
   12. *Mycobacterium avium* intracellular infection
   13. Neuropathies
   14. Myopathies

I. Possible surgical interventions: bone marrow transplant (see page 346)

♦ XIII. Iron deficiency anemia

A. Definition—chronic, slowly progressive decrease in circulating RBCs

B. Possible etiology
   1. Acute and chronic bleeding
   2. Inadequate intake of iron-rich foods
   3. Gastrectomy
   4. Malabsorption syndrome
   5. Vitamin B_6 deficiency
   6. Pregnancy
   7. Menstruation
   8. Alcohol abuse
   9. Drug induced

C. Pathophysiology
   1. Iron deficiency is caused by inadequate absorption or excessive loss of iron
   2. Decreased iron affects formation of Hgb and RBCs
   3. Decreased Hgb and RBCs reduce the capacity of the blood to transport oxygen to cells

D. Possible assessment findings
   1. Palpitations
   2. Dizziness
   3. Sensitivity to cold
   4. Stomatitis
   5. Dyspnea
   6. Weakness and fatigue

7. Pale, dry mucous membranes
8. Papillae atrophy of the tongue
9. Cheilosis
10. Pallor
11. Koilonychia

E. Possible diagnostic test findings
  1. Hematology: decreased Hgb, HCT, iron, ferritin, reticulocytes, red cell indices, transferrin saturation; absent hemosiderin; increased iron-binding capacity
  2. Peripheral blood smear: microcytic and hypochromic RBCs

F. Medical management
  1. Diet: high-iron, high-roughage, high-protein, high ascorbic acid, high-vitamin with increased fluids; avoid teas
  2. Oxygen therapy
  3. Position: semi-Fowler's
  4. Activity: bed rest
  5. Monitoring: VS, UO, and I/O
  6. Laboratory studies: arterial blood gases (ABGs), Hgb, HCT, iron, iron-binding capacity
  7. Transfusion therapy: packed RBCs
  8. Antianemics: ferrous sulfate (Feosol), iron dextran (Imferon)
  9. Vitamins: pyridoxine hydrochloride (vitamin B_6), ascorbic acid (vitamin C)

G. Nursing interventions
  1. Maintain the patient's diet with increased fluids
  2. Force fluids
  3. Administer oxygen
  4. Assess cardiovascular and respiratory status
  5. Keep the patient in semi-Fowler's position
  6. Monitor and record VS, UO, I/O, and laboratory studies
  7. Administer medications, as prescribed
  8. Allay the patient's anxiety
  9. Monitor stool, urine, and emesis for occult blood
  10. Provide rest periods
  11. Provide mouth, skin, and foot care
  12. Protect the patient from falls
  13. Keep the patient warm
  14. Individualize home care instructions
    a. Recognize the signs and symptoms of bleeding
    b. Monitor stools for occult blood
    c. Avoid using hot pads and hot water bottles

H. Possible medical complications
1. Plummer-Vinson syndrome
2. Angina pectoris
3. Congestive heart failure (CHF)

I. Possible surgical interventions: none

♦ **XIV. Pernicious anemia**

A. Definition—chronic, progressive macrocytic anemia caused by a deficiency of intrinsic factor

B. Possible etiology
1. Deficiency of intrinsic factor
2. Gastric mucosal atrophy
3. Genetics
4. Prolonged iron deficiency
5. Autoimmune disease
6. Lack of administration of vitamin B_{12} after small-bowel resection or total gastrectomy
7. Malabsorption
8. Bacterial or parasitic infections

C. Pathophysiology
1. Without intrinsic factor, dietary vitamin B_{12} cannot be absorbed by the ileum
2. Normal DNA synthesis is inhibited, resulting in defective maturation of cells

D. Possible assessment findings
1. Weakness
2. Pallor
3. Dyspnea
4. Palpitations
5. Fatigue
6. Sore mouth
7. Glossitis
8. Weight loss and anorexia
9. Dyspepsia
10. Constipation or diarrhea
11. Mild jaundice of sclera
12. Tingling and paresthesia of hands and feet
13. Paralysis
14. Depression
15. Delirium
16. Gait disturbances
17. Tachycardia

E. Possible diagnostic test findings
1. Schilling test: positive
2. Romberg test: positive
3. Gastric analysis: hypochlorhydria
4. Peripheral blood smear: oval, macrocytic, hyperchromic erythrocytes
5. Bone marrow: increased megaloblasts; few maturing erythrocytes; defective leukocyte maturation
6. Blood chemistry: increased bilirubin, lactate dehydrogenase (LD)
7. Hematology: decreased HCT, Hgb
8. Upper GI series: atrophy of gastric mucosa

F. Medical management
1. Diet: high in iron and protein, with increased intake of vitamin B_{12} and folic acid; restrict highly seasoned, coarse, or extremely hot foods
2. Position: semi-Fowler's
3. Activity: as tolerated
4. Monitoring: VS and neurovital signs
5. Laboratory studies: Hgb, HCT, and bilirubin
6. Treatment: bed cradle
7. Transfusion therapy: packed RBCs
8. Antianemics: ferrous sulfate (Feosol), iron dextran (Imferon)
9. Vitamins: pyridoxine hydrochloride (vitamin B_6), ascorbic acid (vitamin C), cyanocobalamin (vitamin B_{12}), folic acid (Folvite)

G. Nursing interventions
1. Maintain the patient's diet
2. Assess neurologic and respiratory status
3. Keep the patient in semi-Fowler's position
4. Monitor and record VS, laboratory studies, and neurovital signs
5. Administer medications, as prescribed
6. Allay the patient's anxiety
7. Maintain activity, as tolerated
8. Provide treatments: bed cradle
9. Monitor and record amount, consistency, and color of stools
10. Provide mouth care before and after meals
11. Use soft toothbrushes
12. Maintain warm environment
13. Provide foot and skin care
14. Prevent the patient from falling
15. Individualize home care instructions
    a. Recognize the signs and symptoms of skin breakdown
    b. Alter activities of daily living (ADLs) to compensate for paresthesia
    c. Comply with lifelong, monthly injections of vitamin B_{12}
    d. Avoid using heating pads and electric blankets

CLINICAL
ALERT

H. Possible medical complications
1. Chronic renal failure
2. Arrhythmias
3. Gastric cancer
4. GI bleeding
5. CHF
6. Angina
7. Neurogenic bladder
8. CVA

I. Possible surgical interventions: none

◆ XV. Aplastic anemia (pancytopenia)

A. Definition—failure of bone marrow to produce adequate amounts of erythrocytes, leukocytes, and platelets

B. Possible etiology
1. Idiopathic
2. Exposure to chemicals
3. Drug induced: chloramphenicol (Chloromycetin), phenylbutazone (Butazolidin), phenytoin (Dilantin)
4. Chemotherapy
5. Radiation
6. Viral hepatitis

C. Pathophysiology
1. Bone marrow suppression, destruction, or aplasia results in failure of bone marrow to produce an adequate number of stem cells
2. Without an adequate number of stem cells, sufficient amounts of erythrocytes, leukocytes, and platelets cannot be produced
3. Pancytopenia includes leukopenia, thrombocytopenia, and anemia

D. Possible assessment findings
1. Fatigue
2. Dyspnea
3. Multiple infections
4. Elevated temperature
5. Headache
6. Weakness
7. Anorexia
8. Gingivitis
9. Epistaxis
10. Purpura
11. Petechiae

12. Ecchymosis
13. Pallor
14. Palpitations
15. Tachycardia
16. Tachypnea
17. Melena

E. Possible diagnostic test findings
   1. Peripheral blood smear: pancytopenia
   2. Hematology: decreased granulocytes, thrombocytes, RBCs
   3. Fecal occult blood: positive
   4. Urine chemistry: hematuria
   5. Bone marrow biopsy: fatty marrow with reduction of stem cells

F. Medical management
   1. Diet: high-protein, high-calorie, high-vitamin
   2. I.V. therapy: hydration, heparin lock
   3. Oxygen therapy
   4. Position: semi-Fowler's
   5. Activity: as tolerated
   6. Monitoring: VS, UO, and I/O
   7. Laboratory studies: RBCs, WBCs, platelets, and stool for occult blood
   8. Treatments: tepid sponge baths, cooling blankets
   9. Precautions: protective
   10. Transfusion therapy: platelets, packed RBCs
   11. Antibiotics: penicillin G potassium (Pentids), ticarcillin sodium (Ticar), tobramycin sulfate (Nebcin)
   12. Analgesics: ibuprofen (Motrin), acetaminophen (Tylenol)
   13. Antithymocyte globulin (ATG or RATG)
   14. Androgenic steroids: fluoxymesterone (Halotestin), oxymetholone (Anadrol)
   15. Recombinant human granulocyte-macrophage colony stimulating factor (GMCSF)
   16. Hematopoietic growth factor: epoetin alfa (Neupogen)

G. Nursing interventions
   1. Maintain the patient's diet
   2. Force fluids
   3. Administer I.V. fluids
   4. Administer oxygen
   5. Provide TCDB
   6. Assess cardiovascular and respiratory status and fluid balance
   7. Keep the patient in semi-Fowler's position
   8. Monitor and record VS; UO; I/O; laboratory studies; stool, urine, and emesis for occult blood; and specific gravity

9. Administer transfusion therapy, as prescribed
10. Administer medications, as prescribed
11. Allay the patient's anxiety
12. Alternate rest periods with activity
13. Provide cooling blankets and tepid sponge baths
14. Maintain protective precautions
15. Provide mouth care before and after meals
16. Provide skin care

17. Protect the patient from falls
18. Avoid giving the patient intramuscular injections
19. Avoid using hard toothbrushes and straight razors on the patient
20. Monitor for infection, bleeding, and bruising
21. Individualize home care instructions
    a. Recognize the signs and symptoms of bleeding
    b. Avoid contact sports
    c. Wear a medical identification bracelet
    d. Avoid using over-the-counter medications
    e. Monitor stool for occult blood
    f. Use an electric razor
    g. Avoid taking aspirin

H. Possible medical complications
   1. Hemorrhage
   2. Infection
   3. Septicemia
   4. CVA
   5. GI bleeding

I. Possible surgical interventions
   1. Bone marrow transplant (see page 346)
   2. Splenectomy (see page 345)

◆ XVI. Idiopathic thrombocytopenic purpura (ITP)

A. Definition—increased premature destruction of platelets

B. Possible etiology
   1. Unknown
   2. Autoimmune disease
   3. Viral infection

C. Pathophysiology
   1. Antibody-coated platelets are removed from circulation by reticuloendothelial cells of the spleen and liver
   2. Decreased number of circulating platelets cause bleeding

D. Possible assessment findings
   1. Petechiae
   2. Ecchymosis
   3. Epistaxis
   4. Gingivitis
   5. Visual disturbances
   6. Dizziness
   7. Menorrhagia
   8. Hematomas
   9. Increased bleeding after dental extraction
   10. Gastrointestinal bleeding

E. Possible diagnostic test findings
   1. Hematology: decreased Hgb, HCT, platelets; normal PT, PTT; prolonged bleeding time
   2. Urine chemistry: hematuria
   3. Fecal occult blood: positive
   4. Blood chemistry: increased immunoglobulins (IgG), complement fixation
   5. Bone marrow biopsy: increased and abnormal megakaryocytes
   6. Rumpel-Leede capillary fragility tourniquet test: positive with increased capillary fragility

F. Medical management
   1. Diet: soft and bland
   2. I.V. therapy: heparin lock
   3. Activity: bed rest
   4. Monitoring: VS, UO, daily weight, and stool for occult blood
   5. Laboratory studies: Hgb, HCT, and platelets
   6. Precautions: protective
   7. Transfusion therapy: FFP, platelets, packed RBCs, and plasma
   8. IgG antibody: immune globulin I.V. (Gammagard)
   9. Stool softener: docusate sodium (Colace)
   10. Immunosuppressants: azathioprine (Imuran), cyclophosphamide (Cytoxan), vincristine sulfate (Oncovin)
   11. Anabolic steroid: danazol (Cyclomen)
   12. Corticosteroid: prednisone (Deltasone)

G. Nursing interventions
   1. Maintain the patient's diet
   2. Force fluids
   3. Administer I.V. fluids and transfusion therapy
   4. Assess for bruising, bleeding, and infection
   5. Monitor and record VS; UO; I/O; laboratory studies; daily weight; stool, urine, and emesis for occult blood; neurovital signs; pad count; and blood loss

6. Administer medications, as prescribed
7. Allay the patient's anxiety
8. Provide gentle mouth care
9. Protect the patient from falls
10. Avoid giving the patient intramuscular injections, aspirin, enemas, and rectal temperatures
11. Avoid using straight razors, tape, and tourniquets on the patient

CLINICAL ALERT

12. Alternate rest periods with activity
13. Rotate extremities for blood pressure monitoring
14. Individualize home care instructions
    a. Recognize the signs and symptoms of bleeding
    b. Avoid contact sports
    c. Wear a medical identification bracelet
    d. Use electric razors and soft toothbrushes
    e. Avoid sneezing, coughing, nose blowing, straining while defecating, and heavy lifting
    f. Avoid using over-the-counter medications

H. Possible medical complications
   1. Hypersplenism
   2. CVA
   3. Shock
   4. Hemothorax
   5. Peripheral paralysis and paresthesia
   6. Bleeding into diaphragm

I. Possible surgical intervention: splenectomy (see page 345)

◆ XVII. Polycythemia vera

A. Definition—myeloproliferative disorder that results in the increased production of erythrocytes, hemoglobin, myelocytes, and thrombocytes

B. Possible etiology
   1. Unknown
   2. Hypernephroma
   3. Hepatoma
   4. Uterine fibroids
   5. Pheochromocytoma
   6. Lung tumors
   7. Adrenal cancer
   8. Cerebral hemangioblastoma

C. Pathophysiology
   1. Hyperplasia of bone marrow results in increased production of erythrocytes, hemoglobin, granulocytes, and platelets
   2. Overproduction results in increased blood viscosity, increased total blood volume, and severe congestion of all tissues and organs

D. Possible assessment findings
   1. Ruddy complexion
   2. Dusky mucosa
   3. Vertigo
   4. Headaches
   5. Dyspnea and orthopnea
   6. Tachycardia
   7. Ecchymosis
   8. Hepatomegaly and splenomegaly
   9. Increased gastric secretions
   10. Weakness and fatigue
   11. Pruritus
   12. Epistaxis
   13. GI bleeding
   14. Angina

E. Possible diagnostic test findings
   1. Blood chemistry: increased uric acid, unconjugated bilirubin, vitamin B_{12}, alkaline phosphatase, serum aspartate aminotransferase (AST), serum alanine aminotransferase (ALT), LD
   2. Hematology: increased erythrocytes, leukocytes, platelets, HCT, Hgb
   3. Bone marrow biopsy: increased number of immature cell forms, decreased iron in marrow
   4. Urine chemistry: hematuria
   5. Stool specimen: positive for blood
   6. ABGs: normal PaO_2

F. Medical management
   1. Diet: soft, low-iron
   2. I.V. therapy: heparin lock
   3. Activity: as tolerated
   4. Monitoring: VS, UO, CVP, I/O, and neurovital signs
   5. Laboratory studies: Hgb, HCT, WBCs, RBCs, platelets, and unconjugated bilirubin
   6. Treatment: tepid sponge baths
   7. Analgesic: acetaminophen (Tylenol)
   8. Antacids: magnesium and aluminum hydroxide (Maalox), aluminum hydroxide gel (AlternaGEL)
   9. Histamine antagonists: cimetidine (Tagamet), ranitidine (Zantac)

10. Antihistamine: diphenhydramine hydrochloride (Benadryl)
11. Antigouts: colchicine (Colsalide), allopurinol (Zyloprim)
12. Radioactive phosphorus (P32)
13. Phlebotomy
14. Myelosuppressants: busulfan (Myleran), chlorambucil (Leukeran), cyclophosphamide (Cytoxan)
15. Mucosal barrier fortifier: sucralfate (Carafate)

G. Nursing interventions
1. Maintain the patient's diet
2. Force fluids
3. Assess cardiovascular and respiratory status
4. Keep the patient in semi-Fowler's position
5. Monitor and record VS, UO, I/O, laboratory studies, CVP, neurovital signs, and fecal occult blood
6. Administer medications, as prescribed
7. Allay the patient's anxiety
8. Protect the patient from falls
9. Provide treatments: tepid baths and ROM exercises
10. Provide postchemotherapeutic and postradiation nursing care
    a. Provide prophylactic skin, mouth, and perineal care
    b. Monitor dietary intake
    c. Administer antiemetics and antidiarrheals, as prescribed
    d. Monitor for bleeding, infection, and electrolyte imbalance
    e. Provide rest periods
11. Individualize home care instructions
    a. Recognize the signs and symptoms of CHF and thrombophlebitis
    b. Avoid taking hot showers

H. Possible medical complications
1. Hypertension
2. CHF
3. CVA
4. Myocardial infarction (MI)
5. Deep vein thrombosis
6. Hemorrhage
7. Peptic ulcer
8. Gout
9. Acute leukemia

I. Possible surgical interventions: none

♦ XVIII. Disseminated intravascular coagulation (DIC)

A. Definition—body's response to injury or disease in which microthrombi obstruct blood supply of organs and hemorrhage occurs throughout the body

B. Possible etiology
   1. Unknown
   2. Frequent, rapid transfusions
   3. Gram-negative sepsis
   4. Neoplastic disease
   5. Massive burns
   6. Massive trauma
   7. Anaphylaxis
   8. Chronic disease

C. Pathophysiology
   1. Underlying disease causes release of thromboplastic substances that promote the deposition of fibrin throughout the microcirculation
   2. Red blood cells are trapped in fibrin strands and are hemolyzed
   3. Platelets, prothrombin, and other clotting factors are destroyed, leading to bleeding
   4. Excessive clotting activates the fibrinolytic system that inhibits platelet function, causing further bleeding
   5. Acute activation of clotting mechanism results in consumption of plasma-clotting factors that the liver cannot replenish quickly enough
   6. Activation of the thrombin and fibrinolytic system results in simultaneous bleeding and thrombosis

D. Possible assessment findings
   1. Petechiae
   2. Ecchymosis
   3. Prolonged bleeding after venipuncture
   4. Hemorrhage
   5. Oliguria
   6. Anxiety
   7. Restlessness
   8. Purpura
   9. Acrocyanosis
   10. Joint pain
   11. Dyspnea
   12. Hemoptysis
   13. Crackles

E. Possible diagnostic test findings
　1. Hematology: decreased platelets, RBCs, fibrinogen, factor assay (II, V, VII); increased fibrin split products, thrombin, PT, PTT; positive protamine sulfate test
　2. Urine chemistry: hematuria
　3. ABGs: metabolic acidosis
　4. Ophthalmoscopic exam: retinal hemorrhage
　5. Fecal occult blood: positive

F. Medical management
　1. Diet: withhold food and fluids
　2. I.V. therapy: hydration, electrolyte replacement, and heparin lock
　3. Oxygen therapy
　4. Intubation and mechanical ventilation
　5. GI decompression: NG tube
　6. Position: semi-Fowler's
　7. Activity: bed rest and active and passive ROM exercises
　8. Monitoring: VS, UO, I/O, ECG, and hemodynamic variables
　9. Laboratory studies: PT, PTT, platelets, fibrinogen, and fibrin split products
　10. Nutritional support: TPN
　11. Treatment: indwelling urinary catheter
　12. Transfusion therapy: platelets, packed RBCs, FFP, whole blood, volume expanders, and cryoprecipitates
　13. Glucocorticoids: prednisone (Deltasone), hydrocortisone (Cortef)
　14. Analgesics: ibuprofen (Motrin), acetaminophen (Tylenol)
　15. Antacids: magnesium and aluminum hydroxide (Maalox), aluminum hydroxide gel (Gelusil)
　16. Stool softener: docusate sodium (Colace)
　17. Anticoagulant: heparin sodium (Lipo-Hepin)
　18. Hemodialysis
　19. Precautions: seizure
　20. Pulse oximetry

G. Nursing interventions
　1. Withhold food and fluids
　2. Administer I.V. fluids
　3. Administer oxygen
　4. Provide suction and TCDB
　5. Assess cardiovascular and respiratory status and fluid balance
　6. Maintain position, patency, and low suction of NG tube
　7. Irrigate NG tube gently and do not reposition it
　8. Keep the patient in semi-Fowler's position
　9. Monitor and record VS, UO, I/O, laboratory studies, hemodynamic variables, neurovital signs, fecal occult blood, and pulse oximetry

10. Administer TPN
11. Administer medications, as prescribed
12. Allay the patient's anxiety
13. Maintain bed rest
14. Provide gentle mouth and skin care
15. Avoid giving the patient intramuscular injections, enemas, and rectal temperatures

16. Avoid using straight razors and tape on the patient
17. Rotate extremities for blood pressure monitoring
18. Maintain seizure precautions
19. Administer transfusion therapy, as prescribed
20. Maintain endotracheal tube to mechanical ventilator
21. Individualize home care instructions
    a. Recognize the signs and symptoms of occult bleeding
    b. Wear a medical identification bracelet
    c. Avoid straining while defecating
    d. Avoid using over-the-counter medications
    e. Monitor stool for occult blood
    f. Use an electric razor
    g. Avoid using aspirin and enemas

H. Possible medical complications
   1. Acute renal failure
   2. Shock
   3. CVA
   4. Convulsions
   5. Hemothorax
   6. Hemorrhage
   7. Coma

I. Possible surgical interventions: none

♦ XIX. Multiple myeloma

A. Definition—abnormal proliferation of plasma cells in the bone marrow

B. Possible etiology
   1. Unknown
   2. Genetic
   3. Environmental

C. Pathophysiology
   1. Single tumor in bone marrow disseminates into lymph nodes, liver, spleen, kidneys, and bone
   2. Plasma cell tumors produce abnormal amounts of immunoglobulins
   3. Tumor cells trigger osteoblastic activity, leading to bone destruction throughout the body

D. Possible assessment findings

1. Headaches
2. Constant, severe bone pain
3. Pathologic fractures
4. Skeletal deformities of sternum and ribs
5. Renal calculi
6. Multiple infections
7. Hepatomegaly
8. Splenomegaly
9. Loss of height
10. Hemorrhage

E. Possible diagnostic test findings

1. X-ray: diffuse, round, "punched out" bone lesions; osteoporosis, osteolytic lesions of the skull, widespread demineralization
2. Bone scan: increased uptake
3. Bone marrow biopsy: increased number of immature plasma cells
4. Hematology: decreased HCT, WBCs, platelets; increased ESR
5. Blood chemistry: increased calcium, uric acid, BUN, creatinine, globulins, protein; decreased albumin-globulin (A-G) ratio
6. Urine chemistry: increased calcium, uric acid
7. Immunoelectrophoresis: monoclonal spike
8. Bence Jones protein assay: positive

F. Medical management

1. Diet: high-protein, high-carbohydrate, high-vitamin and mineral in small, frequent feedings
2. I.V. therapy: hydration, electrolyte replacement, and heparin lock
3. Activity: as tolerated
4. Monitoring: VS, UO, I/O, and neurovital signs
5. Laboratory studies: HCT, calcium, BUN, creatinine, uric acid, WBCs, protein, platelets, and surveillance cultures
6. Radiation therapy
7. Chemotherapy
8. Precautions: seizure
9. Transfusion therapy: packed RBCs
10. Antibiotics: doxorubicin (Adriamycin), plicamycin (Mithracin)
11. Antigout: allopurinol (Zyloprim)
12. Alkylating agents: melphalan (Alkeran), cyclophosphamide (Cytoxan)
13. Antineoplastics: vinblastine (Velban), vincristine sulfate (Oncovin)
14. Analgesic: meperidine hydrochloride (Demerol)
15. Diuretic: furosemide (Lasix)
16. Glucocorticoid: prednisone (Deltasone)

17. Antacids: magnesium and aluminum hydroxide (Maalox), aluminum hydroxide gel (Gelusil)
18. Androgen: fluoxymesterone (Halotestin)
19. Orthopedic devices: braces, splints, casts
20. Peritoneal and hemodialysis
21. Antiemetic: prochlorperazine (Compazine)

G. Nursing interventions
1. Maintain the patient's diet
2. Force fluids
3. Administer I.V. fluids
4. Provide TCDB
5. Assess renal, cardiovascular, and respiratory status and fluid balance
6. Monitor and record VS, UO, I/O, laboratory studies, specific gravity, daily weight, urine and stool for occult blood, and neurovital signs
7. Administer transfusion therapy, as prescribed
8. Administer medications, as prescribed
9. Allay the patient's anxiety
10. Maintain seizure precautions
11. Provide skin and mouth care
12. Alternate rest periods with activity
13. Monitor for infection and bruising
14. Prevent the patient from falling
15. Provide postchemotherapeutic and postradiation nursing care
    a. Provide prophylactic skin, mouth, and perineal care
    b. Monitor dietary intake
    c. Administer antiemetics and antidiarrheals, as prescribed
    d. Monitor for bleeding, infection, and electrolyte imbalance
    e. Provide rest periods
16. Assess bone pain
17. Move the patient gently
18. Apply and maintain braces, splints, and casts
19. Individualize home care instructions
    a. Provide information about the American Cancer Society
    b. Exercise regularly, with particular attention to muscle-strengthening exercises
    c. Recognize the signs and symptoms of renal calculi, fractures, and seizures
    d. Avoid lifting, constipation, and over-the-counter medications
    e. Monitor self for occult blood
    f. Use braces, splints, and casts

CLINICAL ALERT

  H. Possible medical complications
1. Paraplegia
2. Acute renal failure
3. Hemorrhage
4. Infection
5. Urolithiasis
6. Pathologic fractures
7. Seizures
8. Gout

  I. Possible surgical interventions: none

♦ XX. Hemophilia

  A. Definition
1. Hereditary bleeding disorder
2. Two types
    a. Hemophilia A—most common type caused by deficiency of factor VIII
    b. Hemophilia B—deficiency of factor IX

  B. Possible etiology
1. Inherited as x-linked traits by males primarily
2. Asymptomatic mothers and sisters as carriers

  C. Pathophysiology
1. Hemophilia A: deficiency of factor VIII causes extended clotting time
2. Hemophilia B: deficiency of factor IX causes extended clotting time

  D. Possible assessment findings
1. Large spreading bruises
2. Bleeding into muscles, joints, and soft tissues after minimal trauma
3. Pain in joints
4. Joint swelling and limited ROM
5. Recurrent joint hemorrhages
6. Spontaneous hematuria
7. Spontaneous GI bleeding

  E. Possible diagnostic test findings
1. HCT: decreased
2. Hgb: decreased
3. Coagulation time: prolonged
4. Bleeding time: normal
5. PT and PTT: normal
6. Platelet function and count: normal
7. Factor VIII: missing (Hemophilia A)
8. Factor IX: missing (Hemophilia B)

F. Medical management

1. Activity: as tolerated
2. Monitoring: VS, UO, I/O
3. Laboratory studies: HCT, Hgb, coagulation time, CVP, and PAP
4. I.V. therapy: heparin lock, whole blood, blood components, IV fluids
5. Nonsteroidal antiinflammatory drug (NSAID): ibuprofen (Motrin)
6. Stool softener: docusate sodium (Colace)
7. Treatment: cold compresses
8. Hemostatic: factor VIII concentrate (Hemophilia A) or factor IX concentrate (Hemophilia B)
9. Hemostatic: aminocaproic acid (Amicar)
10. Corticosteroid: hydrocortisone sodium succinate (Solu-Cortef)
11. Vasopressor: desmopressin acetate (DDAVP)

G. Nursing interventions

1. Assess patient for internal bleeding, hematuria, melena, hematemesis, joint space hemorrhages, and muscle hematomas
2. Assess cardiac and respiratory status
3. Monitor and record VS, UO, I/O, and laboratory studies
4. Administer medications, as prescribed
5. Allay patient's anxiety
6. Provide skin and mouth care
7. Administer I.V. fluids, blood, and blood components, as prescribed
8. Turn patient every 2 hours if on bed rest
9. Use padded side rails

CLINICAL
ALERT

10. Assess location and intensity of pain
11. Avoid aspirin and intramuscular injections
12. Apply gentle pressure to external bleeding sites
13. Apply cold compresses, as prescribed
14. Individualize home care instructions
    a. Make patient aware that there is the potential for hemorrhage with dental extractions and surgery
    b. Administer factor VIII or factor IX at first sign of bleeding
    c. Avoid nose blowing, coughing, straining while defecating, and lifting
    d. Maintain regular dental hygiene appointments
    e. Wear joint and muscle splints and orthopedics, as prescribed
    f. Use soft tooth brush
    g. Use cane or crutches, as directed
    h. Use electric razor
    i. Prevent stress on joints
    j. Take warm baths for joint pain unless there is active bleeding
    k. Avoid contact sports

H. Possible medical complications
   1. Ankylosis
   2. Hypovolemia
   3. Shock
   4. Hematuria
   5. GI bleeding
   6. Hematemesis
   7. Melena
   8. Sensitization to antihemolytic factor (AHF)

I. Possible surgical interventions: none

POINTS TO REMEMBER

♦ After bone marrow transplantation, the patient should be placed in protective isolation.

♦ AIDS results from a defect in T-cell mediated immunity that allows development of opportunistic infections.

♦ A patient with pernicious anemia usually has a positive Schilling's test and hypochlorhydria.

♦ The nurse should avoid intramuscular injections, enemas, and rectal temperatures when caring for a patient with bleeding tendencies.

STUDY QUESTIONS

To evaluate your understanding of this chapter, answer the following questions in the space provided; then compare your responses with the correct answers in Appendix B, pages 385 and 386.

1. Which nursing interventions are appropriate after a lymphangiogram? ___
   _____
   _____

2. What should the nurse teach a patient who has had a splenectomy?_____
   _____
   _____

3. Which possible assessment findings are related to the early or acute stage of AIDS? _____

_____

_____

4. What is the recommended diet for a patient with iron deficiency anemia?

_____

_____

5. What is the pathophysiology of ITP? _____

_____

_____

6. What is the pathophysiology of DIC? _____

_____

_____

CRITICAL THINKING AND APPLICATION EXERCISES

1. Observe a bone marrow aspiration. Prepare an oral presentation for your fellow students describing the procedure and patient care before, during, and after the procedure.

2. Develop a chart comparing the major drug classes used for treating bleeding disorders.

3. Interview a patient with AIDS. Evaluate the information for possible risk factors, and identify ways to modify them.

4. Follow a patient with a hematologic or lymphatic disorder from admission through discharge. Develop a patient-specific plan of care, including any needs for follow-up and home care.

Glossary

Anisometropia—condition involving unequal refraction in both eyes

Anuria—absence of urine output

Aqueous humor—transparent liquid contained in the anterior and posterior chambers of the eye

Ascites—fluid in the peritoneal cavity

Astigmatism—a condition in which light rays are refracted over a large diffuse area instead of being sharply focused on the retina

Ataxia—lack of muscular coordination

Bruit—sound of abnormal blood flow heard on auscultation

Cerumen—waxlike substance found in the external ear canal

Crackles—abnormal inspiratory or expiratory breath sounds, usually associated with the presence of fluid

Crepitation—grating sound produced by bone rubbing against bone

Decerebration—abnormal extension and internal rotation of arms and legs

Dysphagia—difficulty in swallowing

Dyspnea—difficult, labored breathing

Ecchymosis—bruise

Epistaxis—bleeding from the nose

Hematemesis—vomiting of blood

Hematuria—blood in the urine

Hemoptysis—expectoration of bloody sputum

Hirsutism—excessive hair growth or unusual distribution of hair

Hyperopia—far-sightedness; rays focus behind the retina

Intermittent claudication—calf pain caused by walking and relieved by rest

Intraocular pressure (IOP)—normal tension within the eyeball

Jugular venous distention—distended neck veins that may indicate increased central venous pressure

Lichenification—thickening and hardening of the epidermis

Lymphadenopathy—enlargement of the lymph nodes

Melena—black, tarry stools

Mineralocorticoid—substance, such as aldosterone, produced by the adrenal cortex that regulates electrolyte and water balance

Myopia—nearsightedness; rays focus in front of the retina; objects seen only when very close to the eye

Neurovital signs—neurologic assessment of pupils, motor and verbal response, level of consciousness, vital signs, pulse pressure, mean arterial pressure, and intracranial pressure

Nevi—moles or birthmarks

Nystagmus—constant involuntary cyclical movement of the eyeball in any direction

Oliguria—urine output of less than 30 ml/hour

Optic atrophy—condition of the eye where the optic disk atrophies because of degeneration of the second cranial nerve

Orthopnea—respiratory distress that is relieved by sitting upright

Pannus—granular tissue that covers and invades articular cartilage

Papilledema—swelling of the optic nerve head

Paroxysmal nocturnal dyspnea—respiratory distress that occurs after lying in a recumbent position for several hours

Petechiae—multiple, small, hemorrhagic areas on the skin

Point of maximal impulse (PMI)—point on the anterior chest wall, located at the midclavicular line at the fifth intercostal space, that the tip of the left ventricle hits during ventricular systole; using light palpation, the nurse can feel a tap with each heartbeat

Polydipsia—excessive thirst

Polyphagia—excessive eating

Polyuria—excessive urination

Presbyopia—visual deficit associated with aging from loss of lens elasticity

Pruritus—itching

Ptosis—drooping of the eyelid

Pyuria—pus in the urine

Renal colic—flank pain that radiates to the groin

Rhonchi—abnormal inspiratory or expiratory breath sounds, usually associated with airway constriction

Steatorrhea—fatty stools

Subluxation—partial dislocation of a joint

Sympathectomy—surgical removal of ganglia to improve blood flow to the skin (usually performed on the lumbar ganglia)

Tachypnea—abnormally fast rate of breathing

Thenar—musculature at the thumb's base

Tinnitus—ringing in the ears

Tophi—urate crystals deposited in areas of diminished blood flow, such as joints and ear lobes

Trophic—integumentary changes (such as hair loss or skin thickening and drying) caused by prolonged tissue ischemia and malnutrition

Vasopressin—antidiuretic hormone

Vertigo—sensation of moving around in space or of objects moving around the person; a result of a disturbance in the equilibratory mechanism of the middle ear

Vesicle—fluid-filled sac

Answers to Study Questions

CHAPTER 1

1. Cardiac output equals stroke volume times heart rate:
$$CO = SV \times HR$$

2. After cardiac catheterization, the nurse should monitor the patient's vital signs and peripheral pulses, check the insertion site for bleeding, maintain a pressure dressing, promote bed rest, force fluids unless contraindicated, and allay the patient's anxiety.

3. The modifiable risk factors for developing cardiovascular disorders include smoking, hypertension, hypercholesterolemia, obesity, physical inactivity, and emotional stress.

4. After vascular grafting, the key assessment is peripheral circulation, which includes checking temperature, color, pulses, and sensations distal to the graft site.

5. The patient with hypertension should be taught to consume a low-sodium, low-calorie, low-cholesterol, low-fat diet with limited intake of alcohol and caffeine.

6. A patient with angina would describe the pain as substernal and crushing or compressing. The pain might radiate to the arms and last for 3 to 5 minutes after exertion, emotional excitement, or exposure to cold.

7. The assessment findings in acute pulmonary edema include dyspnea; paroxysmal cough; blood-tinged, frothy sputum; orthopnea; tachypnea; agitation; restlessness; intense fear; chest pain; syncope; tachycardia; cold, clammy skin; and gallop rhythms, S_3 and S_4.

8. Three assessment findings in PVD are trophic changes, diminished or absent pulses, and temperature changes in the extremities.

CHAPTER 2

1. After bronchoscopy, nursing interventions include assessing the patient's cough and gag reflex, assessing the patient's sputum, determining the patient's respiratory status, withholding the patient's food and fluids until the gag reflex returns, and checking the patient's vasovagal response.

2. A key postoperative assessment for a radical neck dissection is determining the patient's gag and cough reflex plus the patient's ability to swallow.

3. Following a pneumonectomy, the patient should be placed on the back or the side of the surgery.

4. Possible assessment findings in pneumonia include cough, malaise, chills, shortness of breath, dyspnea, elevated temperature,

rales, rhonchi, pleural friction rub, pleuritic pain, and sputum production.
5. The nurse should teach the patient and family that TB is transmitted through droplets produced during coughing.
6. The key assessment finding present in a pneumothorax is diminished or absent breath sounds unilaterally.
7. Home care instructions for the patient with a pulmonary embolism should include avoid smoking, stress, prolonged sitting and standing, constrictive clothing, leg crossing, and oral contraceptives.

CHAPTER 3

1. After an LP, the nurse should keep the patient flat in bed for 24 hours, administer prescribed analgesics, check the insertion site for bleeding, monitor the patient's neurovital signs, and force fluids.
2. Two key postoperative nursing interventions after a craniotomy are to check the patient for signs of increased intracranial pressure and to maintain seizure precautions.
3. When a patient has a seizure, the nurse should observe and record aura incontinence, initial movement, respiratory pattern, duration of the seizure, loss of consciousness, and pupillary changes.
4. The assessment findings in a patient with a cerebellar tumor include poor coordination and impaired equilibrium.

5. Two key nursing interventions for a patient with a spinal cord injury are to assess for autonomic dysreflexia and to check for spinal shock.

CHAPTER 4

1. The primary complication of glaucoma is blindness.
2. Principles of safe eye care include wearing safety glasses during work or sports that may cause eye trauma, wearing sunglasses to protect the eyes from ultraviolet rays, and reading in a well-lighted area.
3. Following eye surgery the patient should be placed in a supine position with the head of the bed elevated. A small pillow should be placed under and at each side of the head.
4. When communicating with a patient with a hearing loss, the nurse should devote full attention to the patient, stand directly in front of the patient, speak slowly, and write the information if necessary.

CHAPTER 5

1. Before an endoscopy, the nurse should withhold food and fluids; obtain written, informed consent; obtain baseline vital signs; and administer sedatives, as prescribed. After the procedure, the nurse should assess the patient's gag and cough reflexes; withhold food and fluids until the gag reflex returns; and assess the patient's vasovagal response.
2. After pancreatic surgery, the patient should learn to monitor

urine glucose and ketones and to recognize the signs of hyperglycemia.

3. Home care instructions for the patient with a hiatal hernia include: follow dietary recommendations and restrictions; eat small, frequent meals; avoid carbonated beverages and alcohol; and maintain an upright position for 2 hours after eating.

4. The patient with a gastric ulcer should eliminate caffeine, alcohol, and spicy or fried foods.

5. The assessment findings in a patient with an intestinal obstruction include nausea, singultus, constipation, cramping pain, abdominal distention, elevated temperature, diminished or absent bowel sounds, weight loss, and vomiting of fecal material.

6. Type A hepatitis virus is transmitted through oral ingestion of fecal-contaminated food and liquids, such as water and milk. Type B hepatitis virus is transmitted by blood and body fluids.

CHAPTER 6

1. After an adrenalectomy, the patient should be taught that hormonal replacement will be lifelong.

2. After a parathyroidectomy, the patient should have a diet high in calcium and vitamin D, with calcium and vitamin D supplements.

3. The possible assessment findings for hypothyroidism include fatigue, weight gain, dry flaky skin, edema, intolerance to cold, coarse hair, alopecia, thick

tongue, swollen lips, mental sluggishness, menstrual disorders, constipation, hypersensitivity to drugs (narcotics, barbiturates, and anesthetics), anorexia, decreased diaphoresis, and hypothermia.

4. Diagnostic tests for Cushing's syndrome include dexamethasone suppression test, X-rays, angiography, CT scan, urine chemistry, blood chemistry, ultrasonography, hematology, and GTT.

5. The acid-base imbalance seen with hyperaldosteronism is metabolic alkalosis.

6. Two key assessment findings for diabetes insipidus are polyuria (greater than 5 L/day) and polydipsia (4 to 40 L/day).

CHAPTER 7

1. In a patient with glomerulonephritis, a urine chemistry test would reveal increased RBCs, WBCs, protein, casts, and specific gravity. A blood chemistry test for the same patient would reveal increased BUN and creatinine but decreased protein, creatinine clearance, C-reactive protein, and albumin.

2. A diet high in calcium, vitamin D, milk, protein, oxalate, and alkali is associated with urolithiasis.

3. The diet therapy for acute renal failure is low-protein, increased carbohydrate, and moderate-calorie with potassium, sodium, and phosphorus intake regulated according to serum levels.

4. Key assessment findings for BPH are urinary frequency, urgency, or hesitancy; burning on urination; and decreased force and amount of stream.

CHAPTER 8

1. After a total hip replacement, the patient's hips should be kept in abduction. Hip flexion should be limited to 90 degrees when the patient is sitting or being turned to the side, as ordered.
2. The patient with an external fixation needs to recognize the signs and symptoms of soft tissue and bone infection.
3. Patients commonly describe the pain of rheumatoid arthritis as morning stiffness and the pain of osteoarthritis as joint stiffness. The discomfort of osteoarthritis lessens with rest and worsens in damp, cold weather.
4. Medications for treating gouty arthritis include uricosuric agents, xanthine-oxidase inhibitors, antigout agents, analgesics, and NSAIDs.
5. Osteomyelitis, an infection causing bone destruction, results from organisms reaching the bone through an open wound or the bloodstream. As the infection progresses, bone fragments die. During healing, new bone cells form over the sequestrum. The result is nonunion.
6. Assessment findings for lumbar HNP include acute lower back pain radiating across the buttock and down the leg; weakness, numbness, and tingling in the foot and leg; pain when walking;

and straightening of the normal lumbar curve with scoliosis away from the affected side. Assessment findings for cervical HNP include neck pain that radiates down the arm to the hand; neck stiffness; weakness, numbness, and tingling in the hand; weakness in the affected upper extremities; and atrophy of the biceps and triceps.

CHAPTER 9

1. The key assessment after a skin graft is to inspect the recipient site for infection, hematoma, and fluid accumulation under the graft.
2. Medications for contact dermatitis include antibiotics, antipruritics, corticosteroids, antihistamines, and antianxiety agents.
3. The assessment findings for second-degree burns include pain; oozing, fluid-filled vesicles; erythema; and a shiny, wet subcutaneous layer after vesicles rupture.
4. Three modifiable risk factors for skin cancer include skin moles, the exposure of the skin to the sun, and skin contact with chemicals.

CHAPTER 10

1. After a lymphangiogram, the nurse should assess the patient's VS and peripheral pulses, inspect the catheter insertion site for bleeding, force fluids, and advise the patient that skin, stool, and urine will have a blue discoloration.

2. After a splenectomy, the patient should be taught about the need for prophylactic antibiotics.

3. In the early, or acute, stage of AIDS, clinical manifestations include fatigue, weakness, anorexia, weight loss, recurrent diarrhea, fever, lymphadenopathy, pallor, night sweats, and malnutrition.

4. Diet therapy for iron deficiency anemia would include a high intake of iron, roughage, protein, and vitamins. Fluids should also be increased.

5. In ITP, antibody-coated platelets are removed from circulation by the reticuloendothelial cells of the spleen and liver. The decrease in the number of circulating platelets causes bleeding.

6. DIC is the body's response to an injury or disease in which microthrombi obstruct the blood supply to organs and hemorrhage occurs throughout the body. Activation of the thrombin and fibrinolytic system results in simultaneous bleeding and thrombosis.

NANDA Taxonomy

The taxonomy developed by the North American Nursing Diagnosis Association (NANDA) is the currently accepted classification system for nursing diagnoses. The list of approved nursing diagnoses is grouped into nine human response patterns. The complete taxonomy is listed below.

PATTERN 1: EXCHANGING

1.1.2.1	Altered nutrition: More than body requirements
1.1.2.2	Altered nutrition: Less than body requirements
1.1.2.3	Altered nutrition: Potential for more than body requirements
1.2.1.1	Risk for infection
1.2.2.1	Risk for altered body temperature
1.2.2.2	Hypothermia
1.2.2.3	Hyperthermia
1.2.2.4	Ineffective thermoregulation
1.2.3.1	Dysreflexia
1.3.1.1	Constipation
1.3.1.1.1	Perceived constipation
1.3.1.1.2	Colonic constipation
1.3.1.2	Diarrhea
1.3.1.3	Bowel incontinence
1.3.2	Altered urinary elimination
1.3.2.1.1	Stress incontinence
1.3.2.1.2	Reflex incontinence
1.3.2.1.3	Urge incontinence
1.3.2.1.4	Functional incontinence
1.3.2.1.5	Total incontinence
1.3.2.2	Urinary retention
1.4.1.1	Altered (specify type) tissue perfusion (renal, cerebral, cardiopulmonary, gastrointestinal, peripheral)
1.4.1.2.1	Fluid volume excess
1.4.1.2.2.1	Fluid volume deficit
1.4.1.2.2.2	Risk for fluid volume deficit
1.4.2.1	Decreased cardiac output
1.5.1.1	Impaired gas exchange
1.5.1.2	Ineffective airway clearance
1.5.1.3	Ineffective breathing pattern
1.5.1.3.1	Inability to sustain spontaneous ventilation
1.5.1.3.2	Dysfunctional ventilatory weaning response
1.6.1	Risk for injury
1.6.1.1	Risk for suffocation
1.6.1.2	Risk for poisoning
1.6.1.3	Risk for trauma
1.6.1.4	Risk for aspiration
1.6.1.5	Risk for disuse syndrome
1.6.2	Altered protection
1.6.2.1	Impaired tissue integrity
1.6.2.1.1	Altered oral mucous membrane
1.6.2.1.2.1	Impaired skin integrity
1.6.2.1.2.2	Risk for impaired skin integrity
1.7.1	Decreased adaptive capacity: Intracranial*
1.8	Energy field disturbance*

PATTERN 2: COMMUNICATING

2.1.1.1	Impaired verbal communication

*Indicates 1 of the 19 new diagnoses recently approved by NANDA.

PATTERN 3: RELATING

3.1.1	Impaired social interaction
3.1.2	Social isolation
3.1.3	Risk for loneliness*
3.2.1	Altered role performance
3.2.1.1.1	Altered parenting
3.2.1.1.2	Risk for altered parenting
3.2.1.1.2.1	Risk for altered parent/infant/child attachment*
3.2.1.2.1	Sexual dysfunction
3.2.2	Altered family processes
3.2.2.1	Caregiver role strain
3.2.2.2	Risk for caregiver role strain
3.2.2.3.1	Altered family process: Alcoholism*
3.2.3.1	Parental role conflict
3.3	Altered sexuality patterns

PATTERN 4: VALUING

4.1.1	Spiritual distress (distress of the human spirit)
4.2	Potential for enhanced spiritual well-being*

PATTERN 5: CHOOSING

5.1.1.1	Ineffective individual coping
5.1.1.1.1	Impaired adjustment
5.1.1.1.2	Defensive coping
5.1.1.1.3	Ineffective denial
5.1.2.1.1	Ineffective family coping: Disabling
5.1.2.1.2	Ineffective family coping: Compromised
5.1.2.2	Family coping: Potential for growth
5.1.3.1	Potential for enhanced community coping*
5.1.3.2	Ineffective community coping*
5.2.1	Ineffective management of therapeutic regimen: Individual
5.2.1.1	Noncompliance (specify)
5.2.2	Ineffective management of therapeutic regimen: Families*
5.2.3	Ineffective management of therapeutic regimen: Community*
5.2.4	Effective management of therapeutic regimen: Individual*
5.3.1.1	Decisional conflict (specify)
5.4	Health-seeking behaviors (specify)

PATTERN 6: MOVING

6.1.1.1	Impaired physical mobility
6.1.1.1.1	Risk for peripheral neurovascular dysfunction
6.1.1.1.2	Risk for perioperative positioning injury*
6.1.1.2	Activity intolerance
6.1.1.2.1	Fatigue
6.1.1.3	Risk for activity intolerance
6.2.1	Sleep pattern disturbance
6.3.1.1	Diversional activity deficit
6.4.1.1	Impaired home maintenance management
6.4.2	Altered health maintenance
6.5.1	Feeding self-care deficit
6.5.1.1	Impaired swallowing
6.5.1.2	Ineffective breast-feeding
6.5.1.2.1	Interrupted breast-feeding
6.5.1.3	Effective breast-feeding
6.5.1.4	Ineffective infant feeding pattern
6.5.2	Bathing or hygiene self-care deficit

*Indicates 1 of the 19 new diagnoses recently approved by NANDA.

6.5.3	Dressing or grooming self-care deficit
6.5.4	Toileting self-care deficit
6.6	Altered growth and development
6.7	Relocation stress syndrome
6.8.1	Risk for disorganized infant behavior*
6.8.2	Disorganized infant behavior*
6.8.3	Potential for enhanced organized infant behavior*

PATTERN 7: PERCEIVING

7.1.1	Body image disturbance
7.1.2	Self-esteem disturbance
7.1.2.1	Chronic low self-esteem
7.1.2.2	Situational low self-esteem
7.1.3	Personal identity disturbance
7.2	Sensory or perceptual alterations (specify visual, auditory, kinesthetic, gustatory, tactile, or olfactory)
7.2.1.1	Unilateral neglect
7.3.1	Hopelessness
7.3.2	Powerlessness

PATTERN 8: KNOWING

8.1.1	Knowledge deficit (specify)
8.2.1	Impaired environmental interpretation syndrome*
8.2.2	Acute confusion*
8.2.3	Chronic confusion*
8.3	Altered thought processes
8.3.1	Impaired memory*

PATTERN 9: FEELING

9.1.1	Pain
9.1.1.1	Chronic pain
9.2.1.1	Dysfunctional grieving
9.2.1.2	Anticipatory grieving
9.2.2	Risk for violence: Self-directed or directed at others
9.2.2.1	Risk for self-mutilation
9.2.3	Posttrauma response
9.2.3.1	Rape-trauma syndrome
9.2.3.1.1	Rape-trauma syndrome: Compound reaction
9.2.3.1.2	Rape-trauma syndrome: Silent reaction
9.3.1	Anxiety
9.3.2	Fear

*Indicates 1 of the 19 new diagnoses recently approved by NANDA.

Common Laboratory Test Values

HEMATOLOGIC TESTS

Erythrocyte sedimentation rate
0 to 20 mm/hour; rates gradually increase with age

Hematocrit
- Adult males: 42% to 52%
- Adult females: 38% to 46%

Hemoglobin
- Adult males: 14 to 18 g/dl
- Adult females: 12 to 16 g/dl

Iron and total iron-binding capacity (TIBC)

	Men	Women
Serum iron	70 to 150 µg/dl	80 to 150 µg/dl
TIBC	300 to 400 µg/dl	300 to 450 µg/dl
Saturation	20% to 50%	20% to 50%

Red blood cell count
- Adult males: 4.5 to 6.2 million/µl of venous blood
- Adult females: 4.2 to 5.4 million/µl of venous blood

Reticulocyte count
0.5% to 2% of total RBC count

White blood cell count
4,100 to 10,900/µl

White blood cell differential
Adult values
- Neutrophils: 47.6% to 76.8%
- Lymphocytes: 16.2% to 43%
- Monocytes: 0.6% to 9.6%
- Eosinophils: 0.3% to 7%
- Basophils: 0.3% to 2%

COAGULATION TESTS

Activated partial thromboplastin time (APTT)
25 to 36 seconds

Bleeding time
- Template: 2 to 8 minutes
- Ivy: 1 to 7 minutes
- Duke: 1 to 3 minutes

Platelet count
130,000 to 370,000/mm^3

Prothrombin time
- Males: 9.6 to 11.8 seconds
- Females: 9.5 to 11.3 seconds

Whole blood clotting time
5 to 15 minutes

ARTERIAL BLOOD GASES

PaO_2
75 to 100 mm Hg

$PaCO_2$
35 to 45 mm Hg

pH
7.35 to 7.42

O_2 Sat
94% to 100%

HCO_3-
22 to 26 mEq/L

O_2Ct
15% to 23%

Total CO_2 content
22 to 34 mEq/L

SERUM ELECTROLYTES

Calcium
4.5 to 5.5 mEq/L (Atomic absorption: 8.9 to 10.1 mg/dl)

Chloride
100 to 108 mEq/L

Magnesium
1.5 to 2.5 mEq/L (atomic absorption: 1.7 to 2.1 mg/dl)

Phosphates
1.8 to 2.6 mEq/L (atomic absorption: 2.5 to 4.5 mg/dl)

Potassium
3.8 to 5.5 mEq/L

Sodium
135 to 145 mEq/L

SERUM ENZYMES

Acid phosphatase
- 0 to 1.1 Bodansky units/ml
- 1 to 4 King-Armstrong units/ml
- 0.13 to 0.63 BLB units/ml

Alanine aminotransferase (ALT)
- Adult males: 10 to 32 units/L
- Adult females: 9 to 24 units/L

Alkaline phosphatase
- 1.5 to 4 Bodansky units/dl
- 4 to 13.5 King-Armstrong units/dl
- Chemical inhibition method: Men, 90 to 239 units/dl; Women < age 45, 76 to 196 units/L; women > age 45, 87 to 250 units/L

Amylase
60 to 180 Somogyi units/dl

Angiotensin-converting enzyme
18 to 67 units/L (adults)

Aspartate aminotransferase (AST)
8 to 20 units/L

Creatine kinase
- Total: Men, 23 to 99 units/L; women, 15 to 57 units/L
- CK-BB: none
- CK-MB: 0 to 7 IU/L
- CK-MM: 5 to 70 IU/L

Hydroxybutyric dehydrogenase (HBD)
- Serum HBD: 114 to 290 units/ml
- LD/HBD ratio: 1.2 to 1.6:1

Lactic dehydrogenase (LD)
- Total: 48 to 115 IU/L
- LD_1: 18.1% to 29% of total
- LD_2: 29.4% to 37.5% of total
- LD_3: 18.8% to 26% of total
- LD_4: 9.2% to 16.5% of total
- LD_5: 5.3% to 13.4% of total

SERUM HORMONES

Aldosterone
1 to 21 ng/dl

Antidiuretic hormone
1 to 5 pg/ml

Chorionic gonadotropin
< 3 mIU/ml

Cortisol (plasma)
7 to 28 µg/dl in the morning to 2 to 18 µg/dl in the afternoon

Estrogens
- Premenopausal women: 24 to 68 pg/ml on days 1 to 10, 50 to 186 pg/ml on days 11 to 20, and 73 to 149 pg/ml on days 21 to 28
- Men: 12 to 34 pg/ml

Free thyroxine (FT$_4$)
0.8 to 3.3 ng/dl

Free triiodothyronine
0.2 to 0.6 ng/dl

Growth hormone
- Men: 1 to 5 ng/ml
- Women: 0 to 10 ng/ml

Insulin
0 to 25 µU/ml

Parathyroid hormone
210 to 310 pg/ml

Prolactin
0 to 23 ng/dl in nonlactating females

Thyroxine (T_4)
5 to 13.5 µg/dl

Triiodothyronine
90 to 239 ng/dl

SERUM LIPIDS AND LIPOPROTEINS

Lipoprotein-cholesterol fractionation
- HDL: 29 to 77 mg/dl
- LDL: 62 to 185 mg/dl

Total cholesterol
- Ideal: < 200 mg/dl
- Borderline high: 200 to 239 mg/dl
- High: > 240 mg/dl

Triglycerides
- Ages 0 to 29: 10 to 140 mg/dl
- Ages 30 to 39: 10 to 150 mg/dl
- Ages 40 to 49: 10 to 160 mg/dl
- Ages 50 to 59: 10 to 190 mg/dl

SERUM PROTEINS AND PIGMENTS

Bilirubin, serum
Adult: direct, < 0.5 mg/dl; indirect, ≤ 1.1 mg/dl

Blood urea nitrogen (BUN)
8 to 20 mg/dl

Creatinine
- Males: 0.8 to 1.2 mg/dl
- Females: 0.6 to 0.9 mg/dl

Proteins
- Total serum protein: 6.6 to 7.9 g/dl (100%)
- Albumin: 3.3 to 4.5 g/dl (53%)
- Alpha$_1$ globulin: 0.1 to 0.4 g/dl (14%)
- Alpha$_2$ globulin: 0.5 to 1 g/dl (14%)
- Beta globulin: 0.7 to 1.2 g/dl (12%)
- Gamma globulin: 0.5 to 1.6 g/dl (20%)

Uric acid
- Men: 4.3 to 8 mg/dl
- Women: 2.3 to 6 mg/dl

SERUM CARBOHYDRATES

Fasting plasma glucose
70 to 100 mg/dl

Lactic acid
0.93 to 1.65 mEq/L

Oral glucose tolerance test (OGTT)
Peak at 160 to 180 mg/dl, 30 to 60 minutes after challenge dose

Two-hour postprandial plasma glucose
< 145 mg/dl

URINALYSIS

Routine urinalysis
- Appearance: clear
- Casts: none, except occasional hyaline casts
- Color: straw
- Crystals: present
- Epithelial cells: none
- Odor: slightly aromatic
- pH: 4.5 to 8.0
- Specific gravity: 1.025 to 1.030
- Sugars: none
- Red blood cells: 0 to 3 per high-power field

Routine urinalysis *(continued)*

- White blood cells: 0 to 4 per high-power field
- Yeast cells: none

Urine concentration test

- Specific gravtiy: 1.025 to 1.032
- Osmolality: > 800 mOsm/kg water

Urine dilution test

- Specific gravity: < 1.003
- Osmolality: < 100 mOsm/kg; 80% of water excreted in 4 hours

URINE CHEMISTRY TESTS

Amylase
10 to 80 amylase units/hour

17-ketosteroids (17-KS)

- Men: 6 to 21 mg/24 hours
- Women: 4 to 17 mg/24 hours

Creatinine clearance

- Men (age 20): 90 ml/minute/1.73 m^2
- Women (age 20): 84 ml/minute/1.73 m^2

Protein
< 150 mg/24 hours

Uric acid
250 to 750 mg/24 hours

Glucose oxidase
Negative

Ketones
Negative

Calcium

- Males: < 275 mg/24 hours
- Females: < 250 mg/24 hours

Phosphate
< 1,000 mg/24 hours

Sodium
30 to 280 mEq/24 hours

Chloride
110 to 250 mEq/24 hours

CEREBROSPINAL FLUID

Glucose
50 to 80 mg/100 ml (two-thirds of blood glucose)

Pressure
50 to 180 mm H_2O

Protein
15 to 45 mg/dl

STOOL TESTS

Lipids
Less than 20% of excreted solids, with excretion of less than 7 g/24 hours

Occult blood
2.5 mg/24 hours

Urobilinogen
50 to 300 mg/24 hours

Selected References

Black, J.M., and Matassarin-Jacobs, E., eds. *Luckmann and Sorensen's Medical-Surgical Nursing: A Psychophysiologic Approach,* 4th ed. Philadelphia: W.B. Saunders Co., 1993.

Davis, J., and Sherer, K. *Applied Nutrition and Diet Therapy,* 2nd ed. Philadelphia: W.B. Saunders Co., 1994.

Fuller, J., and Schaller-Ayers, J. *Health Assessment,* 2nd ed. Philadelphia: J.B. Lippincott Co., 1994.

Govoni, L., and Hayes, J.E. *Drugs and Nursing Implications,* 8th ed. East Norwalk, Conn.: Appleton & Lange, 1995.

Gruendemann, B.J., and Meeker, M.H. *Alexander's Care of the Patient in Surgery.* St. Louis: Mosby–Year Book, Inc., 1995.

Ignatavicius, D. *Medical Surgical Nursing.* Philadelphia: W.B. Saunders Co., 1995.

Kinney, M.R., et al. *AACN's Clinical Reference for Critical-Care Nursing,* 3rd ed. St. Louis: Mosby–Year Book, Inc., 1993.

Nurse's Drug Guide97. Springhouse, Pa.: Springhouse Corp., 1997.

Pagana, K.D., and Pagana, T.J. *Mosby's Diagnostic and Laboratory Test Reference,* 2nd ed. St. Louis: Mosby–Year Book, Inc., 1995.

Patrick, M.L., et al. *Medical Surgical Nursing: Pathophysiological Concepts,* 4th ed. Philadelphia: J.B. Lippincott Co., 1994.

Phipps, W.J., et al. *Medical-Surgical Nursing Concepts and Clinical Practice,* 5th ed. St. Louis: Mosby–Year Book, Inc., 1995.

Porth, C. *Pathophysiology,* 4th ed. Philadelphia: J.B. Lippincott Co., 1994.

Smeltzer, S.C., and Bare, B.G. *Brunner and Suddarth's Textbook of Medical-Surgical Nursing,* 8th ed. Philadelphia: J.B. Lippincott Co., 1996.

Swearingen, P.L., and Keen, J.H. *Manual of Critical Care Nursing,* 3rd ed. St. Louis: Mosby–Year Book, Inc., 1995.

Thompson, J.M., et al. *Clinical Nursing,* 3rd ed. St. Louis: Mosby–Year Book, Inc., 1993.

Ulrich, S.P., et al. *Nursing Care Planning Guides: A Nursing Diagnosis Approach,* 3rd ed. Philadelphia: W.B. Saunders Co., 1994.

Index

i refers to an illustration; t refers to a table

i refers to an illustration; t refers to a table

i refers to an illustration; t refers to a table

i refers to an illustration; t refers to a table

i refers to an illustration; t refers to a table

i refers to an illustration; t refers to a table

i refers to an illustration; t refers to a table

Notes

Notes

About the StudySmart Disk

StudySmart Disk lets you:

- review subject areas of your choice and learn the rationales for the correct answers
- take tests of varying lengths on subjects of your choice
- print the results of your tests to gauge your progress over time.

Recommended system requirements

486 IBM-compatible personal computer (386 minimum)
Windows 3.1 or greater (Windows 95 compatible)
High-density 3½″ floppy drive
8 MB RAM (4 MB minimum)
S-VGA monitor (VGA minimum)
2 MB of available space on hard drive

Installing and running the program

- Start Windows.
- In Program Manager, choose Run from File menu.
- Insert disk, type a:\setup.exe (where a: is the letter of your floppy drive), and click on OK.

For Windows 95 Installation

- Start Windows.
- Select Start button and then Run.
- Insert disk, type a:\setup.exe (where a: is the letter of your floppy drive), and click on OK.

For technical support, call 215-628-7744 Monday through Friday, 9 a.m. to 6 p.m. Eastern Standard Time.

The clinical information and tools in the *StudySmart Disk* are based on research and consultation with nursing, medical, and legal authorities. To the best of our knowledge, this program reflects currently accepted practice; nevertheless, it can't be considered absolute or universal. For individual application, all recommendations must be considered in light of the patient's clinical condition and, before administration of new or infrequently used drugs, in light of the latest package-insert information. The authors and publisher disclaim responsibility for any adverse effects resulting directly or indirectly from the suggested procedures, from any undetected errors, or from the reader's misunderstanding of the program.
